The Extraction and Application of Functional Components in Algae

The Extraction and Application of Functional Components in Algae

Guest Editors

Aurora Silva
Miguel Ángel Prieto Lage
Clara Grosso
Maria Fátima Sá Barroso

MDPI

Basel • Beijing • Wuhan • Barcelona • Belgrade • Novi Sad • Cluj • Manchester

Guest Editors

Aurora Silva
Instituto Superior de Engenharia do Porto
Porto
Portugal

Miguel Ángel Prieto Lage
Department of Analytical Chemistry and Food Science
University of Vigo
Ourense
Spain

Clara Grosso
Instituto Superior de Engenharia Do Porto
Porto
Portugal

Maria Fátima Sá Barroso
Polytechnic Institute of Porto
Porto
Portugal

Editorial Office
MDPI AG
Grosspeteranlage 5
4052 Basel, Switzerland

This is a reprint of the Special Issue, published open access by the journal *Marine Drugs* (ISSN 1660-3397), freely accessible at: https://www.mdpi.com/journal/marinedrugs/special_issues/8G98VL6730.

For citation purposes, cite each article independently as indicated on the article page online and as indicated below:

Lastname, A.A.; Lastname, B.B. Article Title. *Journal Name* **Year**, *Volume Number*, Page Range.

ISBN 978-3-7258-7052-3 (Hbk)
ISBN 978-3-7258-7053-0 (PDF)
https://doi.org/10.3390/books978-3-7258-7053-0

Contents

About the Editors

Aurora Silva

Aurora Silva is a researcher in agrifood science and bioactive natural products. Her research focuses on the extraction, characterization, and biological evaluation of natural compounds, with particular emphasis on antimicrobial, antioxidant, and neuroprotective activities. She has authored and co-authored several peer-reviewed publications indexed in international scientific databases and has collaborated with multidisciplinary national and international research teams. Her work aims at the valorization of natural resources, particularly algae, and the development of sustainable applications of bioactive compounds in food and health-related fields.

Miguel Ángel Prieto Lage

Miguel Ángel Prieto Lage is an associate professor in Food Science and Technology at the University of Vigo, where he leads the Nutrition and Food Group (NuFoG) within the Department of Analytical and Food Chemistry. He is an expert in mathematical modelling and optimization. His research interests include the extraction, characterization, and valorization of bioactive compounds from natural food matrices, with emphasis on sustainable processes and functional food applications. He has authored and co-authored numerous peer-reviewed scientific publications and has been involved in several national and international research projects in the food and health fields.

Clara Grosso

Clara Grosso is an assistant researcher at REQUIMTE/LAQV. Her field of research focuses on natural products from plants and seaweeds, regarding aspects like extraction optimization using green extraction methodologies, identification of secondary metabolites, and assessment of in vitro bioactivities with emphasis on oxidative stress and enzymes related to Alzheimer's disease and depression. She has authored and co-authored several scientific papers and Reprint chapters and edited a Reprint. She has participated in several projects related to natural products valorization for the food and health sectors.

Maria Fátima Sá Barroso

Maria Fátima Sá Barroso is an assistant researcher at ISEP/IPP. Her field of research focuses on the development of electrochemical (bio)sensors applied to food and health fields, namely for the antioxidant detection of food matrices or food wastes. She has authored and co-authored several scientific papers and Reprint chapters. She has participated in several national and international projects related to waste valorization and biosensor development.

Preface

Algae represent one of the most diverse and versatile groups of organisms in the marine environment, including a wide range of macroalgae (seaweeds) and microalgae with remarkable biochemical complexity. Over recent decades, growing scientific and industrial interest has focused on algae as a sustainable and abundant source of functional components with significant biological and technological value. These organisms synthesize a broad spectrum of metabolites, many of which exhibit well-documented bioactivities. Antioxidant, anti-inflammatory, antimicrobial, neuroprotective, antitumor, and metabolic regulatory effects have been reported for numerous algal-derived compounds, highlighting their potential applications in food, pharmaceutical, nutraceutical, cosmetic, and biomedical sectors.

Despite this recognized potential, the structural diversity, complexity, and heterogeneous distribution of bioactive compounds in algal matrices pose considerable challenges for their efficient recovery and characterization. Conventional extraction methods often show low selectivity, high solvent use, and compound degradation. Therefore, algae research increasingly emphasizes green and innovative extraction techniques to improve yields, preserve bioactivity, and reduce environmental impact.

In parallel with extraction advances, significant progress has been made in analytical techniques for the characterization and quantification of algal functional components. These analytical developments are essential not only for validating bioactive potential but also for ensuring quality control, reproducibility, and regulatory compliance in downstream applications.

This reprint brings together a collection of original research articles and review papers published within the Special Issue "The Extraction and Application of Functional Components in Algae". The contributions collectively address key aspects of algal bioactive research, including innovative extraction and purification strategies, analytical characterization of diverse classes of metabolites, and evaluation of biological activities and practical applications. By covering both methodological advances and application-oriented studies, the volume reflects the multidisciplinary nature of contemporary algae research, integrating perspectives from marine biology, chemistry, biotechnology, health, and applied sciences.

The insights presented in this Reprint not only expand current knowledge but also identify remaining challenges and future research directions, including scalability of extraction processes, standardization of analytical protocols, and translation of laboratory findings into commercial products.

Aurora Silva, Miguel Ángel Prieto Lage, Clara Grosso, and Maria Fátima Sá Barroso
Guest Editors

marine drugs

MDPI

Article

Structural Characterization and Anti-Inflammatory Properties of an Alginate Extracted from the Brown Seaweed *Ericaria amentacea*

Maha Moussa [1,2], Serena Mirata [1,3], Lisa Moni [4], Valentina Asnaghi [1,2], Marina Alloisio [4], Simone Pettineo [4], Maila Castellano [4], Silvia Vicini [4], Mariachiara Chiantore [1,2] and Sonia Scarfi [1,2,3,*]

1 Department of Earth, Environment and Life Sciences, University of Genoa, 16132 Genoa, Italy; maha.moussa@edu.unige.it (M.M.); serenamira94@gmail.com (S.M.); valentina.asnaghi@unige.it (V.A.); mariachiara.chiantore@unige.it (M.C.)

2 National Biodiversity Future Center (NBFC), 90133 Palermo, Italy

3 Inter-University Centre for the Promotion of the 3Rs Principles in Teaching & Research, 10129 Turin, Italy

4 Department of Chemistry and Industrial Chemistry (DCCI), University of Genoa, 16146 Genoa, Italy; lisa.moni@unige.it (L.M.); marina.alloisio@unige.it (M.A.); pettineo.simone@gmail.com (S.P.); maila.castellano@unige.it (M.C.); silvia.vicini@unige.it (S.V.)

* Correspondence: soniascarfi@unige.it; Tel.: +39-0103350227

Abstract

Brown algae of the Cystoseira genus are recognized as valuable sources of bioactive compounds, including polysaccharides. Within the framework of current restoration efforts regarding damaged *Ericaria amentacea* populations in the Mediterranean Sea, the valorization of apices derived from ex situ cultivation waste represents a sustainable opportunity for industrial and biomedical applications. In this study, sodium alginate (SA) was extracted from *E. amentacea* apex by-products using a hydrothermal–alkaline method and subsequently chemically characterized. FTIR analysis showed O-H, C-H, and COO- stretching compatible with commercial alginates, while 1H-NMR spectroscopy indicated high β-D-mannuronic acid content with an M/G ratio of 2.33. The extracted SA displayed a molecular weight of 1×10^4 g/mol and a polydispersity index of 3.5. The bioactive properties of the SA extract were investigated in chemico and in vitro. SA exhibited remarkable antioxidant activity, showing significant DPPH and nitric oxide-radical-scavenging capacity. Furthermore, SA demonstrated a strong anti-inflammatory effect in LPS-stimulated macrophages through modulation of several inflammatory mediators (i.e., IL-6, IL-8/CXCL5, MCP-1, and TNF-α). In particular, SA promoted a striking iNOS gene expression inhibition, which, paired with its direct NO-scavenging ability, paves the way for future pharmacological use of *E. amentacea* derivatives, particularly if sustainably obtained from restoration activity waste.

Keywords: brown algae; *Ericaria amentacea*; sodium alginate; biological effects; gene expression

1. Introduction

Macroalgae are widely recognized as a valuable source of bioactive compounds with applications in the food, cosmeceutical, and pharmaceutical industries, as well as in the production of phycocolloids [1,2]. According to the Food and Agriculture Organization (FAO) of the United Nations, global seaweed production reached approximately 34.7 million tons in 2019. Of this total, red and brown seaweed represent the majority, contributing about 53% and 47%, respectively, while green seaweed accounts for only 0.054% [3]. Brown seaweed, in particular, is regarded as a sustainable and renewable biomass source due to its widespread availability and fast growth [4]. Moreover, the bioprocessing of seaweed is considered environmentally friendly, as it is biodegradable and biocompatible, making it suitable for various industrial and biomedical applications [5].

Phycocolloids are polysaccharides associated with the cell walls and intercellular spaces of certain seaweed species [6]. A typical example is alginate, a naturally occurring polysaccharide, first identified by British chemist E.C.C. Stanford in 1881 [7]. It represents the primary structural polysaccharide in brown seaweed, and it is typically found in the cell wall and matrix as a mixture of cationic salts naturally present in seawater. In its native state, alginate occurs as a mixture of alginic calcium, magnesium, and sodium salts, contributing both to the strength and the flexibility of the algal tissue [8].

At the molecular level, alginates are anionic, linear binary copolymers composed of β-D-mannuronic acid (M) and α-L-guluronic acid (G) residues, linked through (1→4) glycosidic bonds. The stereochemical difference between mannuronic and guluronic acid arises from the configuration at the C-5 carbon in the uronic acid ring. These two acids are arranged into three distinct block types: homopolymeric sequences of mannuronic acid (MM-blocks), homopolymeric sequences of guluronic acid (GG-blocks), and heteropolymeric sequences of alternating M and G units (MG-blocks) [9,10]. Mannuronic acid units form β-(1→4) bonds, resulting in linear and flexible M-block segments. In contrast, guluronic acid units are connected by α-(1→4) bonds, introducing steric hindrance around the carboxyl groups, which leads to folded, rigid conformations in the G-block segments [10]. The ratio of mannuronic to guluronic acid (M/G ratio) varies depending on the algal species, the specific tissue, and even the harvesting season [11]. These structural characteristics, particularly the M/G ratio, the block arrangement, and the distribution of M and G units, have a significant impact on the physicochemical properties of alginates. To date, approximately 200 distinct alginate types have been identified, each with varying M/G ratios depending on the source and extraction conditions [12]. The water-soluble form of sodium alginate (SA) is especially valued in the food and pharmaceutical industries due to its ability to form hydrogels in the presence of divalent cations such as Ca^{2+} [13]. In such cases, guluronic acid residues from different polymer chains interact with calcium ions via their carboxylic groups (COO^-), forming a thermally irreversible, water-insoluble three-dimensional network commonly referred to as the "egg-box" model [14]. Owing to their biocompatibility, non-toxicity, biodegradability, and polyelectrolytic nature, alginates are particularly suitable for various biological and biomedical purposes, including anti-inflammatory and antioxidant applications [15].

Inflammation is a fundamental component of the innate immune response, playing a crucial role in protecting the body against pathogenic invasion and tissue injury. Traditionally, it is characterized by vasodilation and leukocyte infiltration, manifesting clinically as erythema, heat, edema, and pain [16]. From an evolutionary standpoint, the inflammatory cascade is an essential defense mechanism designed to eliminate harmful stimuli and initiate tissue repair through a transient, self-regulated process [17]. However, when inflammatory triggers persist and/or the inflammatory response fails to resolve, the process can become chronic. In contrast to acute inflammation, which is typically short-lived and beneficial, chronic inflammation is often subclinical and prolonged, progressively contributing to cellular dysfunction and tissue damage. Furthermore, chronic inflammation is nowadays a broadly recognized feature of several diseases such as diabetes, hypertension, atherosclerosis, and cancer [18]. To counteract inflammation, various synthetic anti-inflammatory agents have been developed. While effective, many of these compounds are associated with adverse side effects. As a result, there is growing interest

 https://doi.org/10.3390/md24010041

in the exploration of naturally derived bioactive compounds (i.e., polysaccharides) with dual anti-inflammatory and antioxidant capabilities.

A key molecular mechanism linking inflammation and cellular damage is oxidative stress, which arises from the overproduction of reactive oxygen species (ROS). Reactive oxygen species (ROS)—including superoxide anion ($\bullet O_2^-$), hydrogen peroxide (H_2O_2), organic peroxide (ROOR′), hydroxyl radical (•OH), and peroxynitrite ($ONOO^-$)—are natural byproducts of cellular metabolism and of exposure to xenobiotics [19,20]. Although ROS play essential roles in intracellular signaling and certain physiological processes, excessive ROS production results in oxidative stress, leading to cellular and molecular damage. Elevated intracellular ROS levels can damage organic macromolecules such as proteins [21], DNA [22], and lipids [23]. When oxidative damage exceeds the cellular antioxidant defense capacity, it impairs key cellular functions and ultimately triggers cell death via apoptosis or necrosis [24].

In the Mediterranean Sea, macroalgal forests are predominantly composed of species belonging to *Cystoseira sensu lato* (s.l.) (Fucales, Phaeophyceae). In the last few decades, these forests have experienced significant decline or local extinction due to anthropogenic pressures and the impacts of climate change [25]. One of the species impacted by this decline is *Ericaria amentacea*, a Mediterranean endemic fucoid alga that colonizes the lower intertidal zone, forming dense monospecific belts. To mitigate its decline, various ex situ restoration activities have been implemented to support the recovery of *E. amentacea* populations along the Mediterranean and Ligurian coasts [26,27]. These restoration efforts generate biological waste, i.e., apical segments of the algal fronds, used to obtain the gametes needed for the cultivation process [28]. In this study, we aimed to extract and characterize, for the first time, sodium alginate polymers from *E. amentacea* using the apical waste material generated during ex situ cultivation for restoration purposes. Furthermore, we investigated the antioxidant and anti-inflammatory properties of these SA extracts by means of in chemico and in vitro cellular tests, showing very promising biological properties.

2. Results

2.1. Chemical Composition

The chemical content of *Ericaria amentacea* sodium alginate (SA) is presented in Table 1. Colorimetric assays revealed that the SA extract contained 44.25% total sugar and 49% uronic acids. In addition, 0.52% proteins and 0.93% polyphenols were detected.

Table 1. Chemical content of *E. amentacea* SA.

Sample	Yield (%)	Total Sugar (%)	Uronic Acid (%)	Total Polyphenols (%)	Protein (%)
SA	3 ± 0.78	44.25 ± 4	49 ± 2.2	0.93 ± 0.08	0.52 ± 0.04

2.2 Chemical Analyses

2.2.1. Fourier-Transform Infrared Spectroscopy

The Fourier-transform infrared (FTIR) spectrum of SA is shown in Figure 1. The chemical structure of this SA exhibited O-H, C-H, and COO- stretching, which are represented by bands at 3301 cm^{-1}, 2926 cm^{-1}, and 1597–1408 cm^{-1}, respectively, according to commercial alginates [29].

2.2.2. NMR Spectroscopy

The characterization of the chemical composition and block distribution of the SA extracted from *E. amentacea* was performed by ^1H NMR spectroscopy. The acquired data showed a typical 400 MHZ-^1H NMR spectrum (Figure 2) with a set of specific signals

https://doi.org/10.3390/md24010041

characteristic of the sodium alginate fraction, confirming the high purity of the extracted polysaccharide. The signal assignment was achieved by comparison with previously reported chemical shifts [30,31].

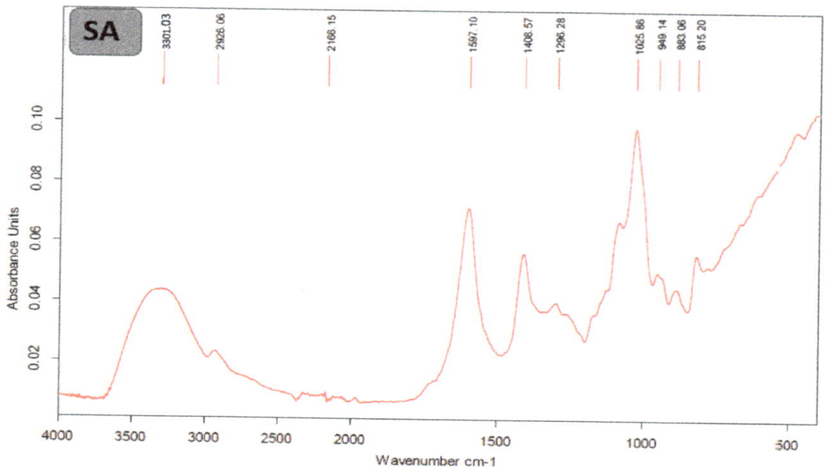

Figure 1. FTIR spectrum of *E. amentacea* SA.

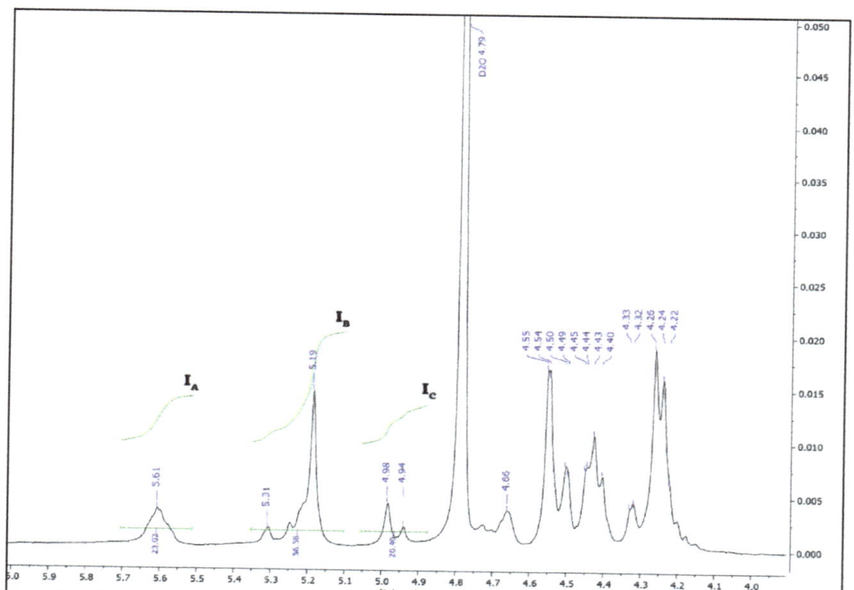

Figure 2. ^{1}H NMR analysis of SA extracted from *E. amentacea* by setting the residual HOD signal in D_2O to 4.79 ppm: signal I_A = guluronic acid anomeric proton (G-1), signal I_B = overlap between the mannuronic acid anomeric proton (M-1) and the H-5 of alternating blocks (GM-5) signal I_C = guluronic acid H-5 position (block GG-5G).

The spectrum revealed signals of the guluronic acid anomeric proton (G-1) at 5.61 ppm (signal I_A) and guluronic acid H-5 (GG-5G) at 4.98 ppm (signal I_C), while the overlap between the mannuronic acid anomeric proton (M-1) and the C-5 of alternating blocks (GM-5) was identified at 5.19 ppm (signal I_B).

 https://doi.org/10.3390/md24010041

The area of the described signals (I_A, I_B, and I_C) was calculated and used to define the M/G ratio, the molar pair frequencies of the monads of mannuronic and guluronic acid (F_M and F_G), and the diad sequences (F_{GG}, F_{MM}, F_{MG}, or F_{GM}). Indeed, the proportions of each block (F_G and F_M) and the homogeneous (F_{GG} and F_{MM}) and heterogeneous (F_{GM} and F_{MG}) blocks of SA extracted from *E. amentacea* were estimated by applying the commonly used equations of Grasdalen et al. [30], summarized as follows:

$$F_G = I_A/(I_B + I_C)$$

$$F_{GG} = I_C/(I_B + I_C)$$

$$F_M = 1 - F_G$$

$$F_{GM} = F_G - F_{GG}$$

$$F_{MM} = F_M - F_{MG}$$

$$M/G = F_M/F_G$$

The chemical composition of SA extracted from *E. amentacea*, as summarized in Table 2, was determined using integral ^{1}H NMR values, as well as the equations mentioned above.

Table 2. Structural characterization of SA extracted from *E. amentacea* harvested in the Ligurian Sea.

Fraction	F_G [1]	F_M [2]	F_{GG} [3]	F_{GM} or F_{MG} [4]	F_{MM} [5]	M/G [6]	η [7]
SA	0.30	0.70	0.26	0.04	0.66	2.33	0.160

[1] F_G—fraction of individual blocks of guluronic acid units; [2] F_M—fraction of individual blocks of mannuronic acid units; [3] F_{GG}—fraction of homogeneous block of guluronic acid; [4] F_{GM} or F_{MG}—fraction of heterogeneous blocks of alternating mannuronic and guluronic acids; [5] F_{MM}—fraction of homogeneous block of mannuronic acid; [6] M/G—ratio between F_M and F_G; [7] η—parameter defined as $\eta = F_{MG}/(F_M \times F_G)$.

2.3. Molecular Weight Determination

Intrinsic viscosity analysis was performed to evaluate the molecular weight of the SA extract. As shown in Table 3, SA was characterized by a weight average molecular mass (M_w) of 1×10^4 g/mol, a number average molecular mass (M_n) of 2.9×10^3 g/mol, and a polydispersity index q (M_w/M_n) of 3.5.

Table 3. Molecular weight, number average molecular weight, polydispersity index, and intrinsic viscosity of SA extracted from *E. amentacea* harvested in the Ligurian Sea.

Sample	M_W (g/mol)	M_n (g/mol)	q (M_w/M_n)	[η] (mL/g)
SA	1×10^4	2.9×10^3	3.5	36.8

2.4. Biological Properties

2.4.1. Antioxidant Potential DPPH Radical-Scavenging Activity

The overall radical-scavenging activity of the SA measured by the DPPH assay revealed an elevated antioxidant potential (Figure 3a). At 1.25 mg/mL and 0.625 mg/mL tested concentrations, in fact, the SA showed a scavenging potential higher than 50%, with 91% and 59% reduction capacities, respectively, and a resulting IC_{50} of 0.410 mg/mL.

- Reducing Fe (III) Power Assay

SA's ability to reduce the Fe^{3+}/ferricyanide complex to the ferrous form was evaluated by following the potassium ferricyanide method (Figure 3b). The reducing power of SA increased with increasing concentrations (from 0.067 to 0.535 mg/mL), obtaining A_{700} values of 1.06 A.U. at 0.535 mg/mL, corresponding to the highest SA concentration used.

https://doi.org/10.3390/md24010041

- NO-Scavenging Activity

The NO-scavenging activity of the SA extract was evaluated by the nitroprusside NO donor assay. The reducing power of SA proved to be dose-dependent (from 0.042 to 0.417 mg/mL). The NO IC_{50} scavenging potential of the SA extract was 0.417 mg/mL (Figure 3c).

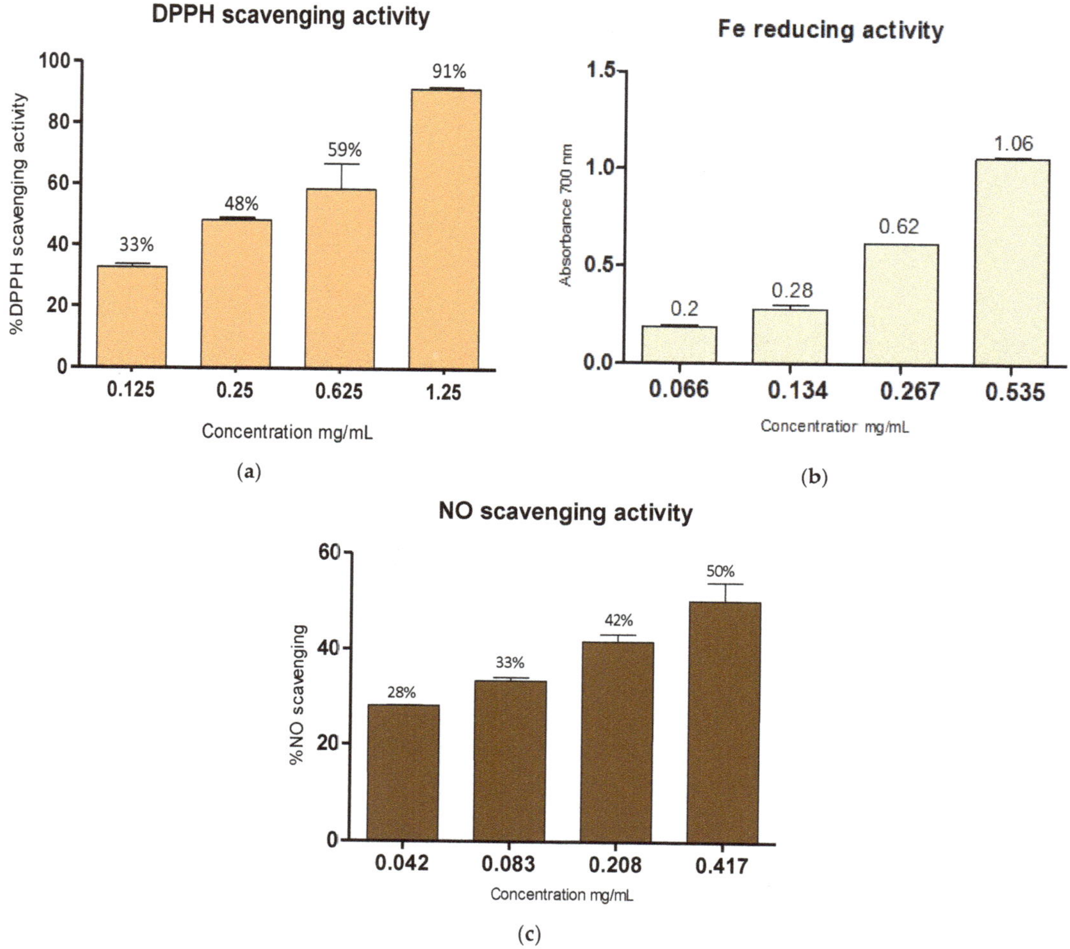

Figure 3. The antioxidant activity of *E. amentacea* SA in spectrophotometric tests. (**a**) ROS scavenging activity by the DPPH assay; (**b**) Fe reducing activity of *E. amentacea* SA; (**c**) NO-scavenging potential of *E. amentacea* SA. Ascorbic acid (AA) and sodium nitroprusside (SN) were used as positive controls, AA in the DPPH and Fe reducing activity assay, SN in the NO assay. Data are the mean ± S.D. of three experiments performed in duplicate.

2.4.2. Anti-Inflammatory Potential

- Cytotoxicity test

The cytotoxicity of SA at various concentrations was evaluated in murine RAW 264.7 macrophages and in human THP-1-derived M0 macrophages to investigate the safe use of these extracts for human health applications. The RAW 264.7 cells and differentiated THP-1 M0 cells were incubated for 24 h with various dilutions of SA (from 0.05 to

https://doi.org/10.3390/md24010041

0.4 mg/mL), and then, the cell viability was evaluated by the MTT test and compared to untreated control cells (Figure 4). Concerning RAW 264.7 murine macrophages, a slight decrease in the cell number (around 30%) for all tested concentrations was observed after SA exposure (Figure 4a) as compared to control cells, probably due to a slower growth rate in the presence of the SA, which was concentration-independent. Conversely, for the differentiated human THP-1 M0 macrophages, the results showed no significant effects on cell growth for all tested concentrations (0.05 and 0.4 mg/mL, Figure 4b). These data indicate that *E. amentacea* SA might be safely used in humans due to the absence of significant toxicity.

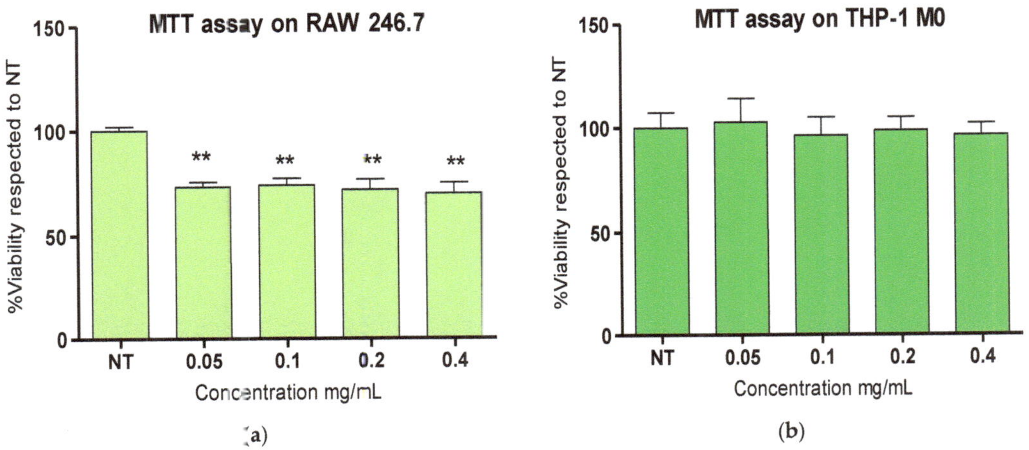

Figure 4. MTT assay for the assessment of in vitro cytotoxicity. (**a**) In vitro cytotoxicity of SA at various (from 0.05 to 0.4 mg/m/L) concentrations evaluated on RAW 264.7 murine macrophages. (**b**) In vitro cytotoxicity of SA at the same concentrations evaluated on human differentiated THP-1 M0 macrophages. The results are expressed as a percentage of viability with respect to the control (untreated cells) and are the mean ± SD of three experiments performed in five replicates. ANOVA was significant (i.e., $p < 0.05$) in (**a**), with ** $p < 0.01$ vs. NT in Tukey post-test.

- Gene expression analysis for LPS-activated RAW 264.7 macrophages

RAW 264.7 cells were stimulated with 100 ng/mL of pro-inflammatory bacterial endotoxin (LPS). The expression of inflammatory cytokines and mediators, such as interleukin 1β (IL-1β); interleukin 6 (IL-6); the murine homologue of human IL-8 cytokine, i.e., C-X-C Motif Chemokine Ligand 5 (CXCL5); tumor necrosis factor (TNF-α); and cyclooxygenase-2 (COX-2), was evaluated by qPCR to assess the in vitro anti-inflammatory potential of the *E. amentacea* SA at 0.2 and 0.4 mg/mL concentrations.

All investigated cytokines and inflammatory mediators were significantly overexpressed in murine macrophages following 8 or 24 h of LPS treatment (Figure 5a,b), as compared to untreated controls. After 8 h of LPS stimulation, the SA at the lowest concentration (0.2 mg/mL) exhibited inhibition potentials of 17% and 12% on the overexpression of IL-6 and CXCL5, respectively, as compared to LPS alone (Figure 5a). On the other hand, the highest SA concentration (0.4 mg/mL) led to the inhibition of the IL-6 gene by 26%. Instead, a significant gene expression increase in IL-1β, exceeding that of LPS alone, was detected after both SA treatments, while no significant effects were detected in either SA treatment on the COX-2 and TNF-α gene expression profiles after the 8 h LPS stimulation.

After 24 h, the lowest SA concentration (0.2 mg/mL) led to a significant inhibition of IL-6, TNF-α, and CXCL5 overexpression, as compared to LPS alone, by 25%, 39%, and 20%, respectively (Figure 5b). On the other hand, at the highest SA concentration (0.4 mg/mL),

https://doi.org/10.3390/md24010041

we observed the inhibition of IL-1β and CXCL5 overexpression, as compared to LPS alone, by 15% and 40%, respectively. No inhibitory effects were detected in the induced COX-2 gene overexpression by either SA concentration. In conclusion, a mild but significant inhibition of IL-6, CXCL5, and TNF-α gene expression was achieved in inflamed murine macrophages following *E. amentacea* SA treatment. Parallel experiments were performed in RAW 264.7 cells using 0.4 mg/mL of commercial low and medium molecular weight SA (CL and CM, respectively) and are reported in Figure S1. In this case, at 8 h (panel A) in the presence of LPS, both CL and CM significantly stimulated IL-1β, IL-6, and CXCL5 expression as compared to LPS alone, with no significant effect on TNF-α and COX-2 stimulation. This trend was also maintained at 24 h (panel B), with the only difference observed in TNF-α being slight inhibition caused by both alginates as compared to LPS alone. These data reveal significantly different behaviors between the *E. amentacea*-extracted SA and the two commercially available SAs, with the former showing potential, although mild, anti-inflammatory activity in activated murine macrophages not paralleled by the latter.

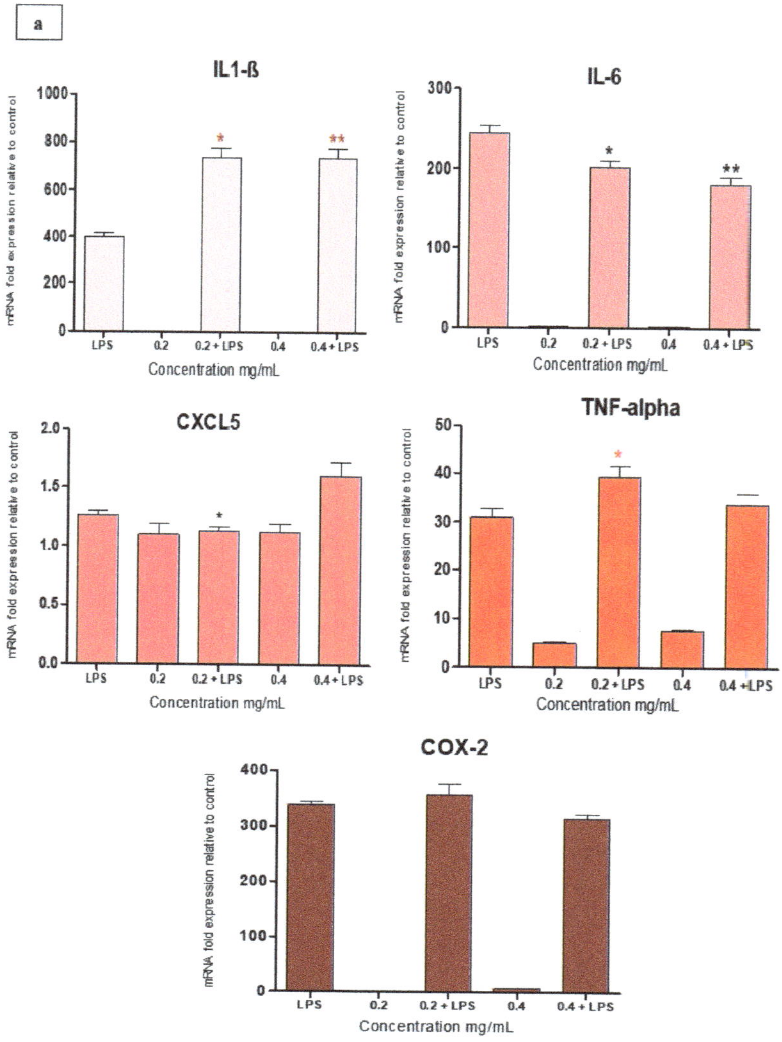

Figure 5. *Cont.*

https://doi.org/10.3390/md24010041

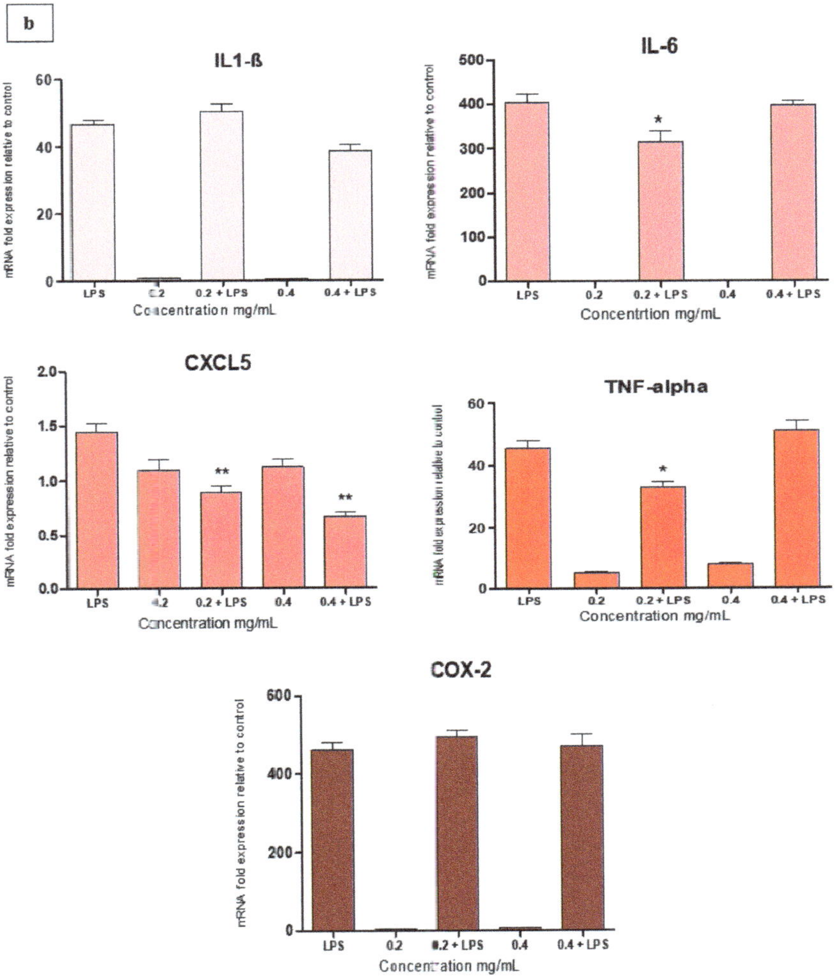

Figure 5. *E. amentacea* SA inhibition of gene expression in LPS-activated RAW 264.7 macrophages. Gene expression measured by qPCR analysis of IL-1β, IL-6, CXCL5, TNF-α, and COX-2, after incubation for 8 h (**a**) and 24 h (**b**), with or without LPS (100 ng/mL), and in the presence or absence of 0.2 and 0.4 mg/mL SA. Data are normalized on the GAPDH housekeeping gene and expressed as mRNA fold increase compared to control, untreated cells. Results are the mean ± SD of three experiments performed in duplicate. ANOVA was significant in each histogram ($p < 0.05$), with * $p < 0.05$, and ** $p < 0.01$ vs. LPS in Tukey post-test.

- Gene expression analysis of LPS-activated THP-1 M0

Differentiated human THP-1 M0 macrophages were stimulated with 100 ng/mL of LPS. The expression of inflammatory cytokines, i.e., IL-1β, IL-6, IL-8, monocyte chemoattractant protein-1 (MCP-1), and TNF-α, was evaluated by qPCR to assess the anti-inflammatory potential of the *E. amentacea* SA at a 0.4 mg/mL concentration.

All inflammatory cytokines were significantly upregulated after 24 h of LPS incubation (Figure 6), and SA treatment resulted in the significant inhibition of IL-6, IL-8, MCP-1, and TNF-α, as compared to LPS alone, by 46%, 46%, 81%, and 23%, respectively. Similarly to the results obtained from RAW 264.7 macrophages, also in THP-1 M0 cells, no inhibitory effects were detected in the LPS-stimulated IL-1β gene overexpression. Also in this case,

https://doi.org/10.3390/md24010041

parallel experiments were performed on THP-1 M0 macrophages by using 0.4 mg/mL of commercial CL and CM SA (Figure S2), and the results showed very different behavior with respect to the *E. amentacea* SA extract. In particular, no inhibitory effect on LPS-overexpressed cytokines was observed in the presence of CL SA, except for a light decrease in MCP-1, while a slight but significant inhibition of all cytokines was observed in the case of the CM treatment, as compared to LPS alone, indicating a mild anti-inflammatory effect on activated human macrophages caused by the medium molecular weight SA.

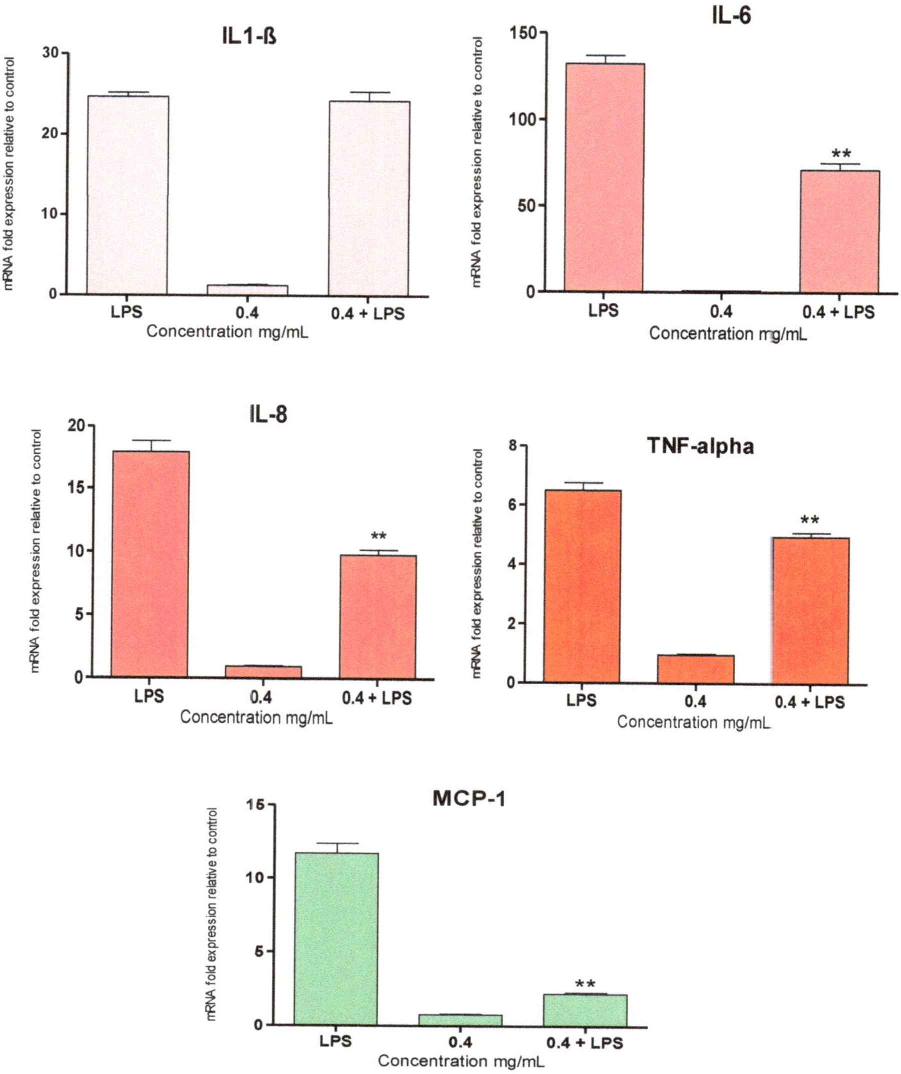

Figure 6. *E. amentacea* SA inhibition of gene expression in THP-1 M0 macrophages. Gene expression measured by qPCR analysis of IL-1β, IL-6, IL-8, TNF-α, and MCP-1 after THP-1 M0 macrophage incubation, with or without LPS (100 ng/mL), and in the presence or absence of 0.4 mg/mL SA for 24 h. Data are normalized on the HPRT-1 housekeeping gene and expressed as mRNA fold increase compared to control, untreated cells. Results are the mean $\pm$ SD of three experiments performed in duplicate. ANOVA was significant in each histogram ($p < 0.05$), with ** $p < 0.01$ vs. LPS in Tukey post-test.

https://doi.org/10.3390/md24010041

- NO-Scavenging activity and iNOS gene expression in LPS-Activated RAW 264.7 Macrophages

RAW 264.7 macrophages were stimulated with LPS (100 ng/mL), and the NO production was evaluated after incubation in the presence or absence of the *E. amentacea* SA at 0.2 and 0.4 mg/mL (Figure 7). LPS stimulation led to significant NO overproduction in RAW 264.7 macrophages (17.35 and 40.01 nmol/mL/mg protein after 8 and 24 h incubation; Figure 7a and b, respectively) compared to control cells, in which the production was undetectable. After 8 h of incubation, NO production was significantly inhibited (by 45.5% and 52%) by both the 0.2 and 0.4 mg/mL SA concentrations, respectively. Similarly, the LPS-stimulated NO overproduction was significantly inhibited by the two SA concentrations after 24 h of incubation by 44.7% and 34%, respectively.

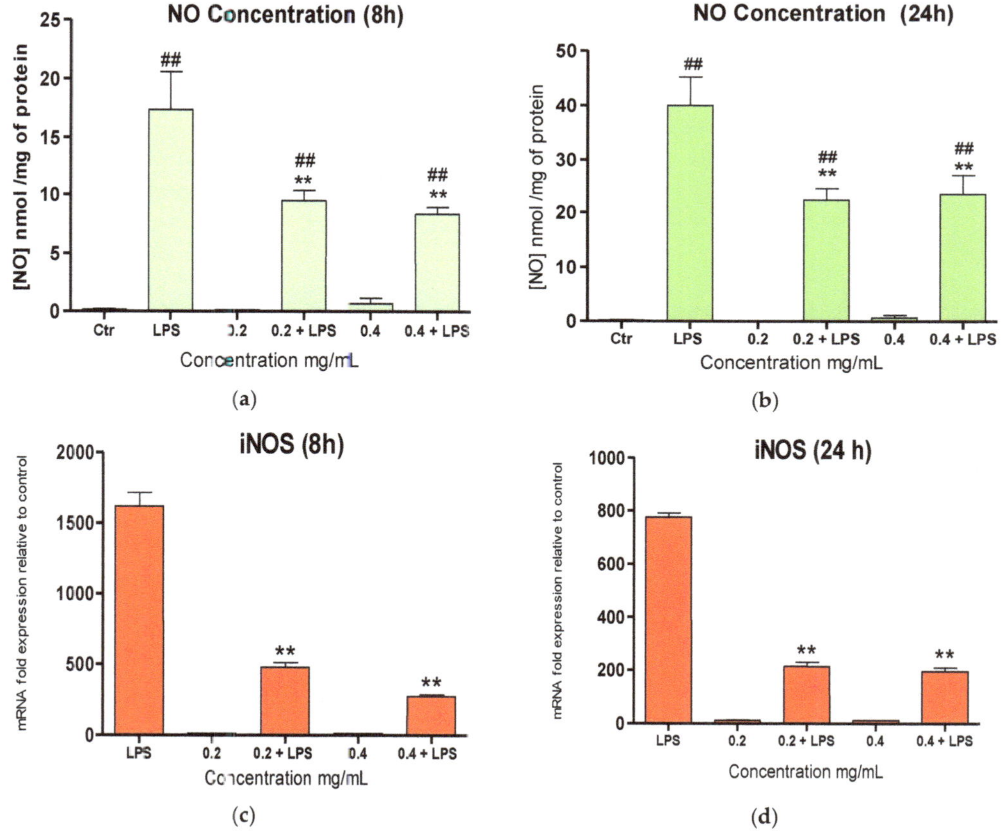

Figure 7. NO-scavenging activity and iNOS gene expression in cellular assay. (**a**,**b**) Intracellular NO production measured by Griess assay in RAW 264.7 murine macrophages incubated for 8 h (**a**) and 24 h (**b**) with LPS (100 ng/mL) in the presence or absence of 0.2 and 0.4 mg/mL of SA. The results are expressed as a percentage of NO production, with respect to control, untreated cells, and are the mean ± SD of two assays performed in triplicate. (**c**,**d**) Gene expression measured by qPCR analysis of iNOS after RAW 264.7 cell incubation, for 8 h (**c**) and 24 h (**d**), with or without 100 ng/mL LPS and in the presence or absence of 0.2 and 0.4 mg/mL SA. Data are normalized on the GAPDH housekeeping gene and expressed as mRNA fold increases compared to control, untreated cells. Results are the mean ± SD of three experiments performed in duplicate. ANOVA was significant in each histogram ($p < 0.05$), with ** $p < 0.01$ vs. LPS in Tukey post-test and ## $p < 0.01$ vs. negative control in Tukey post-test.

 https://doi.org/10.3390/md24010041

In relation to this important inhibition of NO production at the biochemical level, we also aimed to quantify the enzyme responsible for its production, the inducible NO synthase (iNOS). The gene expression level was quantified after LPS stimulation in the presence and absence of the *E. amentacea* SA (Figure 7c,d). Indeed, a strong impairment of inducible NO synthase expression was achieved in inflamed murine macrophages following the SA treatment. In detail, after 8 h, we observed inhibitions of 70% and 83% on the overexpression of the iNOS gene, as compared to LPS alone (Figure 7c), in the presence of 0.2 and 0.4 mg/mL SA, respectively. Following this trend, also after 24 h, both SA concentrations maintained a significant 70% inhibition of iNOS overexpression, as compared to LPS alone (Figure 7d). Parallel experiments were performed using 0.4 mg/mL of commercial CL and CM SA in the presence of LPS, also in this case measuring NO release and iNOS gene expression in RAW 264.7 macrophages. The results are shown in Figure S3. In detail, concerning NO release, no inhibition of this molecular species was observed after the 8 h treatment in the presence of LPS and CL, while a significant increase was observed in the presence of LPS and CM SA as compared to LPS alone. Conversely, at 24 h, the two commercial SAs caused a slight decrease in NO production as compared to LPS alone. Furthermore, concerning the iNOS gene expression, at both 8 and 24 h, the two commercial SAs caused a significant decrease, as compared to overexpression caused by LPS alone, although this inhibition was significantly lower than that obtained in the presence of the *E. amentacea* SA extract.

3. Discussion

For the first time, the structural characterization of sodium alginate (SA) isolated from *E. amentacea* end-products, specifically from apices wasted by a cultivation step during an algal forest restoration, is reported. The extraction yield of the *E. amentacea* SA was about 3.05% (*w*/*w*), which is close to the 5.43% reported by Zrid and collaborators [32] for alginate extracted from another species of the same complex, *Cystoseira humilis*. This yield was lower by about three-fold than that obtained with other species of *Cystoseria* complex, such as *Gongolaria barbata* SA (9.9% [33]) and *Ericaria sedoides* (11% [34]) harvested from the Tunisian coasts. Moreover, the obtained yield was much lower compared with other species, such as *Cystoseira crinita* (20.18% [15]), *Cystoseira compressa* (21.65% [35]), *Laminaria digitate* (36% [36]), *Macrocystis pyrifera* (18–45% [37]), *Laminaria ochroleuca* (50% [38]), *Durvillaea antarctica* (53%), *Ecklonia cava* (35–38%) [39], *Durvillaea potatorum* (55% [40]). As demonstrated in Table 1, SA contained 44.25% total sugars and 49% uronic acids, with the presence of some impurities like proteins (0.53%) and phenolic compounds (0.93%). All of these results were in accordance with the literature concerning SA extracted from other algal species, such as *Padina perindusiata*, *G. barbata*, and *C. compressa* [33,35,41]. This broad disparity in the extraction yields and chemical composition of all of these brown seaweeds might be explained by some differences in the extraction procedures but also by the seasonal trends and ecological factors, as well as the species' own characteristics [33,37]. In our case, the use of the seaweed apices after gamete release induction for the ex situ cultivation step for algal restoration purposes may also explain the lower SA yield from the present *E. amentacea* samples. Indeed, the seaweed apices could present lower SA content either because they are younger formations and/or because they need a different structural plasticity/flexibility, as compared to the stiffness of the mature thalli.

The calculated M/G ratio of the *E. amentacea* SA was 2.33, indicating that this polymer is primarily composed of 70% mannuronic acid (F_M = 0.7) and 30% guluronic acid (F_G = 0.3). Similar results have been reported in studies on other algal species. For instance, SA extracted from *D. potatorum*, *Saccorhiza polyschides*, and *D. antarctica* exhibited mannuronic/guluronic (M/G) ratios of 2.125, 2.14, and 2.15, respectively [38]. This ratio

 https://doi.org/10.3390/md24010041

was lower than those reported in the literature for SA extracted from *Turbinaria turbinata* (M/G = 2.66), *Durvillaea willana* (M/G = 2.57), *Fucus guiryi* (M/G = 4.41), *Sargassum cinereum* (M/G = 4.5), and *Dictyota dichotoma* (M/G = 4.8) [29,38,42]. These values are considered high, as several algal SAs typically exhibit M/G ratios ranging between 0.45 and 1.86 [15]. According to the literature, M/G ratios are influenced by factors such as algal maturity, seasonal environmental conditions, and the extraction method used [11]. In addition, the various biological activities of SA polysaccharides are often closely related to their physical properties in aqueous media. The physicochemical characteristics of alginate depend not only on the M/G ratio but more fundamentally on the molar frequencies of uronic acid pairings—specifically, the homopolymeric block structures (F_{MM}; F_{GG}) and the alternating blocks ($F_{MG}/_{GM}$). These structural parameters significantly influence the chemical and physical behavior of alginates, as the stiffness of the polymer chain increases in the order MM-block < MG-block < GG-block. Therefore, this allows for the classification of alginates as high-M ($F_M > 0.7$), low-M ($F_M < 0.6$), and intermediate-M (F_M, 0.6–0.7) [43]. Based on our results, the alginate extracted from the *E. amentacea* algal apices yielded an intermediate-M ($F_M = 0.7$), which contained a higher homopolymeric fraction ($F_{MM} = 0.66$; $F_{GG} = 0.26$) compared to heteropolymeric blocks ($F_{GM}/_{MG} = 0.04$), with a predominance of MM-blocks ($\eta = 0.190$), allowing for more flexibility compared to seaweed thalli [44]. A complete description of the alginate monomer sequence is not possible only through diad analysis (F_{GG}, F_{MM}, F_{GM}, and F_{MG}), as described previously. Nevertheless, the η parameter, defined as $\eta = F_{MG}/(F_M \times F_G)$, can be used to predict the sequence distributions in algal alginates. Therefore, values of $\eta < 1$ indicate the abundance of MM and GG homopolymeric block types, whereas $\eta = 1$ reveals completely random cases, and $1 < \eta < 2$ illustrates alternate-like cases of MG and GM [30,45]. The calculated η value for the extracted alginate was 0.190 ($\eta < 1$), indicating a polymer structure predominantly composed of homopolymeric block sequences.

Structural characteristics of SA might be tied to the functional and ecological roles of *E. amentacea* apices. In fact, *E. amentacea* is typically found in shallow, intertidal, or upper subtidal habitats, where it is constantly exposed to strong hydrodynamic forces such as waves, currents, and tidal fluctuations. In such environments, mechanical flexibility is critical to preventing structural damage. The apical regions are younger, actively growing tissues that must maintain structural integrity while still being pliable enough to withstand water movement. Higher MM content in alginate allows these tissues to bend and flex without breaking, acting almost like a shock absorber against mechanical stress. Moreover, the apices are also sites of cell division and elongation, requiring a less rigid and more hydrated cell wall to accommodate expansion [46,47]. Mannuronic acid-rich alginate forms softer, more elastic gels, which likely facilitate cell wall remodeling during growth and morphogenesis. Indeed, it is important to note that the composition and structure of alginate can vary along different parts of the algal body. The stipe or basal regions may contain more guluronic acid-rich alginate (a lower M/G ratio), which forms stiffer, more rigid gels (due to GG-block dominance), contributing to mechanical strength and anchorage. In contrast, the apex may maintain a mannuronic-rich composition specifically to preserve tissue flexibility, which is essential for both growth and hydrodynamic performance in exposed shallow-water habitats [15,48,49]. From a biotechnological perspective, the structural characteristics of SA are generally very useful for many bioengineering applications, particularly for the production of soft hydrogels and flexible membranes. The high mannuronic acid (M) content leads to the formation of softer, more elastic gels that can better accommodate dynamic environments, ideal for tissue engineering, wound healing, and drug delivery systems where mechanical adaptability, moisture retention,

 https://doi.org/10.3390/md24010041

and biocompatibility are critical [50,51]. These hydrogels can closely mimic the natural extracellular matrix, supporting cell growth and migration [52,53].

The estimated molecular weight (M_W) for our SA extract was remarkably low compared to those reported in previous investigations on alginates from fucales, such as *E. sedoides*, *C. compressa*, and *G. barbata*, which had M_W values of 1×10^5, 1.4×10^5, and 2×10^5, respectively [33–35]. SA polydispersity index q was around 3.5, indicating a partially hydrolyzed alginate, probably a result of the extraction process [33]. The SA intrinsic viscosity (37 mL/g) was ten times lower compared to other *Cystoseiraceae* species, which were in the range of 283–860 mL/g [33]. These results may be related to our extraction process, which differs from the standard protocol usually used to purify sodium alginate (SA). We employed a hydrothermal–alkaline extraction, starting with a thermal treatment (2 h at 120 °C) typically used for fucoidan polysaccharides, followed by a precipitation with $CaCl_2$ and alkaline treatment to recover the alginate. This approach is sustainable, as it allows for the simultaneous extraction of both fucoidan and alginate polymers from the by-products of ex situ algal cultivation for restoration purposes. Thus, our extract cannot be considered crude alginate due to partial degradation; however, it also cannot be strictly classified as an oligosaccharide since this is generally between 200 and 4000 Da [54]. Furthermore, we used the apical (new growth) parts of the algae for restoration, which may also explain the lower molecular weight, as younger tissues contain lower M_W alginate compared to older parts [15].

The antioxidant potential of seaweed extracts makes them promising candidates for nutritional, pharmacological, and medical applications [55]. For this reason, the antioxidant activity of *E. amentacea* SA extract was evaluated using three different in chemico assays: overall radical-scavenging activity, Fe^{3+} reducing power, and nitric oxide (NO) scavenging activity. The DPPH assay is widely used to assess the free radical-scavenging ability of compounds and is a reliable method for evaluating the reducing properties of antioxidant substances [56]. The SA polysaccharide demonstrated a concentration-dependent antiradical activity. At the highest concentration (1.25 mg/mL), it showed a scavenging potential exceeding 90%, while at the lowest (0.125 mg/mL), the activity remained slightly above 30%. This result is comparable to that reported by Hentati et al. [35], who studied the DPPH scavenging activity of SA extracted from *C. compressa* and found approximately 46% activity at 0.5 mg/mL. However, this is lower than the scavenging activity observed for SA extracted from *G. barbata*, which reached 74% at the same concentration [33]. Moreover, the *E. amentacea* SA extract showed an IC_{50} value of approximately 0.41 mg/mL, which is lower (more potent) than the alginate extracted from *E. sedoides* (IC_{50} = 2 mg/mL [34]) and also lower than that of *C. compressa*, which showed an IC_{50} of around 0.56 mg/mL [35]. In general, the DPPH radical-scavenging effect of antioxidant polysaccharides is closely related to their hydrogen-donating ability. The mechanism of DPPH scavenging has been associated with several antioxidant processes, including chain inhibition, prevention of continued hydrogen abstraction, hydrogen donation, and direct radical scavenging [57]. According to the literature, mannuronic acid units form β-(1→4) bonds, resulting in linear and flexible M-block segments. In contrast, guluronic acid units are connected by α-(1→4) bonds, introducing steric hindrance around the carboxyl groups, which leads to folded, rigid conformations in the G-block segments [10]. Based on this information, the high mannuronic acid content of the extracted SA from *E. amentacea* may show higher chain flexibility, thereby exposing more –OH and $–COO^-$ groups in M-blocks and enhancing radical-scavenging activity. In addition, low-molecular-weight alginates obtained by heat treatment have been reported to exhibit higher antioxidant activity than non-treated alginates [58], which is consistent with the lower molecular weight observed in our SA extract. These findings suggest that this *E. amentacea* SA extract possesses promising

https://doi.org/10.3390/md24010041

antioxidant properties, making it a potential bioactive molecule for pharmaceutical and nutraceutical applications.

Following the evaluation of the overall antioxidant capacity of the SA polysaccharide, its specific scavenging activity against highly reactive oxygen species (ROS) was investigated. This approach aimed to identify which ROS might be most effectively influenced at the intracellular level by the pharmacological application of *E. amentacea* SA. This analysis is particularly relevant, as ROS are commonly produced during oxidative stress and are closely associated with both acute and chronic inflammatory conditions. The Fe^{3+}-reducing power of the SA extract was assessed using the potassium ferricyanide method. The reducing power of SA increased with concentration, ranging from 0.067 to 0.535 mg/mL, and reached an absorbance (A_{700} nm) of 1.06 at 0.535 mg/mL. This result is consistent with findings reported by Hentati et al. [35], who observed an A_{700} of approximately 1.0 at 0.5 mg/mL of SA extracted from *C. compressa*. Additionally, the reducing power observed in our study was higher than that reported by Sellimi et al. [33], who measured an A_{700} of 0.7 at the same concentration of SA extracted from *G. barbata*. These findings demonstrate that the *E. amentacea* SA can act as an effective electron donor, reacting with free radicals to convert them into more stable, non-reactive species and thereby interrupting radical chain reactions.

Additionally, the nitric oxide (NO) scavenging activity of the SA polysaccharide was evaluated. NO radicals are known to cause significant molecular damage both intracellularly and extracellularly under conditions of oxidative stress. Moreover, they function as secondary messengers in key signal transduction pathways, contributing to the propagation of the inflammatory response [59]. The extracted SA exhibited an in chemico NO-scavenging activity of 50% at a concentration of 0.417 mg/mL. Although no prior studies were found in the literature evaluating NO-scavenging activity specifically for SA, similar activities were reported for ethanol and DMSO extracts of *E. amentacea*, with calculated IC_{50} values of 0.546 mg/mL and 1.293 mg/mL, respectively [60]. However, in that case, the effect was mostly due to the presence of polyphenols and meroditerpenes species in those extracts, in the absence of polysaccharides. Notably, also in in vitro experiments, in the LPS-stimulated RAW 264.7 cellular model, after only 8 h, more than 40% inhibition of NO release in the extracellular medium was observed in the presence of the SA extract and maintained over time (i.e., up to 24 h). However, this inhibitory activity was not concentration-dependent, reaching a maximum at 0.2 mg/mL SA and not increasing at higher amounts. Moreover, the in vitro cellular tests also showed a pronounced inhibition of LPS-induced iNOS gene overexpression in RAW 264.7 murine macrophages, responsible for the massive production of NO during the inflammatory response, with over 70% suppression at both 8 and 24 h incubation times in the presence of SA. Conversely, by using two different commercial SAs characterized by low and medium molecular weights (CL and CM), we could not obtain the same remarkable inhibition of both NO production and iNOS expression. In fact, only a slight effect for the two commercial SA was observed (~20% NO release at 24 h and iNOS overexpression at 8 and 24 h, respectively). These different results could indicate that the inhibitory effect on this important inflammatory pathway could be due to the specific chemical composition of each SA and/or to the different molecular weight and tridimensional conformation of the various SA polymers. These effects are particularly noteworthy since, in addition to exerting direct antioxidant activity by scavenging NO excess produced by this enzyme, *E. amentacea* SA can also inhibit the upstream expression of iNOS at the mRNA level, thereby reducing both its transcription and protein production. This dual mechanism has the potential to effectively diminish the damage caused by excessive NO. These results are in accordance with those reported for some alginate oligosaccharides [61,62], indicating a similar effect compared to our low-M_w SA

https://doi.org/10.3390/md24010041

hydrothermal extract. Overall, these data demonstrate the very promising activity of the *E. amentacea* SA, which could pave the way for the use of this seaweed-derived product as a tool to reduce inflammatory foci, where the NO overproduction often leads to significant tissue damage if not counteracted by pharmacological intervention [63].

Inflammation plays a key role in the development of several pathological conditions, including cancer, obesity, and cardiovascular diseases [64,65]. Toll-like receptors (TLRs), particularly TLR4, are central to the molecular mechanisms underlying these conditions [66]. When activated by lipopolysaccharide (LPS), TLR4 triggers signaling pathways that lead to the activation of the transcription factor NF-κB, as well as several kinases, such as Akt, MAPK, and PI3K. This cascade results in the increased synthesis of inflammation-related mediators, including prostaglandin E2 (PGE_2) and nitric oxide (NO), produced by the pro-inflammatory enzymes COX-2 and iNOS, respectively, and pro-inflammatory cytokines [67,68]. As a consequence, excessive or chronic inflammation may have detrimental effects on the body. In this context, polymers such as alginate have been widely studied for their anti-inflammatory properties, owing to their high biocompatibility [69–71]. In addition to its notable antioxidant and NO-scavenging activity, SA extracted from *E. amentacea* demonstrated significant anti-inflammatory effects. These effects were observed in both RAW 264.7 murine macrophages and differentiated human THP-1 M0 macrophages following LPS treatment for 8 and 24 h. Notably, in both cell lines, the SA extract at 24 h significantly reduced the expression levels of key pro-inflammatory cytokines, including IL-6, IL-8/CXCL5, and TNF-α, which are crucial mediators in propagating inflammatory signals and recruiting immune cells to the site of inflammation. The anti-inflammatory potential of our SA extract was especially evident in human THP-1 M0 macrophages, where the suppression effect of IL-6, IL-8, MCP-1, and TNF-α was even more prominent than in murine macrophages.

Conversely, by using the same dose of SA for a shorter incubation time in the presence of LPS (8 h), we observed inhibitory effects only on some inflammatory mediators in RAW 264.7 murine macrophages. Specifically, the expression levels of IL-6, CXCL5 (i.e., the functional homolog of human IL-8 in mice), and iNOS were significantly suppressed, whereas IL-1β and TNF-α expression levels showed an increase, while COX-2 remained unaffected by the presence of *E. amentacea* SA. Thus, there is a limitation in the anti-inflammatory potential of the new SA extract, which is indeed absent for LPS-induced IL1-β and COX-2, where no efficacy could be claimed. At the same time, parallel experiments performed on commercial CL and CM SA showed the very low anti-inflammatory potential of these two polymers as compared to the *E. amentacea* SA extract. The inhibitory effect was only observed by use of the medium-molecular-weight SA (CM) versus IL-6, IL-8, TNF-α, and MCP-1 cytokine overexpression, indicating different degrees of efficacy of the various SA obtained from marine organisms. Our results indicate that this inhibitory potential likely depends both on the different monomer chemical composition, as well as on the average molecular weight of the polysaccharide extracted, since our SA shows a significantly lower M_w as compared to the commercial ones. Notably, all SAs tested in this study failed to exert any inhibition of COX-2 overexpression and also caused a significant IL-1β increase in the presence of LPS early stimulation (8 h) in murine macrophages, indicating that these polysaccharides may act at different levels of the various cytokine induction pathways, with different results for each cytokine. Furthermore, the two commercial SAs caused a significant increase in IL-1β and IL-6 at 24 h in LPS-stimulated murine macrophages, and these results are partially comparable to those reported by Yang and Jones [72], who demonstrated that SA stimulated RAW 264.7 macrophages, increasing the levels of pro-inflammatory cytokines IL-1β, IL-6, IL-12, and TNF-α and activating innate immune responses through NF-κB signaling. This pro-inflammatory effect was attributed

 https://doi.org/10.3390/md24010041

to an SA containing high proportions of M- and MG-blocks. Similar observations have been reported in other studies [15]. While these findings partially align with our results, we observed a contrasting outcome, in that *E. amentacea* SA at the same incubation time significantly inhibited the expression of IL-6, CXCL5, and iNOS, and even more at longer incubation times. Indeed, at 24 h of incubation, where most cytokines were significantly inhibited by the *E. amentacea* SA, both in murine and human macrophages, our findings are in contrast with previous reports that suggest that high mannuronic acid content in SA enhances its immunogenicity and promotes immunostimulatory effects [73,74]. In fact, the SA used in this study, composed of 70% mannuronic acid and 30% guluronic acid, exhibited significant anti-inflammatory and antioxidant activities in two macrophage cellular models. Since our *E. amentacea* SA showed a lower average molecular weight than other alginates, we may at least partially attribute the anti-inflammatory effect exerted on immune cells to this difference, other than the presence of other components in the SA extracts from other marine organisms, as compared to the one we obtained through a hydrothermal process from this brown seaweed. Notably, it is frequently reported that brown algae alginate extracts retain low levels of phenolic compounds [34,35,42,75,76] and that achieving completely phenolic-free alginate from brown seaweed is technically challenging [42]. Thus, although sodium alginate represents the largely predominant component of the *E. amentacea* extract and is likely to play a major role in the biological effects observed, a partial contribution of residual polyphenols cannot be excluded.

These in vitro results for *E. amentacea* SA in immune cells also demonstrate promising therapeutic potential for in vivo systems, where dampening these signals is essential to extinguishing inflammatory foci and reducing the possibility of the chronicization of the process since all the above-mentioned cytokines are involved in feeding and propagating the inflammation at the tissue level [77]. Notably, the ability of the SA extract to inhibit a wide range of critical inflammatory mediators—including cytokines and NO synthase—suggests that its mechanism of action may occur upstream in the inflammatory signaling cascade. This could involve interference with key signals, like an intracellular ROS increase, for example, which is known to activate transduction pathways that lead to macrophage activation and subsequent changes in gene expression profiles during the inflammatory response [78]. Similar to our findings in vitro, other authors have reported the anti-inflammatory effects of alginate in in vivo studies. Indeed, various forms of alginate, from oligosaccharides to microspheres or hydrogels, have already been used to alleviate ulcerative colitis and joint inflammatory disorder symptoms with promising lenitive and anti-inflammatory outcomes [63,79–81]. Furthermore, alginate has been shown to exert local anti-inflammatory effects, and it is already in use for rectal administration in the treatment of chronic hemorrhoids, proctosigmoiditis, and chronic anal fissures following surgical interventions in the rectal region [82]. Additionally, alginate has been reported to promote mucous membrane regeneration, suppress gastric inflammation, and support the restoration of intestinal microbial flora. These polymers have also demonstrated beneficial effects in treating inflammation of the gastric and esophageal mucosa, as well as radiation-induced stomatitis [83]. Notably, the SA extracted from *E. amentacea* would add the remarkable NO-scavenging effect and inhibition of iNOS production to the already known properties of polysaccharides, increasing the pharmacological success of alginate therapies in all the above-mentioned diseases. Thus, many possibilities for employment seem to lie ahead for this SA extract obtained from *E. amentacea* Mediterranean brown seaweed

https://doi.org/10.3390/md24010041

4. Materials and Methods

4.1. Chemicals

Ethanol, $CaCl_2$ Na_2CO_3, HCl, NaOH, phenol, H_2SO_4, glucose, uronic acid, carbazole, Bradford reagent, Folin–Ciocalteu reagent, D2O, 2,2-diphenyl-1-picrylhydrazyl (DPPH), ascorbic acid, Na_2HPO_4, potassium ferricyanide, trichloroacetic acid, $FeCl_3$, sodium nitroprusside, Griess reagent, $NaNO_2$, 3-(4,5-dimethyl-2-yl)-2,5-diphenyltetrazolium bromide (MTT), lipopolysaccharide (LPS), SDS, DTT, glycerol, and TRIS-HCl, alginic acid low viscosity, and alginic acid medium viscosity were purchased from Sigma-Aldrich (Milan, Italy). DMEM medium, fetal bovine serum (FBS), and RPMI 1640 medium were acquired from Microtech srl (Naples, Italy). Phorbol-12-myristate 13-acetate (PMA) was purchased from PeproTech EC (London, UK). RNeasy Mini Kit was obtained from Qiagen (Milan, Italy). cDNA Synthesis Kit and 4× CAPITAL™ qPCR Green Master Mix were acquired from biotechrabbit GmbH (Henningsdorf, Germany).

4.2. Raw Material

In the Ligurian Sea (Northwestern Mediterranean), apices of *Ericaria amentacea* were harvested in the midlittoral zone, on exposed rocky shores, in Bogliasco, Genoa (NW Italy, 44 2°2′40.37″ N–9°4035.14″ E), in the summer of 2023. After retrieval, the apices were stored in plastic bags kept in cold conditions and immediately transported to the DISTAV laboratory at the University of Genoa. The biomass was thoroughly washed with sterilized seawater to remove sand particles and epiphytes. In the culture facility, the apices were used to seed restoration units following the protocol by Falace et al. [28]. After the release of gametes, the waste biomass from the ex situ culture step was dried at 55 °C for 22 h in the dark to prevent any possible degradation associated with light. The dried sample material was ground using a blender, passed through a 0.5 mm sieve, and kept in plastic bags at −20 °C until use.

4.3. Sodium Alginate Extraction

E. amentacea sodium alginate was extracted by hydrothermal–alkaline extraction [35,84] with some editing (Figure 8). Initially, 10 g of dried apex seaweed powder underwent mild depigmentation and delipidation in EtOH (80% v/v, 24 h). Afterward, the residue was subjected to a thermal treatment at 120 °C for 1 h in an autoclave (Vapor matrc 770, Asal srl, Milan, Italy). The extraction was performed in duplicate, and solids were separated from the liquid by centrifugation (3040 rpm, 13 min). A solution of 35% $CaCl_2$ was added to the supernatant, corresponding to 1% $CaCl_2$ final concentration, and kept at 4 °C overnight. Subsequently, the wet pellet obtained after centrifugation was treated with 100 mL of Na_2CO_3 (3% (w/v), pH = 11) at 60 °C for 2 h under stirring (the supernatant was stocked at −20 °C for fucoidan extraction). After centrifugation at 4000 rpm for 25 min at 4 °C, the supernatant was treated with 2 volumes of 96% ice-cold ethanol (−20 °C) for 15 min, with slight manual stirring, for polysaccharides precipitation. The precipitate was separated by centrifugation (4000 rpm, 45 min, 4 °C), resolubilized in deionized water and then acidified with 6 M HCl to precipitate the alginic acid at a pH value of $1.5 \leq pH \leq 3$. The pellet formed after centrifugation (4000 rpm, 30 min, 4 °C) was resuspended in 40 mL of deionized water and neutralized (pH = 7.5) with an aqueous NaOH (1 M) solution. The obtained sodium alginate (SA) was finally precipitated with two volumes of ice-cold ethanol (96%) for 15 min, and the resulting suspension was centrifuged at 4000 rpm for 45 min at 4 °C. Finally, the polysaccharide pellet was solubilized (50 g/L) and lyophilized to obtain the SA. The yield was calculated using the equation below:

$$\text{Yield of SA (\%)} = (\text{weight of SA}/\text{weight of seaweed dried biomass}) \times 100$$

https://doi.org/10.3390/md24010041

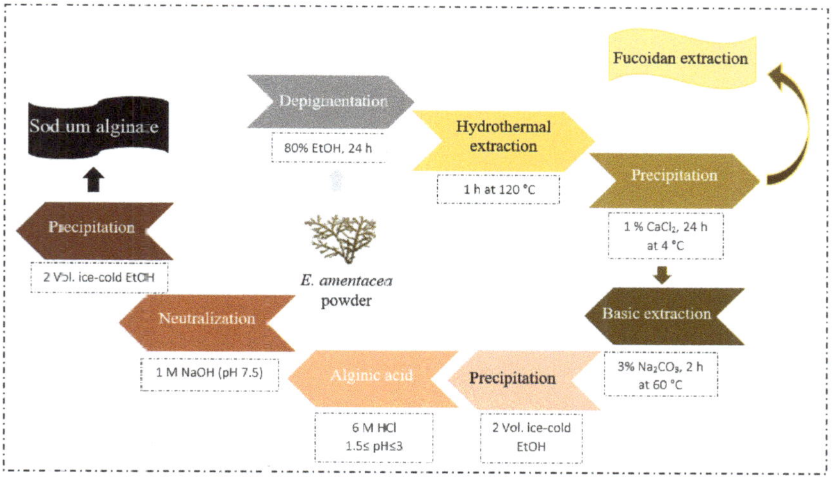

Figure 8. Processing steps for the extraction of alginate from *E. amentacea* dry seaweed biomass.

4.4. Physicochemical Characterization

4.4.1. Centesimal Composition

Total sugars in SA were measured by the phenol-H_2SO_4 method [85], using glucose as a standard. Meanwhile, uronic acids were determined using the carbazole method [86] and glucuronic acid as a standard. The quantification of protein and polyphenol contents was accomplished using the Bradford [87] and Folin–Ciocalteu methods [88], respectively.

4.4.2. Spectral Analyses

- Fourier-transform infrared spectroscopy

The Fourier-transform infrared (FTIR) spectra of the SA were analyzed to identify the possible functional groups as a variation in functional groups in the standard, using a Bruker Vertex 70 spectrometer (Bruker, Milan, Italy). The spectrum was recorded over the range 4000–400 cm^{-1} with 128 scans at a resolution of 2 cm^{-1} by using the platinum ATR: a single reflection diamond ATR sampling accessory.

- NMR spectroscopy

SA was dissolved in D_2O (99.9% D) at a concentration of 6 g/L. After dissolution, the sample was freeze-dried, resulting in sodium alginate with exchangeable protons replaced by deuterium. In total, this step was performed 3 times. Before analysis, the SA-lyophilized sample was dissolved again in D_2O (99.9% D) at a concentration of 8.5 g/L. NMR spectra were obtained at 80 °C using a Jeol JNM-ECZ400R (Akishima, Tokyo, Japan) (400 MHz for ^1H) with a Royal HFX probe. All NMR spectra were analyzed using the software MestReNova (Mestrelab Research® v. 14.2) (Santiago de Compostela, Spain). A spectral width of 4000 Hz was used to acquire the data obtained under the following acquisition parameters: acquisition mode = 2 s, pulse 90° = 8 µsec, scans = 64, recovery = 5 s (for a complete return after the 90° pulse).

4.4.3. Molecular Weight, Viscosity, and Polydispersity Determination

The molecular weight of extracted alginate was determined using intrinsic viscosity [η] measurements obtained via a capillary viscometer. The viscosimetric average molecular

https://doi.org/10.3390/md24010041

weight, M_v, was estimated using the Mark–Houwink–Sakurada equation, which relates the intrinsic viscosity to the molecular weight of the polymer:

$$[\eta] = kM_v^{\alpha}$$

where k (cm^3/g) and α are parameters obtained from the literature and depend on the polymer–solvent system and temperature.

A known amount of polymer was dissolved in a 0.1 mol/L NaCl solution, as most of the Mark–Houwink parameters reported in the literature for alginate were determined using measurements in this aqueous medium to prevent polyelectrolyte expansion in solution.

For measurements at 20 °C, with alginate in solution of 0.1 mol/L NaCl, K assumes a value of 4.85×10^{-3} cm^3/g and α of 0.97 [89].

The weight average molecular mass, M_w, and the number average molecular mass, Mn, were then calculated by means of empirical equations with constants reported in [90], and the polydispersity index q (M_w/Mn) was determined.

4.5. Biological Activities

4.5.1. Antioxidant Activity

- DPPH radical-scavenging activity

The DPPH (2,2-diphenyl-1-picrylhydrazyl) radical-scavenging capacity of SA was evaluated by Kirby and Schmidt's method [91]. Briefly, 500 µL of the samples at different concentrations (from 0.125 to 1.25 mg/mL) was mixed with ethanol (99%, 375 µL) and a DPPH solution in ethanol (125 µL, 0.02% (*w*/*v*)). The solution was incubated for 30 min at room temperature in the dark. The absorbance was read at λ = 517 nm using a NanoDrop One/Onec spectrophotometer (ThermoFisher, Milan, Italy). Ascorbic acid was used as a positive standard, and then, the DPPH scavenging activity was estimated following the equation below:

$$\text{DPPH radical-scavenging activity } \% = ((A_{control} + A_{blank}) - A_{sample})/Acontrol \times 100$$

where $A_{control}$, A_{blank}, and A_{sample} are, respectively, the absorbance of the control reaction (absence of sample), the blank (without DPPH solution), and the SA extracts in the DPPH solution. The procedure was carried out in duplicate.

- Reducing Fe (III) Power Assay

The ability of sodium alginate to reduce iron (III) was determined using the method reported by Sampath Kumar et al. [92]. SA dilutions (0.067–0.535 mg/mL) were mixed with 250 µL of 200 mM phosphate buffer (pH 6.6) and 250 µL of 1% potassium ferricyanide. The mixture was incubated at 50 °C for 30 min, and then, 250 µL of 10% (*w*/*v*) trichloroacetic acid was added. The mixture was then centrifuged at 10,000 rpm for 10 min. In total, 500 µL of the supernatant was mixed with 500 µL of deionized water and 100 µL of 0.1% (*w*/*v*) $FeCl_3$. After 10 min, the absorbance was measured at λ = 700 nm using a NanoDrop One/Onec spectrophotometer. The procedure was performed in duplicate. The negative control was produced by replacing the samples with water, while the positive control consisted of ascorbic acid. Results were expressed as absorbance of Fe^{2+} at 700 nm at different concentrations.

- NO-Scavenging Activity

NO-scavenging activity was determined using the assay reported by Xu et al. [93]. Various dilutions of SA (from 0.042 to 0.417 mg/mL) in 250 µL of phosphate buffer (0.1 M, pH 7.4) were added to 500 µL of 5 mM sodium nitroprusside and 250 µL of phosphate

 https://doi.org/10.3390/md24010041

buffer (pH 7.4). To produce NO, samples were incubated under the light of a lamp at room temperature for 30 min. Afterward, an equal volume of Griess reagent was added to the mixture. After incubation at room temperature for 10 min in the dark, the absorbance was measured at 546 nm through a NanoDrop One/Onec spectrophotometer. For the calibration curve, $NaNO_2$ scalar dilutions were used (1–5–10–50 μM).

4.5.2. Anti-Inflammatory Activity

- Cell culture

The murine RAW 264.7 cell line and the human THP-1 cell line were acquired from the American Type Culture Collection (LGC Standards srl, Milan, Italy). RAW 264.7 cells were cultured in high-glucose D-MEM with L-glutamine, supplemented with 10% FBS (Microtech srl, Naples, Italy). THP-1 cells were maintained in RPMI 1640 supplemented with 10% FBS (Microtech). Cell incubation was carried out in 5% CO_2 atmosphere, 95% humidity, and 37 °C temperature for both cell types.

- Cytotoxicity assay

Cell viability was assessed with the MTT (3-(4,5-dimethyl-2-yl)-2,5- diphenyltetrazolium bromide) reduction assay, as reported in Pozzolini et al. [90]. Seeding of RAW 264.7 macrophages was carried out at a density of 2.5×10^4 cells/well in 96-well plates. THP-1 monocytes were seeded at a density of 5×10^4 cells/well in 96-well plates, and differentiation into M0 macrophages was performed by treatment with 20 ng/mL of phorbol myristate acetate (PMA) for 48 h. Both cell lines were treated by adding SA at different concentrations (0.05, 0.1, 0.2, and 0.4 mg/mL) for 24 h at 37 °C. Experiments were performed in quintuplicate.

- NO-Scavenging in LPS-Treated RAW 264.7 Macrophages

RAW 264.7 macrophages were seeded at 1×10^6 cells/well in 6-well plates for 24 h. Cells were then challenged with bacterial lipopolysaccharide (LPS, 100 ng/mL) in the presence or absence of SA (0.2 and 0.4 mg/mL) or low and medium viscosity alginic acid (CL and CM, respectively, 0.4 mg/mL) for 8 and 24 h. Afterward, the nitrite content of the cell media was measured by the Griess assay [94], while cells were lysed in 300 μL of lysis buffer (2% SDS, 100 mM DTT, 10% glycerol, and 50 mM TRIS-HCl, adjusted to pH 6.8). The lysates were heated at 100 °C for 10 min, and the quantification of protein concentration was performed by the Bradford assay [87]. Nitrite production in each sample was then calculated using a standard $NaNO_2$ curve and normalized on the protein content.

- Gene expression analysis of inflammatory mediators

RAW 264.7 macrophages were plated at a density of 1×10^6 cells/ well in 6-well plates. Instead, THP-1 monocytes were seeded at a density of 5×10^5 cells/well in 6-well plates and differentiated into M0 macrophages by treatment with 20 ng/mL PMA for 48 h. Both cell types were challenged with LPS (100 ng/mL) in the presence or absence of SA (0.2 and 0.4 mg/mL for RAW 264.7 macrophages and 0.4 mg/mL for THP-1 M0 cells), or of CL or CM at 0.4 mg/mL for both cell lines, for 8 and 24 h. At the end of each incubation, the RNA was extracted using the RNeasy Mini Kit (Qiagen, Milan, Italy), according to the manufacturer's instructions. Quality and quantity of RNA were analyzed using a NanoDrop One/Onec spectrophotometer. The cDNA was synthesized from 1 μg of RNA by using a cDNA Synthesis Kit (biotechrabbit GmbH, Henningsdorf, Germany). Gene expression of the inflammatory mediators interleukin 1 β(IL-1β), interleukin-6 (IL-6), interleukin-8 (IL-8), tumor necrosis factor (TNF-α), cyclooxygenase-2 (COX-2), and monocyte chemoattractant protein-1 (MCP-1) was quantified by qPCR for THP-1 M0 cells. Moreover, the gene expressions of IL-1β, IL-6, TNF-α, COX-2, inducible NO synthase

 https://doi.org/10.3390/md24010041

(iNOS), and C-X-C Motif Chemokine Ligand 5 (CXCL5) were also quantified in RAW 264.7 macrophages. Gene expression values were normalized on HPRT-1 and GAPDH housekeeping genes for THP-1 M0 cells and RAW 264.7 macrophages, respectively.

Each qPCR reaction was performed in 10 μL of 4× master mix (biotechrabbit GmbH), 0.2 μM of each primer, and 5 ng of cDNA. All samples were analyzed in triplicate. The following thermal conditions were used: initial denaturation at 95 °C for 3 min, followed by 45 cycles with denaturation at 95 °C for 15 s, and annealing and elongation at 60 °C for 60 s. The fluorescence was measured at the end of each elongation step. All primers (Table 4) were designed using the Beacon Designer 7.0 software (Premier Biosoft International, Palo Alto, CA, USA) and obtained from TibMolBiol (Genova, Italy). Data analyses were obtained using the DNA Engine Opticon 3 Real-Time Detection System Software program (3.03 version), and in order to calculate the relative gene expression compared to an untreated (control) calibrator sample, the comparative threshold Ct method was used within the Gene Expression Analysis for iCycler iQ Real Time Detection System software v3.1 (Bio-Rad, Milan, Italy).

Table 4. List of primer pairs used in the qPCR analyses. h- indicates human genes, m- indicates murine genes.

Gene	GenBank (a.n.)	Forward	Reverse	Product Size (bp)
h-IL-1β	NM_000576.3	TgATggCTTATTACAGTggCAATg	gTAgTggTggTCggAgATTCg	140
h-IL-6	NM_001318095.2	CAgATTTgAggTAgTgAggAAC	CgCAgAATgAgATgAgTTgTC	194
h-IL-8	NM_000584.4	AATTCATTCTCTgTggTATC	CCAggAATCTTgTATTgC	127
h-MCP-1	NM_002982	CTTCTgTgCCTgCTgCTC	CTTgCTgCTggTgATTCTTC	156
h-TNF-α	NM_000594.4	gTgAggAggACgAACATC	gAGCCAgAAgAggTTgAg	113
h-HPRT-1	NM_000194.3	ggTCAggCAgTATAATCCAAAg	TTCATTATAgTCAAgggCATATCC	144
m-IL-1β	NM_008361.4	gCAgCACATCAACAAgAg	CAgCAggTTATCATCATCATC	184
m-IL-6	NM_031168.2	ACCTgTCTATACCACTTC	gCATCATCgTTgTTCATA	117
m-CXCL5	NM_009141.3	TgCTTAACCgTAACTCCAA	ATCCAgACAgACCTCCTT	129
m-iNOS	NM_010927.4	CCgCCgCTCTAATACTTA	TTCATCAAggAATTATACAggAA	121
m-TNF-α	NM_013693.3	CCACCATCAAggACTCAA	ATCTTATCCAgCCTCATTCT	120
m-COX-2	NM_011198.5	CCAgCAAAgCCTAgAgCAAC	AgCACAAAACCAggATCAgg	127
m-GAPDH	NM_001289726.1	TCTCCCTCACAATTTCCATCCCAg	gggTgCAGCgAACTT TATTgATgg	99

4.6. Statistical Analysis

Statistical analyses were performed using one-way ANOVA and a paired Tukey's post-test to assess significant differences (GraphPad Software, Inc., San Diego, CA, USA). * p <0.05 and ** $p < 0.01$ were considered significant.

5. Conclusions

Sodium alginate (SA) isolated from seaweed apices discarded from an ex situ cultivation procedure during the restoration of *Ericaria amentacea* in the Ligurian Sea was characterized using spectroscopic and intrinsic viscosity methods, including FTIR and ^{1}H NMR. These marine polymers were characterized by low molecular weight compared to other alginates and exhibited notable antioxidant properties, as demonstrated by various chemical assays. Additionally, SA showed significant anti-inflammatory activity by modulating LPS-induced inflammatory mediators, including IL-6, IL-8/CXCL5, MCP-1, and TNF-α gene expression, in both human THP-1 M0 macrophages and RAW 264.7 murine macrophages. Furthermore, we showed the remarkable NO radical-scavenging capacity and a significant gene expression inhibition of iNOS, the enzyme responsible for its production in macrophages, suggesting possible pharmacological use of *E. amentacea* SA in counteracting the damaging effects of exacerbated inflammation at the tissue

https://doi.org/10.3390/md24010041

level. These findings highlight the potential of *E. amentacea* polysaccharides, especially when sustainably sourced from restoration procedure waste, for future industrial and biomedical applications.

Supplementary Materials: The following supporting information can be downloaded at https://www.mdpi.com/article/10.3390/md24010041/s1: Figure S1: Commercial acid alginic L and M (CL and CM respectively) inhibition of gene expression in LPS-activated RAW 264.7 macrophages.; Figure S2: Commercial acid alginic L and M (CL and CM respectively) inhibition of gene expression in THP-1 M0 macrophages.; Figure S3: NO scavenging activity and iNOS gene expression in cellular assay.

Author Contributions: Conceptualization, M.M.; methodology, M.M. and S.S.; validation, M.M. and S.S.; formal analysis, M.M.; investigation, M.M., S.M., L.M., V.A., M.A., S.P., M.C. (Maila Castellano) and S.V.; resources, S.S., M.C. (Mariachiara Chiantore), L.M., V.A., M.A. and S.V.; data curation, M.M. and S.S.; writing—original draft preparation, M.M.; writing—review and editing, S.S., M.C. (Maila Castellano), S.M., L.M., V.A., M.A., S.P., M.C. (Mariachiara Chiantore) and S.V.; visualization, M.M.; supervision, S.S. and M.C. (Mariachiara Chiantore); project administration, S.S. and M.C. (Mariachiara Chiantore); funding acquisition, S.S. and M.C. (Mariachiara Chiantore) All authors have read and agreed to the published version of the manuscript.

Funding: This study was funded by the project "National Biodiversity Future Center—NBFC", funded under the National Recovery and Resilience Plan (NRRP), Mission 4 Component 2 Investment 1.4—Call for tender No. 3138 of 16 December 2021, rectified by Decree n. 3175 of 18 December 2021 of the Italian Ministry of University and Research, funded by the European Union—NextGenerationEU; Award Number: Project code CN_00000033, Concession Decree No. 1034 of 17 June 2022, adopted by the Italian Ministry of University and Research, CUP D33C22000960007. This study was also supported by the European Union's HORIZON EUROPE Research and Innovation Programme under grant agreement No 101084180, project NOVAFOODIES (Demonstration of innovative functional food production systems based on a sustainable value chain of marine and freshwater raw materials for conscientious European consumers). The views and opinions expressed are, however, those of the authors only and do not necessarily reflect those of the European Union or the European Research Executive Agency.

Institutional Review Board Statement: Not applicable.

Data Availability Statement: All data are reported within this manuscript.

Acknowledgments: We would like to thank Maroua Chehoui for her valuable advice on the extraction of sodium alginate. We declare that Generative AI (ChatGPT v5.0) was used to assist with rephrasing sentences to improve clarity and correct grammatical errors. All scientific content, analyses, and interpretations were performed solely by the authors.

Conflicts of Interest: The authors declare no conflicts of interest.

Abbreviations

The following abbreviations are used in this manuscript:

ANOVA	Analysis of variance
COX-2	Cyclooxygenase-2
CXCL5	C-X-C Motif Chemokine Ligand 5
DNA	Deoxyribonucleic acid
DPPH	2,2-diphenyl-1-picrylhydrazyl
FTIR	Fourier-transform infrared
GAPDH	Glyceraldehyde 3-phosphate dehydrogenase
HPRT-1	Hypoxanthine-guanine phosphoribosyltransferase 1
IL-1β	Interleukin 1 beta

https://doi.org/10.3390/md24010041

IL-6	Interleukin 6
IL-8	Interleukin 8
iNOS	Inducible nitric oxide synthase
LPS	Lipopolysaccharide
MCP-1	Monocyte chemoattractant protein-1
MTT	3-(4,5-dimethyl-2-yl)-2,5- diphenyltetrazolium bromide
NMR	Nuclear Magnetic Resonance
NO	Nitric oxide
PMA	Phorbol myristate acetate
qPCR	Quantitative polymerase chain reaction
RNA	Ribonucleic acid
ROS	Reactive oxygen species
SA	Sodium alginate
TNF-α	Tumor necrosis factor alpha
UV	Ultraviolet

References

1. Draget, K.I.; Moe, S.T.; Skjåk-Bræk, G.; Smidsrød, O. Alginates. In *Food Polysaccharides and Their Applications*; Stephen, A.M., Phillips, G.O., Williams, P.A., Eds.; CRC Press: Boca Raton, FL, USA, 2006; pp. 159–178.
2. Stengel, D.B.; Connan, S. Marine algae: A source of biomass for biotechnological applications. In *Natural Products from Marine Algae: Methods and Protocols*; Springer: New York, NY, USA, 2015; pp. 1–37. [CrossRef]
3. FAO. *Capture and Global Production Databases*; FAO United Nations: Rome, Italy, 2021.
4. Twigg, G.; Fedenko, J.; Hurst, G.; Stanley, M.S.; Hughes, A.D. A review of the current potential of European brown seaweed for the production of biofuels. *Energy Sustain. Soc.* **2024**, *14*, 21. [CrossRef]
5. Mahmoud, M.S.; Mohamed, S.A. Calcium alginate as an eco-friendly supporting material for Baker's yeast strain in chromium bioremediation. *HBRC J.* **2017**, *13*, 245–254. [CrossRef]
6. Rinaudo, M. Main properties and current applications of some polysaccharides as biomaterials. *Polym. Int.* **2008**, *57*, 397–430. [CrossRef]
7. Stanford, E.C.C. Improvements in the Manufacture of Useful Products from Seaweeds. British Patent 142, 12 January 1881.
8. Kloareg, B.; Quatrano, R.S. Structure of the cell walls of marine algae and ecophysiological functions of the matrix polysaccharides. *Oceanogr. Mar. Biol. Annu. Rev.* **1988**, *26*, 259–315.
9. Larsen, B.; Salem, D.M.; Sallam, M.A.; Mishrikey, M.M.; Beltagy, A.I. Characterization of the alginates from algae harvested at the Egyptian Red Sea coast. *Carbohydr. Res* **2003**, *338*, 2325–2336. [CrossRef] [PubMed]
10. Yang, J.S.; Xie, Y.J.; He, W. Research progress on chemical modification of alginate: A review. *Carbohydr. Polym.* **2011**, *84*, 33–39. [CrossRef]
11. Hachemi-Benmalek, N.; Nouani, A.; Benchabane, A. Valorization of brown algae (*Cystoseira caespitosa*) from local region in Algeria for sodium alginate extraction and their application in the immobilization of microbial pectinases. *Alger. J. Environ. Sci. Technol.* **2019**, *5*, 1155–1162.
12. Lee, K.Y.; Mooney, D.J. Alginate: Properties and biomedical applications. *Prog. Polym. Sci.* **2012**, *37*, 106–126. [CrossRef]
13. Li, Y.; Hu, M.; Du, Y.; Xiao, H.; McClements, D.J. Control of lipase digestibility of emulsified lipids by encapsulation within calcium alginate beads. *Food Hydrocoll.* **2011**, *25*, 122–130. [CrossRef]
14. Hecht, H.; Srebnik, S. Structural characterization of sodium alginate and calcium alginate. *Biomacromolecules* **2016**, *17*, 2160–2167. [CrossRef]
15. Kokova, V.; Lukova, P.; Baldzhieva, A.; Katsarov, P.; Delattre, C.; Molinié, R.; Apostolova, E. Extraction structural characterization, and in vivo anti-inflammatory effect of alginate from *Cystoseira crinita* (Desf.) Borry harvested in the Bulgarian Black Sea. *Mar. Drugs* **2023**, *21*, 245. [CrossRef]
16. Ricker, M.A.; Haas, W.C. Anti-inflammatory diet in clinical practice: A review. *Nutr. Clin. Pract.* **2017**, *32*, 318–325. [CrossRef]
17. Ferrero-Miliani, L.; Nielsen, O.H.; Andersen, P.S.; Girardin, S. Chronic inflammation: Importance of NOD2 and NALP3 in interleukin-1β generation. *Clin. Exp. Immunol.* **2007**, *147*, 227–235. [CrossRef] [PubMed]
18. Sanada, F.; Taniyama, Y.; Muratsu, J.; Otsu, R.; Shimizu, H.; Rakugi, H.; Morishita, R. Source of chronic inflammation in aging. *Front. Cardiovasc. Med.* **2018**, *5*, 12. [CrossRef] [PubMed]
19. Valentine, J.S.; Wertz, D.L.; Lyons, T.J.; Liou, L.L.; Goto, J.J.; Gralla, E.B. The dark side of dioxygen biochemistry. *Curr. Opin. Chem. Biol.* **1998**, *2*, 253–262. [CrossRef] [PubMed]

20. Circu, M.L.; Aw, T.Y. Reactive oxygen species, cellular redox systems, and apoptosis. *Free Radic. Biol. Med.* **2010**, *48*, 749–762. [CrossRef]
21. Stadtman, E.R.; Levine, R.L. Protein oxidation. *Ann. N. Y. Acad. Sci.* **2000**, *899*, 191–208. [CrossRef]
22. Marnett, L.J. Oxyradicals and DNA damage. *Carcinogenesis* **2000**, *21*, 361–370. [CrossRef]
23. Ylä-Herttuala, S. Oxidized LDL and atherogenesis. *Ann. N. Y. Acad. Sci.* **1999**, *874*, 134–137. [CrossRef]
24. Nordberg, J.; Arnér, E.S. Reactive oxygen species, antioxidants, and the mammalian thioredoxin system. *Free Radic. Biol. Med.* **2001**, *31*, 1287–1312. [CrossRef]
25. Falace, A.; Marletta, G.; Savonitto, G.; Candotto Carniel, F.; Srijemsi, M.; Bevilacqua, S.; Alongi, G. Is the South-Mediterranean canopy-forming *Ericaria giacconei* (= *Cystoseira hyblaea*) a loser from ocean warming? *Front. Mar. Sci.* **2021**, *8*, 760637. [CrossRef]
26. De La Fuente, G.; Chiantore, M.; Asnaghi, V.; Kaleb, S.; Falace, A. First ex situ outplanting of the habitat-forming seaweed *Cystoseira amentacea* var. *stricta* from a restoration perspective. *PeerJ* **2019**, *7*, e7290. [CrossRef]
27. Clausing, R.J.; De La Fuente, G.; Falace, A.; Chiantore, M. Accounting for environmental stress in restoration of intertidal foundation species. *J. Appl. Ecol.* **2023**, *60*, 305–318. [CrossRef]
28. Falace, A.; Kaleb, S.; De La Fuente, G.; Asnaghi, V.; Chiantore, M. Ex situ cultivation protocol for *Cystoseira amentacea* var. *stricta* (Fucales, Phaeophyceae) from a restoration perspective. *PLoS ONE* **2018**, *13*, e0193011. [CrossRef]
29. Belattmania, Z.; Kaidi, S.; El Atouani, S.; Katif, C.; Bentiss, F.; Jama, C.; Vasconcelos, V. Isolation and FTIR-ATR and ^{1}H NMR characterization of alginates from the main alginophyte species of the Atlantic coast of Morocco. *Molecules* **2020**, *25*, 4335. [CrossRef] [PubMed]
30. Grasdalen, H.; Larsen, B.; Smidsrød, O. A PMR study of the composition and sequence of uronate residues in alginates. *Carbohydr. Res.* **1979**, *68*, 23–31. [CrossRef]
31. Ilmi, Z.N.; Wulandari, P.A.C.; Husen, S.A.; Winarni, D.; Alamsjah, M.A.; Awang, K.; Pudjiastuti, P. Characterization of alginate from *Sargassum duplicatum* and the antioxidant effect of alginate–okra fruit extracts combination for wound healing on diabetic mice. *Appl. Sci.* **2020**, *10*, 6082. [CrossRef]
32. Zrid, R.; Bentiss, F.; Ali, R.A.B.; Belattmania, Z.; Zarrouk, A.; Elatouani, S.; Sabour, B. Potential uses of the brown seaweed *Cystoseira humilis* biomass: 1-Sodium alginate yield, FT-IR, ^{1}H NMR and rheological analyses. *J. Mater. Environ. Sci.* **2016**, *7*, 613–620.
33. Sellimi, S.; Younes, I.; Ayed, H.B.; Maalej, H.; Montero, V.; Rinaudo, M.; Nasri, M. Structural, physicochemical and antioxidant properties of sodium alginate isolated from a Tunisian brown seaweed. *Int. J. Biol. Macromol.* **2015**, *72*, 1358–1367. [CrossRef]
34. Hadj Ammar, H.; Hafsa, J.; Le Cerf, D.; Bouraoui, A.; Majdoub, H. Antioxidant and gastroprotective activities of polysaccharides from the Tunisian brown algae (*Cystoseira sedoides*). *J. Tunis. Chem. Soc.* **2016**, *18*, 80–88.
35. Hentati, F.; Delattre, C.; Ursu, A.V.; Desbrières, J.; Le Cerf, D.; Gardarin, C.; Pierre, G. Structural characterization and antioxidant activity of water-soluble polysaccharides from the Tunisian brown seaweed *Cystoseira compressa*. *Carbohydr. Polym.* **2018**, *198*, 589–600. [CrossRef]
36. Manns, D.; Nielsen, M.M.; Bruhn, A.; Saake, B.; Meyer, A.S. Compositional variations of brown seaweeds *Laminaria digitata* and *Saccharina latissima* in Danish waters. *J. Appl. Phycol.* **2017**, *29*, 1493–1506. [CrossRef]
37. Westermeier, R.; Murúa, P.; Patiño, D.J.; Muñoz, L.; Ruiz, A.; Müller, D.G. Variations of chemical composition and energy content in natural and genetically defined cultivars of *Macrocystis* from Chile. *J. Appl. Phycol.* **2012**, *24*, 1191–1201. [CrossRef]
38. Kaidi, S.; Bentiss, F.; Jama, C.; Khaya, K.; Belattmania, Z.; Reani, A.; Sabour, B. Isolation and structural characterization of alginates from the kelp species *Laminaria ochroleuca* and *Saccorhiza polyschides* from the Atlantic Coast of Morocco. *Colloids Interfaces* **2022**, *6*, 51. [CrossRef]
39. Draget, K.; Smidsrod, O.; Skjak-Bræk, G. Alginates from algae. In *Biopolymers Online*; Wiley-VCH Verlag GmbH & Co. KGaA: Weinheim, Germany, 2005; pp. 1–30. [CrossRef]
40. Lorbeer, A.J.; Charoensiddhi, S.; Lahnstein, J.; Lars, C.; Franco, C.M.; Bulone, V.; Zhang, W. Sequential extraction and characterization of fucoidans and alginates from *Ecklonia radiata*, *Macrocystis pyrifera*, *Durvillaea potatorum*, and *Seirococcus axillaris*. *J. Appl. Phycol.* **2017**, *29*, 1515–1526. [CrossRef]
41. García-Ríos, V.; Ríos-Leal, E.; Robledo, D.; Freile-Pelegrín, Y. Polysaccharides composition from tropical brown seaweeds. *Phycolog. Res.* **2012**, *60*, 305–315. [CrossRef]
42. El-Sheekh, M.; Kassem, W.M.; Alwaleed, E.A.; Saber, H. Optimization and characterization of brown seaweed alginate for antioxidant, anticancer, antimicrobial, and antiviral properties. *Int. J. Biol. Macromol.* **2024**, *278*, 134715. [CrossRef] [PubMed]
43. Panikkar, R.; Brasch, D.J. Composition and block structure of alginates from New Zealand brown seaweeds. *Carbohydr. Res.* **1996**, *293*, 119–132. [CrossRef]
44. Kelly, B.J.; Brown, M.T. Variations in the alginate content and composition of *Durvillaea antarctica* and *D. willana* from southern New Zealand. *J. Appl. Phycol.* **2000**, *12*, 317–324. [CrossRef]
45. Rioux, L.E.; Turgeon, S.L.; Beaulieu, M. Characterization of polysaccharides extracted from brown seaweeds. *Carbohydr. Polym.* **2007**, *69*, 530–537. [CrossRef]

 https://doi.org/10.3390/md24010041

46. Krumhansl, K.A.; Demes, K.W.; Carrington, E.; Harley, C.D. Divergent growth strategies between red algae and kelps influence biomechanical properties. *Am. J. Bot.* **2015**, *102*, 1938–1944. [CrossRef]
47. Beuder, S.; Braybrook, S.A. Brown algal cell walls and development. *Semin. Cell Dev. Biol.* **2023**, *134*, 103–111. [CrossRef]
48. Craigie, J.S.; Morris, E.R.; Rees, D.A.; Thom, D. Alginate block structure in phaeophyceae from Nova Scotia: Variation with species, environment and tissue-type. *Carbohydr. Polym.* **1984**, *4*, 237–252. [CrossRef]
49. Gheorghita Puscaselu, R.; Lobiuc, A.; Dimian, M.; Covasa, M. Alginate: From food industry to biomedical applications and management of metabolic disorders. *Polymers* **2020**, *12*, 2417. [CrossRef]
50. Jiao, W.; Chen, W.; Mei, Y.; Yun, Y.; Wang, B.; Zhong, Q.; Chen, W. Effects of molecular weight and guluronic acid/mannuronic acid ratio on the rheological behavior and stabilizing property of sodium alginate. *Molecules* **2019**, *24*, 4374. [CrossRef]
51. Deng, Y.; Yang, N.; Okoro, O.V.; Shavandi, A.; Nie, L. Alginate-based composite and its biomedical applications. In *Properties and Applications of Alginates*; IntechOpen: London, UK, 2021. [CrossRef]
52. Rey-Rico, A.; Klich, A.; Cucchiarini, M.; Madry, H. Biomedical-grade, high mannuronic acid content (BioMVM) alginate enhances the proteoglycan production of primary human meniscal fibrochondrocytes in a 3-D microenvironment. *Sci. Rep.* **2016**, *6*, 28170. [CrossRef]
53. Zhang, S.; Dong, J.; Pan, R.; Xu, Z.; Li, M.; Zang, R. Structures, properties, and bioengineering applications of alginates and hyaluronic acid. *Polymers* **2023**, *15*, 2149. [CrossRef] [PubMed]
54. Zhang, X.; Liu, L.; Zhang, C.; Zhu, Y.; Zhao, H.; Zhao, L. Adsorption mechanisms of alginate oligosaccharides with specific degree of polymerizations on a novel ion-exchange resin: Experiments and simulations. *Chem. Eng. J.* **2023**, *460*, 141717. [CrossRef]
55. El-Sheekh, M.M.; El-Shenody, R.A.E.K.; Bases, E.A.; El Shafay, S.M. Comparative assessment of antioxidant activity and biochemical composition of four seaweeds, Rocky Bay of Abu Qir in Alexandria, Egypt. *Food Sci. Technol.* **2020**, *41*, 29–40. [CrossRef]
56. Duan, X.J.; Zhang, W.W.; Li, X.M.; Wang, B.G. Evaluation of antioxidant property of extract and fractions obtained from a red alga, *Polysiphonia urceolata*. *Food Chem.* **2006**, *95*, 37–43. [CrossRef]
57. Yu, H.; Liu, X.; Xing, R.; Liu, S.; Li, C.; Li, P. Radical scavenging activity of protein from tentacles of jellyfish *Rhopilema esculentum*. *Bioorg. Med. Chem. Lett.* **2005**, *15*, 2659–2664. [CrossRef]
58. Ye, S.; Xie, C.; Agar, O.T.; Barrow, C.J.; Dunshea, F.R.; Suleria, H.A.R. Alginates from brown seaweeds as a promising natural source: A review of its properties and health benefits. *Food Rev. Int.* **2024**, *40*, 2682–2710. [CrossRef]
59. Weidinger, A.; Kozlov, A.V. Biological activities of reactive oxygen and nitrogen species: Oxidative stress versus signal transduction. *Biomolecules* **2015**, *5*, 472–484. [CrossRef] [PubMed]
60. De La Fuente, G.; Fontana, M.; Asnaghi, V.; Chiantore, M.; Mirata, S.; Salis, A.; Scarfì, S. The remarkable antioxidant and anti-inflammatory potential of the extracts of the brown alga *Cystoseira amentacea var. stricta*. *Mar. Drugs* **2020**, *19*, 2. [CrossRef]
61. Zhou, R.; Shi, X.Y.; Bi, D.C.; Fang, W.S.; Wei, G.B.; Xu, X. Alginate-derived oligosaccharide inhibits neuroinflammation and promotes microglial phagocytosis of β-amyloid. *Mar. Drugs* **2015**, *13*, 5828–5846. [CrossRef] [PubMed]
62. Fernando, I.S.; Jayawardena, T.U.; Sanjeewa, K.A.; Wang, L.; Jeon, Y.J.; Lee, W.W. Anti-inflammatory potential of alginic acid from Sargassum horneri against urban aerosol-induced inflammatory responses in keratinocytes and macrophages. *Ecotoxicol. Environ. Saf.* **2018**, *160*, 24–31. [CrossRef]
63. Sharma, J.N.; Al-Omran, A.; Parvathy, S.S. Role of nitric oxide in inflammatory diseases. *Inflammopharmacology* **2007**, *15*, 252–259. [CrossRef]
64. Calder, P.C.; Albers, R.; Antoine, J.M.; Blum, S.; Bourdet-Sicard, R.; Ferns, G.A.; Zhao, J. Inflammatory disease processes and interactions with nutrition. *Br. J. Nutr.* **2009**, *101*, 1–45. [CrossRef]
65. Pawelec, G.; Goldeck, D.; Derhovanessian, E. Inflammation, ageing and chronic disease. *Curr. Opin. Immunol.* **2014**, *29*, 23–28. [CrossRef] [PubMed]
66. McInturff, J.E.; Modlin, R.L.; Kim, J. The role of toll-like receptors in the pathogenesis and treatment of dermatological disease. *J. Investig. Dermatol.* **2005**, *125*, 1–8. [CrossRef]
67. Bianchi, M.E.; Manfredi, A.A. How macrophages ring the inflammation alarm. *Proc. Natl. Acad. Sci. USA* **2014**, *111*, 2866–2867. [CrossRef] [PubMed]
68. Levy, E.; Xanthou, G.; Petrakou, E.; Zacharioudaki, V.; Tsatsanis, C.; Fotopoulos, S.; Xanthou, M. Distinct roles of TLR4 and CD14 in LPS-induced inflammatory responses of neonates. *Pediatr. Res.* **2009**, *66*, 179–184. [CrossRef]
69. Kammerlander, G.; Eberlein, T. An assessment of the wound healing properties of Algisite M dressings. *Nurs. Times* **2003**, *99*, 54–56.
70. Ohsumi, H.; Hirata, H.; Nagakura, T.; Tsujii, M.; Sugimoto, T.; Miyamoto, K.; Uchida, A. Enhancement of perineurial repair and inhibition of nerve adhesion by viscous injectable pure alginate sol. *Plast. Reconstr. Surg.* **2005**, *116*, 823–830. [CrossRef]
71. Hori, Y.; Winans, A.M.; Huang, C.C.; Horrigan, E.M.; Irvine, D.J. Injectable dendritic cell-carrying alginate gels for immunization and immunotherapy. *Biomaterials* **2008**, *29*, 3671–3682. [CrossRef]
72. Yang, D.; Jones, K.S. Effect of alginate on innate immune activation of macrophages. *J. Biomed. Mater. Res. A* **2009**, *90*, 411–418. [CrossRef] [PubMed]

 https://doi.org/10.3390/md24010041

73. Otterlei, M.; Østgaard, K.; Skjåk-Bræk, G.; Smidsrød, O.; Soon-Shiong, P.; Espevik, T. Induction of cytokine production from human monocytes stimulated with alginate. *J. Immunother.* **1991**, *10*, 286–291. [CrossRef]
74. Son, E.H.; Moon, E.Y.; Rhee, D.K.; Pyo, S. Stimulation of various functions in murine peritoneal macrophages by high mannuronic acid-containing alginate (HMA) exposure in vivo. *Int. Immunopharmacol.* **2001**, *1*, 147–154. [CrossRef]
75. Viswanathan, S.; Nallamuthu, T. Extraction of sodium alginate from selected seaweeds and their physicochemical and biochemical properties. *Int. J. Pharm. Sci. Res.* **2014**, *3*, 10998–11003.
76. Rashedy, S.H.; Abd El Hafez, M.S.; Dar, M.A.; Cotas, J.; Pereira, L. Evaluation and characterization of alginate extracted from brown seaweed collected in the Red Sea. *Appl. Sci.* **2021**, *11*, 6290. [CrossRef]
77. Michalak, K.P.; Michalak, A.Z. Understanding chronic inflammation: Couplings between cytokines, ROS, NO, Ca^{2+}, HIF-1α, Nrf2 and autophagy. *Front. Immunol.* **2025**, *16*, 1558263. [CrossRef] [PubMed]
78. Iles, K.E.; Forman, H.J. Macrophage signaling and respiratory burst. *Immunol. Res.* **2002**, *26*, 95–105. [CrossRef]
79. Mirshafiey, A.; Rehm, B.H. Alginate and its comonomer mannuronic acid: Medical relevance as drugs. In *Alginates: Biology and Applications*; Springer: Berlin/Heidelberg, Germany, 2009; pp. 229–260. [CrossRef]
80. Wu, A.; Gao, Y.; Kan, R.; Ren, P.; Xue, C.; Kong, B.; Tang, Q. Alginate oligosaccharides prevent dextran-sulfate-sodium-induced ulcerative colitis via enhancing intestinal barrier function and modulating gut microbiota. *Foods* **2023**, *12*, 220. [CrossRef]
81. Du, Y.; Jiang, Y.; Song, Y.; Chen, J.; Wu, Y.; Guo, R.; Huang, Y. Alginate/silk fibroin/Zn^{2+} composite microspheres for site-specific delivery for enhanced ulcerative colitis therapy. *Chem. Eng. J.* **2024**, *495*, 153441. [CrossRef]
82. Abramowitz, L.; Weyandt, G.H.; Havlickova, B.; Matsuda, Y.; Didelot, J.M.; Rothhaar, A.; Wiesel, P. The diagnosis and management of haemorrhoidal disease from a global perspective. *Aliment. Pharmacol. Ther.* **2010**, *31*, 1–58. [CrossRef] [PubMed]
83. Hasegawa, T.; Takahashi, T.; Inada, Y.; Yamada, C.; Tanaka, Y. Reparative effects of sodium alginate (Alloid G) on radiation stomatitis. *Nippon Acta Radiol.* **1989**, *49*, 1047–1051. [PubMed]
84. Rajauria, G.; Ravindran, R.; Garcia-Vaquero, M.; Rai, D.K.; Sweeney, T.; O'Doherty, J. Purification and molecular characterization of fucoidan isolated from *Ascophyllum nodosum* brown seaweed grown in Ireland. *Mar. Drugs* **2023**, *21*, 315. [CrossRef] [PubMed]
85. DuBois, M.; Gilles, K.A.; Hamilton, J.K.; Rebers, P.T.; Smith, F. Colorimetric method for determination of sugars and related substances. *Anal. Chem.* **1956**, *28*, 350–356. [CrossRef]
86. Bitter, T.; Muir, H.M. A modified uronic acid carbazole reaction. *Anal. Biochem.* **1962**, *4*, 330–334. [CrossRef]
87. Bradford, M.M. A rapid and sensitive method for the quantitation of microgram quantities of protein utilizing the principle of protein–dye binding. *Anal. Biochem.* **1976**, *72*, 248–254. [CrossRef]
88. Biju, J.; Sulaiman, C.T.; Sateesh, G.; Reddy, V.R.K. Total phenolics and flavonoids in selected medicinal plants in Kerala. *Int. J. Pharm. Pharm. Sci.* **2014**, *6*, 406–408.
89. Masuelli, M.A.; Illanes, C.O. Review of the characterization of sodium alginate by intrinsic viscosity measurements: Comparative analysis between conventional and single-point methods. *Int. J. Biomater. Sci. Eng.* **2014**, *1*, 1–11.
90. Clementi, F.; Mancini, M.; Moresi, M. Rheology of alginate from *Azotobacter vinelandii* in aqueous dispersions. *J. Food Eng.* **1998**, *36*, 51–62. [CrossRef]
91. Kirby, A.J.; Schmidt, R.J. The antioxidant activity of Chinese herbs for eczema and of placebo herbs—I. *J. Ethnopharmacol.* **1997**, *56*, 103–108. [CrossRef]
92. Sampath Kumar, N.S.; Nazeer, R.A.; Jaiganesh, R. Purification and identification of antioxidant peptides from the skin protein hydrolysate of two marine fishes, horse mackerel (*Magalaspis cordyla*) and croaker (*Otolithes ruber*). *Amino Acids* **2012**, *42*, 1641–1649. [CrossRef] [PubMed]
93. Xu, Y.; Zhao, H.; Zhang, M.; Li, C.J.; Lin, X.Z.; Sheng, J.; Shi, W. Variations of antioxidant properties and NO scavenging abilities during fermentation of tea. *Int. J. Mol. Sci.* **2011**, *12*, 4574–4590. [CrossRef]
94. Pozzolini, M.; Vergani, L.; Ragazzoni, M.; Delpiano, L.; Grasselli, E.; Voci, A.; Giovine, M.; Scarfì, S. Different reactivity of primary fibroblasts and endothelial cells towards crystalline silica: A surface radical matter. *Toxicology* **2016**, *361*, 12–23. [CrossRef] [PubMed]

 https://doi.org/10.3390/md24010041

marine drugs

Article

Integrative Metabolomics, Pharmacoinformatics and Experimental Studies Reveal the Neuroprotective Potential of *Caulerpa racemosa* Metabolites Against Alzheimer's Disease

Nita Handayani [1,*], Dhecella Winy Cintya Ningrum [2], Adha Fauzi Hendrawan [3], Anis Yuniati [1], Raffaele Romano [4], Lucia De Luca [4], Antonello Santini [5,*] and Fahrul Nurkolis [6,7,8]

1 Department of Physics, Faculty of Science and Technology, Universitas Islam Negeri (UIN) Sunan Kalijaga Yogyakarta, Yogyakarta 55281, Indonesia
2 Master's Program in Pharmaceutical Science, Faculty of Pharmacy, Universitas Gadjah Mada, Yogyakarta 55281, Indonesia
3 Department of Medicine, Faculty of Medicine, Public Health, and Nursing, Universitas Gadjah Mada, Yogyakarta 55281, Indonesia; adhafauzihendrawan2004@mail.ugm.ac.id
4 Department of Agricultural Sciences, University of Napoli Federico II, Piazza Carlo di Borbone 1, 80055 Portici, NA, Italy
5 Department of Pharmacy, University of Napoli Federico II, Via Domenico Montesano 49, 80131 Napoli, Italy
6 Master of Basic Medical Science, Faculty of Medicine, Universitas Airlangga, Surabaya 60286, Indonesia; fahrul.nurkolis.mail@gmail.com
7 Medical Research Center of Indonesia, Surabaya 60286, Indonesia
8 Institute for Research and Community Service, State Islamic University of Sunan Kalijaga (UIN Sunan Kalijaga), Yogyakarta 55281, Indonesia
* Correspondence: nita.handayanii@uin-suka.ac.id (N.H.); asantini@unina.it (A.S.); Tel.: +62-812-2722-3305 (N.H.)

Abstract: Alzheimer's disease (AD) is a multifactorial neurodegenerative disorder characterized by cholinergic dysfunction, oxidative/nitrosative stress, and neuroinflammation. Marine green algae *Caulerpa racemosa* are rich in neuroactive lipids and fatty acid derivatives with reported antioxidant and anti-inflammatory properties. However, their integrated mechanistic potential against AD remains largely underexplored. This study aimed to elucidate the neuroprotective mechanisms of *C. racemosa* metabolites against AD using integrative metabolomics, network pharmacology, molecular docking, and in vitro validation assays. Untargeted LC–HRMS profiling was performed to identify major metabolites in the ethanolic extract of *C. racemosa*. Neuroprotective targets were predicted via TargetNet, STRING, and Cytoscape (MCODE, CytoNCA). Functional enrichment was conducted using KEGG, GO (BP, MF, CC), and ClueGO. Molecular docking (CB-Dock2) validated compound–target interactions with ACHE, CHRM1, NOS1, and NOS2. Antioxidant (DPPH) and cholinesterase (AChE/BChE) inhibitory activities were evaluated in vitro. Metabolomic profiling identified lipid-dominant metabolites—oleamide, hexadecanamide, palmitoyl ethanolamide, α-linolenic acid, α-eleostearic acid, and 9-oxo-octadecadienoic acid. Network analysis revealed key AD-related hubs (ACHE, CHRM1, NOS1, NOS2) enriched in cholinergic regulation, arachidonic-acid metabolism, oxidative stress response, and nitric oxide signaling. Docking showed moderate multi-target affinities (−6.0 to −8.4 kcal/mol), with α-linolenic acid, α-eleostearic acid, and oxidized C18 lipids exhibiting the strongest interactions—particularly with ACHE and NOS isoforms. In vitro assays showed moderate antioxidant activity (IC_{50} = 120.97 ± 10.93 μg/mL) and cholinesterase inhibition (AChE IC_{50} = 136.48 ± 1.70 μg/mL; BChE IC_{50} = 145.98 ± 3.28 μg/mL), aligning with predicted multi-target interactions. *C. racemosa* extract exhibits neuroprotective potential through a synergistic combination of cholinergic modulation, antioxidant activity, NOS-mediated nitrosative stress reduction, and suppression of arachidonic-acid inflammatory pathways. These findings support *C. racemosa* as a promising marine-derived multi-target candidate for AD intervention, warranting further mechanistic and in vivo evaluation.

Keywords: *Caulerpa racemosa*; Alzheimer's disease; metabolomics; network pharmacology; molecular docking; acetylcholinesterase; nitric oxide synthase; neuroinflammation; antioxidant activity; marine functional food

1. Introduction

Alzheimer's disease (AD) represents one of the most devastating neurodegenerative disorders, characterized by progressive cognitive decline and neuronal loss driven by oxidative stress, amyloid-β aggregation, cholinergic dysfunction, and neuroinflammation [1,2]. Despite decades of research, currently available treatments such as donepezil, rivastigmine, and memantine only provide symptomatic relief rather than halting disease progression [3]. Therefore, the search for novel, multi-targeted, and naturally derived neuroprotective agents has gained increasing momentum. Among natural sources, marine algae have emerged as prolific reservoirs of bioactive metabolites with diverse pharmacological properties relevant to AD therapy, including antioxidant, anti-inflammatory, and acetylcholinesterase inhibitory activities [4,5].

Marine green algae, particularly *Caulerpa racemosa* (sea grapes), are rich in bioactive lipids, fatty acids, and amides such as oleamide, hexadecanamide, and α-linolenic acid [6]. These metabolites have been associated with neuronal protection through modulation of cholinergic transmission, nitric oxide synthase (NOS) pathways, and synaptic plasticity [7]. Recent advances in marine pharmacology highlight that marine-derived fatty acids and amides can simultaneously act on acetylcholinesterase (AChE), muscarinic receptors (CHRM1), and nitric oxide synthase isoforms (NOS1/NOS2), offering a multi-target approach to combat AD pathology [8]. In particular, oleamide and α-linolenic acid, both of which are found in marine algae, have shown promising inhibitory effects against cholinesterase enzymes and attenuation of neuroinflammation, aligning with findings from recent studies in *Marine Drugs* emphasizing marine algal metabolites as multifunctional agents in AD management [9].

Integrative metabolomics combined with network pharmacology and molecular docking has become a powerful strategy to elucidate bioactive compound–target interactions within complex biological systems [10]. Such approaches enable the identification of key molecular targets and pathways mediating neuroprotection. In this study, we employed LC–HRMS-based metabolomic profiling of *C. racemosa* extract, followed by in silico network pharmacology and molecular docking to predict its interaction with AD-related targets. Furthermore, in vitro assays were performed to validate its antioxidant and cholinesterase inhibitory potential. This integrative approach offers novel insights into the mechanistic landscape of *C. racemosa* as a marine-derived candidate for the prevention or adjunctive management of Alzheimer's disease.

2. Results

2.1. Metabolomic Profiling of Caulerpa Racemosa Extract

Untargeted LC–HRMS analysis of the *Caulerpa racemosa* ethanolic extract revealed a diverse metabolite profile dominated by bioactive fatty acid amides and unsaturated fatty acids (Table 1). Nine major compounds were identified with high confidence scores (mzCloud $\geq$ 95%), including hexadecanamide, oleamide, stearamide, α-eleostearic acid, palmitoleic acid, 9-oxo-10(E),12(E)-octadecadienoic acid, α-linolenic acid, palmitoyl ethanolamide, and 2,4-dihydroxyheptadec-16-en-1-yl acetate. Among these, *oleamide* and *α-linolenic acid* have been previously reported as neuroactive lipids with known roles in modulating sleep–wake cycles, cholinergic transmission, and anti-inflammatory responses. The retention times of 16–24 min and molecular weights ranging from 254 to 350 Da suggest these compounds belong to long-chain lipids with potential to cross the blood–brain barrier, a critical pharmacokinetic feature for neuroprotective agents. The strong match with known MS/MS spectral libraries supports their reliability for downstream pharmacoinformatic analyses.

Table 1. *Caulerpa racemosa* extract compounds (filtered from mzCloud best match > 95) via LC-HRMS.

Name	Formula	Calculated Molecular Weight	RT [min]	Area (Max.)	mzCloud Best Match
Hexadecanamide	$C_{16}H_{33}NO$	255.25505	21.71	132,989,235.55	98.6
Oleamide	$C_{18}H_{35}NO$	281.27056	21.54	104,636,468.21	98.3
Stearamide	$C_{18}H_{37}NO$	283.28606	23.77	82,837,237.90	97.3
α-Eleostearic acid	$C_{18}H_{30}O_2$	278.22365	16.92	82,954,091.16	95.3
Palmitoleic acid	$C_{16}H_{30}O_2$	254.22351	16.65	37,079,182.87	95.9
9-Oxo-10(E),12(E)-octadecadienoic acid	$C_{18}H_{30}O_3$	294.21853	17.87	31,871,173.23	97.7
α-Linolenic acid	$C_{18}H_{30}O_2$	278.22365	19.99	29,136,008.89	97.4
Palmitoyl ethanolamide	$C_{18}H_{37}NO_2$	299.28127	20.29	16,462,133.15	97.3
2,4-dihydroxyheptadec-16-en-1-yl acetate	$C_{19}H_{36}O_4$	350.24193	17.68	13,159,097.66	95.9

2.2. Network Pharmacology and Protein–Protein Interaction

To elucidate the molecular targets associated with Alzheimer's disease (AD), overlapping gene sets between *C. racemosa* metabolites and AD-related genes were analyzed using Venn diagram mapping (Figure 1A). The intersection revealed a substantial overlap of neurodegeneration-related targets, indicating that several metabolites potentially modulate core signaling pathways involved in AD pathology. The protein–protein interaction (PPI) network constructed through the STRING database (Figure 1B) displayed a highly interconnected topology, highlighting key nodes such as ACHE, CHRM1, NOS1, and NOS2. These proteins are central to cholinergic neurotransmission and nitric oxide signaling, two pathways known to deteriorate during AD progression. Cluster analysis using the MCODE algorithm (Figure 1C) identified three major functional modules, suggesting that the active compounds from *C. racemosa* may simultaneously regulate oxidative stress responses, neurotransmitter balance, and inflammatory cascades.

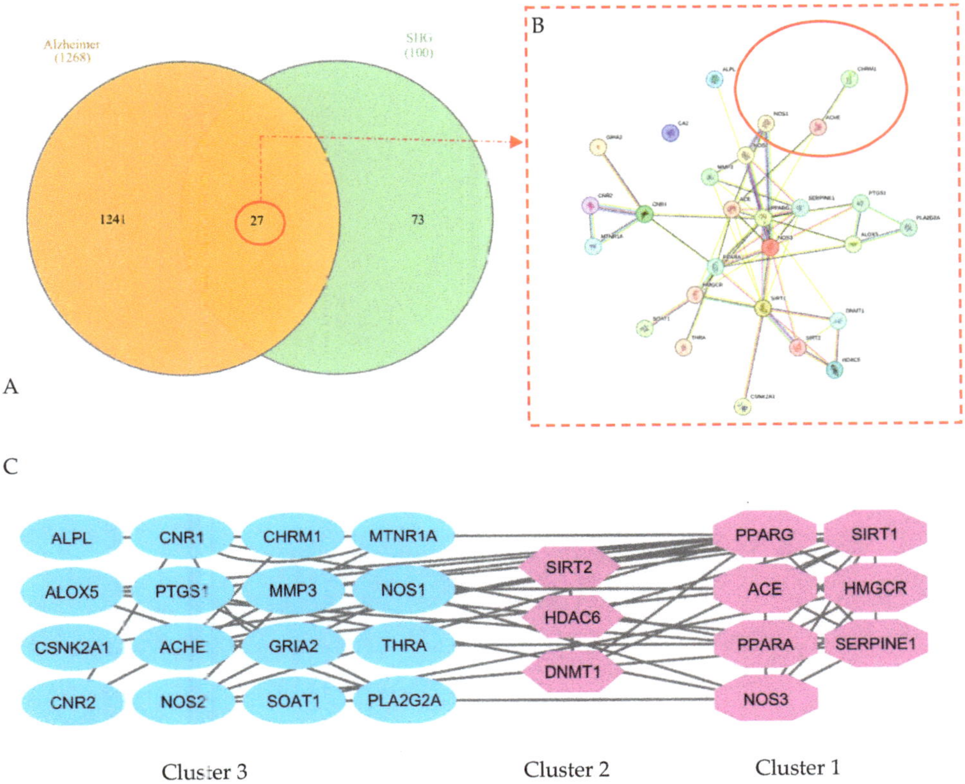

Figure 1. Venn diagram analysis (**A**); protein–protein interaction of potential targets of compounds in Alzheimer's (**B**); clustering by molecular complex detection (MCODE) (**C**). SHG: Sea grapes extract compounds.

2.3. *Functional Enrichment and Biological Process Clustering*

Cluster 3, identified as the most biologically significant, was further analyzed using ClueGO for Gene Ontology (GO) enrichment (Figure 2A–C). The results demonstrated that the predominant biological processes included response to oxidative stress, synaptic signaling, nitric oxide biosynthesis, and acetylcholine catabolic regulation. The clustering of sub-biological processes further reinforced the hypothesis that *C. racemosa* metabolites act through multi-targeted mechanisms, particularly modulating enzymes associated with neurotransmitter degradation (ACHE/BChE) and neuroinflammation (NOS1/NOS2). The distribution of functional terms underscores the integrative mode of action characteristic of natural compounds compared to single-target drugs.

Building on the ClueGO biological-process results above, the PPI analysis in Figure 3 shows that these functions are supported by a tightly connected target core. The initial network (16 nodes, 10 edges) was refined by degree centrality (DC > 0.00) to 12 highly connected hubs without losing edges, indicating stable interprotein cooperation. Key nodes ACHE, NOS1/NOS2, PTGS1, ALOX5, PLA2G2A, GRIA2, CHRM1, CNR1/CNR2, MTNR1A, and MMP3—suggest a multi-target mode where cholinergic degradation (ACHE), nitric oxide–linked oxidative/nitrosative stress (NOS1/NOS2), and arachidonic-acid neuroinflammation (PTGS1/ALOX5/PLA2G2A) converge with synaptic signaling receptors (GRIA2, CHRM1) and neuromodulators, reinforcing the earlier hypothesis of integrated neuroprotective control.

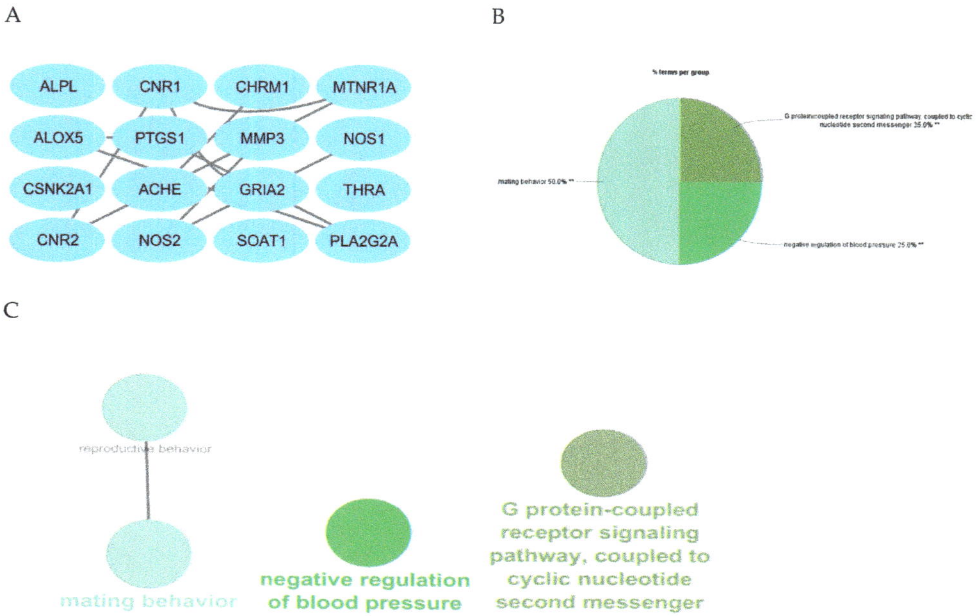

Figure 2. Chosen cluster (cluster of 3) (**A**), Percentage of terms of biological process (**B**), and Subcluster of biological process genes (**C**).

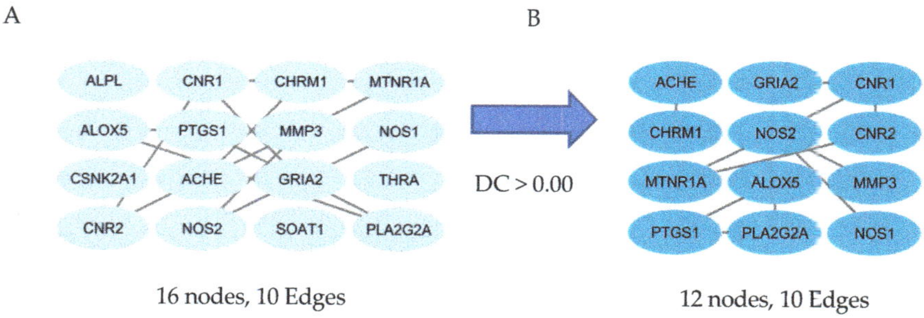

Figure 3. Interprotein interaction using CytoNCA, screening proteins based on degree centrality (DC) score threshold > 0.00. (**A**) the initial protein–protein interaction network before filtering, and (**B**) the filtered core network based on the degree centrality (DC) threshold.

Consistent with this hub architecture, Figure 4A (KEGG) highlights neuroactive ligand–receptor interaction and arachidonic acid metabolism as top pathways, with additional enrichment in circadian entrainment, calcium signaling, long-term depression, and neurodegeneration routes (e.g., Alzheimer's/ALS), indicating simultaneous synaptic and inflammatory regulation. Figure 4B (GO Molecular Function) further specifies the mechanisms as oxidoreductase and nitric-oxide–related activities, carboxylic ester hydrolase/cholinesterase functions, phospholipase A2 activity, and glutamate/acetylcholine receptor activities, matching the main hubs from Figure 3. Figure 4C (GO Cellular Component) localizes these targets to neuron projections, dendrites, synapses, AMPA receptor complexes, and postsynaptic density, showing that *C. racemosa* metabolites likely act at excitatory synaptic sites where oxidative stress and neuroinflammation shape plasticity, setting up the next section of results on how these pathway-level effects translate into therapeutic implications.

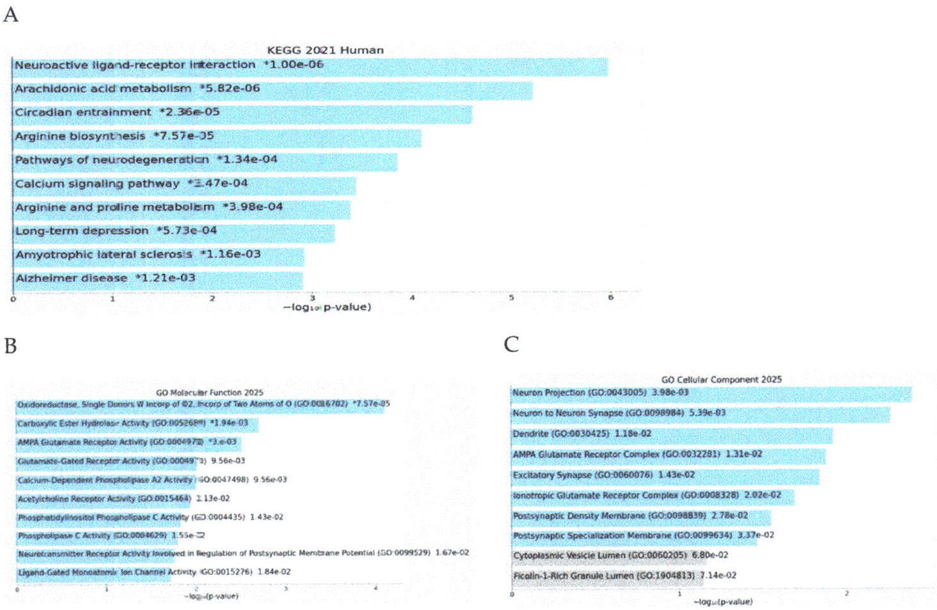

Figure 4. Enrichment analysis of key target proteins. KEGG pathway analysis (**A**); Molecular Function (**B**); and Cellular Components (**C**).

2.4. Molecular Docking Analysis

Molecular docking analysis is shown in Table 2, where it summarizes the docking affinities of *C. racemosa* metabolites against four Alzheimer's-related targets (ACHE, CHRM1, NOS2, NOS1), where more negative Vina scores indicate stronger predicted binding. Overall, all tested compounds showed moderate interactions across the panel (−6.0 to −8.4 kcal/mol), supporting a multi-target profile consistent with the earlier network and enrichment findings. Among them, unsaturated fatty acids and oxidized lipid derivatives tended to perform better than simple amides, suggesting that double bonds and oxygenated groups may enhance target complementarity within both neurotransmission and oxidative-inflammatory proteins.

Table 2. The Vina score (kcal/mol) of the molecular docking parameter for the *Caulerpa racemosa* compounds against selected Alzheimer's diseases protein.

Compounds	ACHE (PDB ID: 4EY7)	CHRM1 (PDB ID: 6WJC)	NOS2 (PDB ID: 1NSI)	NOS1 (PDB ID: 3NOS)
Hexadecanamide	−7.5	−6.5	−6.5	−6.0
Oleamide	−7.7	−6.9	−6.6	−6.4
Stearamide	−7.8	−6.5	−6.7	−6.1
α-Eleostearic acid	−8.3	−6.8	−7.5	−7.0
Palmitoleic acid	−7.6	−6.7	−6.8	−6.2
9-Oxo-10(E),12(E)-octadecadienoic acid	−8.1	−7.4	−7.3	−6.7
α-Linolenic acid	−8.4	−7.2	−7.3	−6.7
Palmitoyl ethanolamide	−7.5	−6.6	−6.7	−6.6

Table 2. *Cont.*

Compounds	ACHE (PDB ID: 4EY7)	CHRM1 (PDB ID: 6WJC)	NOS2 (PDB ID: 1NSI)	NOS1 (PDB ID: 3NOS)
2,4-dihydroxyheptadec-16-en-1-yl acetate	−7.6	−6.6	−6.7	−6.2
Donepezil or Control	−11.8	−8.2	−10.7	−9.4

Target-wise, the strongest natural-compound binding was observed for ACHE, led by α-linolenic acid (−8.4), α-eleostearic acid (−8.3), and 9-oxo-octadecadienoic acid (−8.1), indicating notable potential to interfere with cholinesterase activity. For CHRM1, the best affinity was shown by 9-oxo-octadecadienoic acid (−7.4) and α-linolenic acid (−7.2), aligning with synaptic receptor modulation inferred from Figure 4. In the oxidative-stress axis, α-eleostearic acid displayed the strongest binding to NOS2 (−7.5), while α-eleostearic acid and α-linolenic acid were again highest for NOS1 (both −7.0/−6.7 range), reinforcing their relevance to nitric-oxide-related neuroinflammation. Importantly, the control drug donepezil showed substantially stronger docking across all targets (e.g., −11.8 for ACHE), which is expected for a single-target optimized pharmaceutical; however, the natural compounds' consistent mid-range affinities across multiple proteins support the proposed broad, synergistic mechanism rather than a one-protein dominant effect.

Table 3 shows that α-linolenic acid binds along a hydrophobic channel in the ACHE active gorge, stabilized mainly by van der Waals/hydrophobic contacts with residues such as Trp286, Tyr337, Phe338, Tyr341, Phe297, Val294, and Ser293, and lying near the catalytic region (His447 and the Glu202/Ser203/Ala204 pocket), supporting its docking score in Table 2 and suggesting potential interference with substrate access. Donepezil occupies the same gorge more deeply and extensively, sharing key residues (Trp286, Tyr337, Tyr341, Phe297, Val294/Ser293, His447) but achieving tighter, broader interactions that explain its much stronger affinity. Overall, the residue overlap indicates a common binding corridor, while the simpler lipid scaffold of α-linolenic acid likely limits anchoring strength, reinforcing that *C. racemosa* metabolites may contribute moderate ACHE inhibition within a broader multi-target neuroprotective mechanism.

Table 3. Selected amino acid interaction of *Caulerpa racemosa* metabolites against Alzheimer's diseases.

α-Linolenic acid vs. ACHE

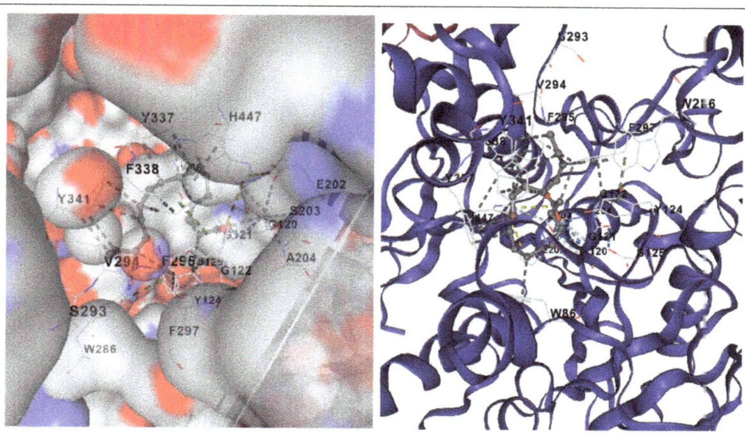

Table 3. *Cont.*

Donepezil vs. ACHE

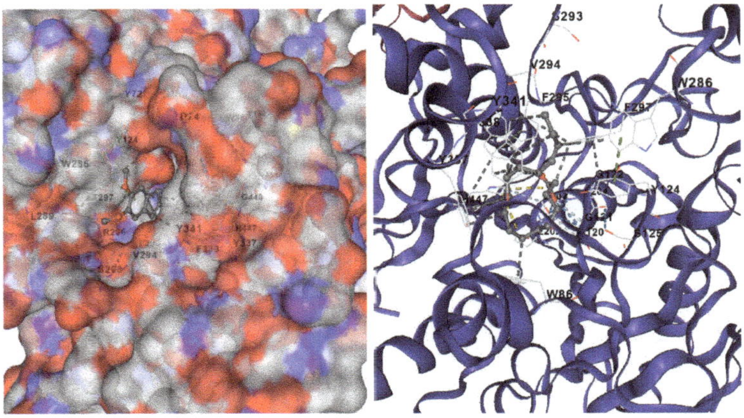

2.5. *In Vitro Antioxidant and Cholinesterase Inhibitory Activities of C. racemosa Extract*

Table 4 reports the IC_{50} values of the sea grape (*C. racemosa*) extract in antioxidant and cholinesterase assays, benchmarking against standard controls. The extract showed measurable but weaker activity than the references in all tests: DPPH scavenging IC_{50} was 120.97 ± 10.93 µg/mL versus Trolox at 99.04 ± 2.15 µg/mL, indicating moderate antioxidant capacity. For enzyme inhibition, the extract yielded IC_{50} values of 136.48 ± 1.70 µg/mL for AChE and 145.98 ± 3.28 µg/mL for BChE, whereas physostigmine was notably stronger (82.34 ± 1.45 and 83.81 ± 0.55 µg/mL, respectively). The superscript differences (a vs. b) suggest these reductions in potency are statistically significant.

Table 4. IC_{50} (µg/mL) values of sea grape extract and controls.

No	Assay	Sample	Control	IC_{50} Extract (µg/mL)	IC_{50} Control (µg/mL)
1	DPPH Antioxidant	Sea grape extract	Trolox	120.97 ± 10.93 ^{a}	99.04 ± 2.15 ^{b}
2	AChE Inhibition	Sea grape extract	Physostigmine	136.48 ± 1.70 ^{a}	82.34 ± 1.45 ^{b}
3	BChE Inhibition	Sea grape extract	Physostigmine	145.98 ± 3.28 ^{a}	83.81 ± 0.55 ^{b}

Values are presented as mean ± SD (n = 3). Superscript letters "a" and "b" indicate statistically significant differences between the extract and control groups at $p < 0.05$.

When integrated with the in silico findings, these IC_{50} trends are expected, docking predicted mid-range affinities across multiple targets rather than drug-like single-target strength. Thus, the extract's moderate cholinesterase inhibition and antioxidant effect likely reflect additive or synergistic contributions from several metabolites (e.g., fatty acids and amides) acting concurrently. This supports the broader mechanism proposed earlier—sea grape metabolites may not outperform classical inhibitors individually, but could provide neuroprotective benefit through combined anti-oxidative and multi-pathway cholinergic/anti-inflammatory modulation.

3. Discussion

The metabolomic profile of *Caulerpa racemosa* ethanolic extract in this study is dominated by fatty-acid amides (oleamide, hexadecanamide, stearamide) and unsaturated/oxidized fatty acids (α-linolenic acid, α-eleostearic acid, palmitoleic acid, 9-oxo-octadecadienoic acid), which is consistent with prior LC–HRMS and phytochemical works showing sea grapes as lipid-rich macroalgae with strong antioxidant-associated constituents [11]. Recent untargeted metabolomics on *C. racemosa* likewise reported broad lipid and secondary metabolite diversity, supporting the reliability of top-hit lipid signatures, while multiple antioxidant studies on *C. racemosa* extracts confirm that these chemical classes track with measurable radical-scavenging activity [12,13]. Taken together, our LC–HRMS findings extend previous chemical evidence by pinpointing specific neuroactive lipid candidates within the extract that are pharmacokinetically plausible for CNS action (Figure 5).

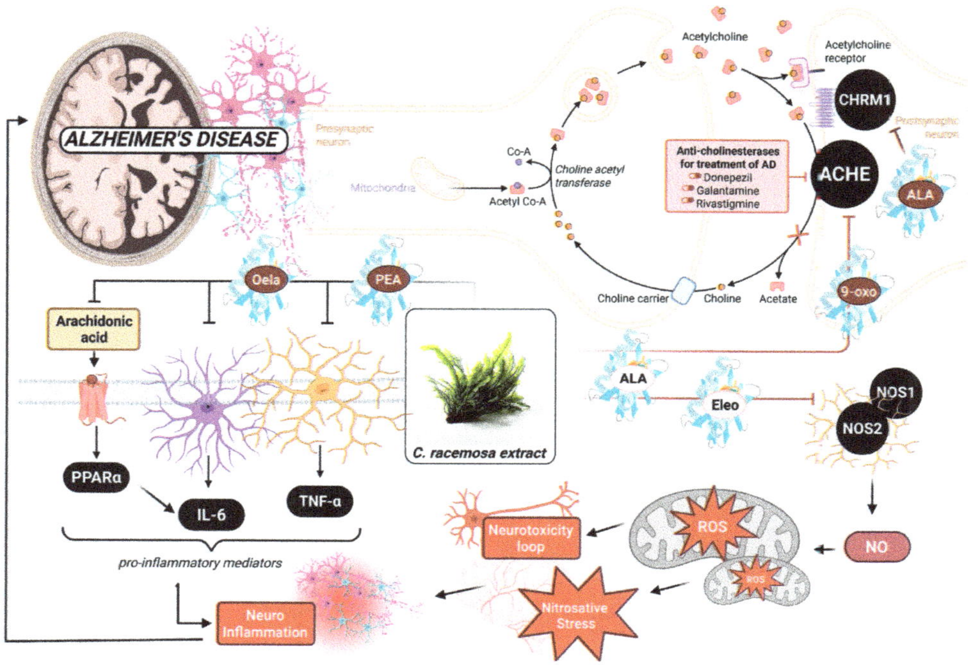

Figure 5. Proposed multi-target neuroprotective mechanisms of *Caulerpa racemosa* metabolites against Alzheimer's disease. This integrative schematic illustrates how key metabolites identified in *C. racemosa*—including oleamide (Oela), palmitoyl ethanolamide (PEA), α-linolenic acid (ALA), α-eleostearic acid (Eleo), and 9-oxo-octadecadienoic acid (9-oxo)—interact with major Alzheimer's disease (AD) pathological pathways. The metabolites demonstrate potential modulation of the cholinergic system by inhibiting acetylcholinesterase (ACHE) and supporting muscarinic acetylcholine receptor function (CHRM1), thereby enhancing acetylcholine availability at synapses. In parallel, the compounds exhibit predicted interactions with nitric oxide synthase isoforms (NOS1 and NOS2), reducing nitric oxide–mediated nitrosative stress and reactive oxygen species (ROS) generation. Additionally, *C. racemosa* lipids interfere with arachidonic-acid–driven pro-inflammatory cascades by influencing PPAR-α–linked signaling, suppressing IL-6 and TNF-α production, and attenuating neuroinflammation. Collectively, the multi-pathway interactions depicted in the figure support a synergistic mechanism in which cholinergic preservation, oxidative/nitrosative stress reduction, and lipid-mediated anti-inflammatory activity converge to mitigate neuronal damage and interrupt the neurotoxicity loop characteristic of AD progression. Created with BioRender.com license by Author (F.N.) (accessed on 10 October 2025).

Network pharmacology and PPI analyses showed that the metabolites converge on ACHE, CHRM1, NOS1, and NOS2, with enrichment in neuroactive ligand receptor interaction, arachidonic-acid metabolism, oxidative-stress response, and synaptic signaling.

This hub architecture mirrors established AD biology in which cholinergic breakdown co-evolves with nitric-oxide-related oxidative/nitrosative stress and lipid-driven neuroinflammation [14,15]. The presence of both cholinergic (ACHE/CHRM1) and redox-inflammatory (NOS1/NOS2; PTGS1/ALOX5/PLA2G2A) cores supports a multi-target strategy that has been repeatedly highlighted as more suitable for AD than single-node blockade, because synaptic loss is reinforced by feedback loops between ROS/RNS damage and microglia-mediated inflammation [16,17].

At the metabolite level, oleamide and palmitoyl ethanolamide (PEA) provide direct mechanistic bridges to earlier neurodegeneration research. Oleamide is a documented neuroactive fatty-acid amide that reverses scopolamine-induced cognitive impairment and restores cholinergic function, which aligns with its moderate docking to ACHE/CHRM1 in our dataset and the enrichment of synaptic receptor pathways [18]. PEA, an endogenous ALIAmide, has a proven ability to reduce reactive astrogliosis/microglial activation, suppress pro-inflammatory cytokines, and improve learning and memory in amyloid-based AD models via PPAR-α and related lipid-signaling targets [19–21]. Our identification of oleamide and PEA in *C. racemosa* suggests that sea-grape lipids may reproduce endogenous pro-homeostatic signaling that dampens neuroinflammation while supporting cholinergic tone.

The strongest docking affinities were observed for α-linolenic acid (ALA), α-eleostearic acid, and oxidized C18 derivatives, particularly toward ACHE and NOS isoforms, implying that unsaturation/oxygenation enhances complementarity to both neurotransmission and oxidative-stress proteins. This pattern is strongly supported by previous studies of ALA's multi-axis protection in AD models, where ALA reduces Aβ-induced oxidative stress and nitric-oxide elevation, restores antioxidant defenses, attenuates neuroinflammation, and improves memory, while also regulating APP processing and neuronal apoptosis pathways [22,23]. Our findings demonstrate that ALA and donepezil share overlapping residue interactions within the AChE catalytic gorge, suggesting a partially common binding trajectory. The comparatively weaker anchoring of ALA, consistent with its lipid-based chemical scaffold, supports a mechanism of partial cholinesterase inhibition. This inhibitory profile may alleviate cholinergic symptoms while simultaneously permitting complementary disease-modifying activity mediated through NOS regulation and modulation of inflammatory lipid signaling pathways.

Finally, the in vitro data validate the system's interpretation emerging from in silico results. The extract showed moderate antioxidant and AChE/BChE inhibitory activities lower than classical controls but consistent with predicted mid-range docking across multiple targets. Similar magnitudes of antioxidant capacity have been reported for *C. racemosa* extracts in earlier studies, reinforcing that sea-grape chemistry yields real redox buffering rather than purely computational promise [13]. When integrated, our findings support an AD-relevant mechanism where *C. racemosa* lipids (i) partially preserve acetylcholine signaling via ACHE/CHRM1 modulation, (ii) reduce oxidative/nitrosative stress through NOS1/NOS2 interaction and antioxidant reinforcement, and (iii) suppress arachidonic-acid and glial inflammatory cascades via PEA/oleamide-linked lipid mediators, collectively yielding a synergistic neuroprotective profile appropriate for the multifactorial pathology of Alzheimer's disease.

4. Materials and Methods

4.1. Preparation of Green Algae Extract

The green algae (*Caulerpa racemosa*) were obtained from a cultivation pond located in Jepara Regency, Central Java, Indonesia, with authorization from the pond owner. The botanical identification and authentication of the species were verified at the State Islamic

University of Sunan Kalijaga, Yogyakarta, Indonesia. The confirmation process employed the National Center for Biotechnology Information (NCBI) Taxonomy ID and the Integrated Taxonomic Information System (ITIS) Report ID, corresponding to *C. racemosa* (ID: 6968). Fresh biomass of *Caulerpa racemosa* was thoroughly washed with sterile seawater to remove impurities and epiphytic microorganisms. The cleaned material was then dried at 40 °C until the moisture content was reduced below 10%, followed by grinding into a fine powder. A total of 100 g of the dried powder was macerated with 1 L of 70% ethanol for 48 h at room temperature in a closed container, with occasional stirring to ensure optimal solvent–matrix interaction. After maceration, the mixture underwent ultrasonic-assisted extraction using a sonicator operating at 40 kHz for 30 min to enhance the solubilization of bioactive compounds. The filtrate was collected through Whatman No. 1 filter paper and concentrated under reduced pressure using a rotary evaporator at 45 °C to obtain a viscous greenish-brown extract [24].

4.2. Metabolomic Analysis

Untargeted metabolomic profiling of the sea grape extract was performed using liquid chromatography–high-resolution mass spectrometry (LC-HRMS) [25]. A 50 µL aliquot of the extract was diluted with 96% ethanol to a final volume of 1500 µL. The mixture was vortexed at 2000 rpm for 2 min, followed by centrifugation at 6000 rpm for 2 min. The resulting supernatant was filtered through a 0.22 µm syringe filter and transferred into an LC vial. The prepared sample was then placed in an autosampler for LC-HRMS analysis. The LC–HRMS system consisted of a Thermo Scientific Dionex Ultimate 3000 RSLCnano HPLC equipped with a microflow meter. The mobile phases used were: solvent A (0.1% formic acid in water) and solvent B (0.1% formic acid in acetonitrile). Chromatographic separation was achieved using a Hypersil™ GOLD aQ analytical column (50 × 1 mm, 1.9 µm particle size) with a flow rate of 40 µL/min and a total run time of 30 min. The column temperature was maintained at 30 °C. Mass spectrometric detection was conducted on a Thermo Scientific Q Exactive instrument operating in both positive and negative ionization modes. Full-scan spectra were acquired at a resolution of 70,000, with data-dependent MS/MS scans collected at 17,500 resolution for 30 min. Data processing and compound identification were carried out using Compound Discoverer software 3.4 integrated with the mzCloud MS/MS Library.

4.3. In Silico Analysis

4.3.1. Identification of Potential Targets

The simplified molecular-input line-entry system (SMILES) codes of the investigated compounds were retrieved from the PubChem (https://pubchem.ncbi.nlm.nih.gov/, accessed on 17 September 2025) [26] and ChemSpider (https://www.chemspider.com/, accessed on 17 September 2025) [27] databases. Prediction of potential protein or gene targets was performed using the TargetNet platform (http://targetnet.scbdd.com/, accessed on 17 September 2025) [28], applying a probability threshold greater than 0.6 to ensure target reliability. To identify Alzheimer's disease (AD)-related targets, the GeneCards (https://www.genecards.org/, accessed on 17 September 2025) and NCBI (https://www.ncbi.nlm.nih.gov/, accessed on 17 September 2025) [29] databases were queried using the keyword "Alzheimer's." The sets of compound-related and disease-related targets were compared using a Venn diagram to determine their intersection, representing the overlapping targets potentially involved in the pharmacological action of the compounds against AD [30].

4.3.2. Network Analysis

The intersecting targets were imported into the STRING database (https://string-db.org/, accessed on 17 September 2025) [31] to evaluate protein–protein interactions (PPIs) and visualize their functional associations. The interaction network was then clustered using the MCODE plug-in in Cytoscape 3.10.3 to identify highly interconnected modules that may represent key biological complexes involved in AD pathology. Functional enrichment of each cluster was performed using the ClueGO plug-in, which integrates Gene Ontology (GO) and pathway information. Subsequently, the CytoNCA plug-in was applied to assess topological parameters, with Degree Centrality used as the selection criterion for hub genes. Targets with degree values greater than zero were subjected to Kyoto Encyclopedia of Genes and Genomes (KEGG) pathway and Gene Ontology analyses using the Enrichr database (https://maayanlab.cloud/Enrichr/, accessed on 17 September 2025) [32]. This analysis enabled the identification of genes significantly involved in AD-related biological processes and signaling pathways, which were subsequently selected for molecular docking validation [33].

4.3.3. Molecular Docking Simulation

To validate the binding interaction between the bioactive compounds and the identified AD-related targets, molecular docking analysis was conducted. The three-dimensional crystal structures of the target proteins were obtained from the Protein Data Bank (PDB) (http://www.rcsb.org/pdb/home/home.do, accessed on 19 September 2025) [34]. The 3D structures of the selected compounds and target proteins were uploaded into the CB-DOCK2 web server (https://cadd.labshare.cn/cb-dock2/, accessed on 19 September 2025) [35], which performs automated docking based on cavity detection and binding site prediction. The docking outcomes were ranked according to binding affinity scores, with the lowest binding energy indicating the most stable and favorable ligand–receptor interaction. These results provided structural insights into the molecular mechanisms underlying the potential therapeutic action of the compounds against Alzheimer's disease.

4.4. In Vitro Experiments

4.4.1. Antioxidant Activity via DPPH Inhibition Assay

The antioxidant potential of green algae extracts was determined through DPPH radical scavenging, following the methods described by Nurkolis et al., 2023 [36]. In the DPPH assay, various concentrations of the green algae extract (35, 70, 105, 140, and 175 µg/mL) were mixed with 3 mL of DPPH solution in a testing vial. The mixture was then incubated for 30 min at room temperature under dark conditions. The reduction in DPPH radical concentration was quantified by measuring the absorbance at 517 nm.

The percentage of inhibition was calculated using the following equation:

$$\% \text{ Inhibition} = 100 - \left(\frac{\text{A0} - \text{A1}}{\text{A0}}\right) \times 100\% \quad (1)$$

where A0 represents the absorbance of the control (blank), and A1 denotes the absorbance of the test sample or standard.

4.4.2. AChE and BChE Inhibitory Assay

The in vitro inhibitory activities of the extract against acetylcholinesterase (AChE) and butyrylcholinesterase (BChE) were determined using a modified Ellman's colorimetric method in a 96-well microplate format [37,38]. The assay is based on the enzymatic hydrolysis of acetylthiocholine iodide (ATCI) or butyrylthiocholine chloride (BTChCl) by AChE or BChE, respectively, releasing thiocholine, which reacts with 5,5′-dithiobis-

(2-nitrobenzoic acid) (DTNB) to yield the yellow-colored 5-thio-2-nitrobenzoate anion detectable at 412 nm. The reaction mixture contained 140 μL of 0.1 M phosphate buffer (pH 8.0), 20 μL of 10 mM DTNB solution, and 20 μL of the test sample or standard inhibitor (physostigmine for AChE and rivastigmine for BChE). After gentle mixing, 10 μL of enzyme solution (AChE from *Electrophorus electricus* or BChE from equine serum, at a final activity of 0.02–0.06 U/mL) was added, followed by a 10 min pre-incubation at room temperature (25–28 °C) to allow reversible binding between the enzyme and inhibitor. The enzymatic reaction was initiated by adding 10 μL of 1.0 mM substrate solution (ATCI for AChE or BTChCl for BChE), resulting in a total volume of 200 μL per well.

The change in absorbance was recorded kinetically at λ = 412 nm every 30–60 s for 5–10 min using a microplate reader. Each assay was performed in triplicate. Blanks (without enzyme) and negative controls (without inhibitor) were included in each plate to correct for non-enzymatic background and baseline activity. The reaction rate (ΔA/min) for each well was calculated from the linear portion of the kinetic curve, and the percentage inhibition was determined using the equation:

$$\%\ \text{Inhibition} = 100 - \left(\frac{\text{slope}_{\text{sample}}}{\text{slope}_{\text{control}}} \times 100 \right) \tag{2}$$

The concentration of the extract or compound that inhibited 50% of enzymatic activity (IC_{50}) was obtained from nonlinear regression analysis of the concentration–response curve fitted to a four-parameter logistic (4PL) model. Selectivity between AChE and BChE inhibition was expressed as the Selectivity Index (SI = IC_{50} (BChE)/IC_{50}(AChE)), where a value greater than 1 indicates preferential inhibition of AChE. All solutions were freshly prepared prior to the assay. The final DMSO concentration was kept below 0.5% *v/v* to prevent solvent-induced inhibition. For extracts with intense color or reducing properties, interference control wells containing sample, DTNB, and buffer (without enzyme and substrate) were included to correct background absorbance. The enzymatic activities were verified by reference inhibitors, with each plate's positive control IC_{50} values remaining within the laboratory's historical acceptance range, ensuring reproducibility and assay robustness.

4.5. Data Analysis and Management

All experimental results were obtained from at least three independent assays, each performed in triplicate to ensure reproducibility. Raw absorbance data were exported from the microplate reader and processed to obtain reaction rates (ΔA/min) through linear regression of absorbance versus time within the linear range of enzyme kinetics. The percentage inhibition at each concentration was calculated relative to the control group, and the IC_{50} values were determined by nonlinear regression fitting of the dose–response curves to a four-parameter logistic (4PL) model using GraphPad Prism version 10.6.1 (GraphPad Software, Boston, MA, USA).

The results were expressed as IC_{50} values (mean ± standard deviation, SD) with 95% confidence intervals (CI). Statistical comparisons between two independent groups (e.g., extract versus positive control, or between AChE and BChE inhibitory activity) were performed using the independent *t*-test after confirming data normality with the Shapiro–Wilk test and homogeneity of variances using Levene's test. Differences were considered statistically significant at $p < 0.05$.

5. Conclusions

5.1. Conclusion

This study concludes that *Caulerpa racemosa* ethanolic extract contains a distinct lipid-dominated metabolite profile, primarily fatty acid amides and unsaturated/oxidized fatty acids such as oleamide, palmitoyl ethanolamide, α-linolenic acid, and α-eleostearic acid, with plausible relevance to Alzheimer's disease (AD). Integrated network pharmacology and PPI analysis showed these metabolites converge on key AD hubs (ACHE, CHRM1, NOS1, NOS2) and related inflammatory-synaptic nodes, enriched in oxidative-stress response, cholinergic regulation, nitric oxide signaling, and arachidonic-acid metabolism.

Molecular docking demonstrated consistent moderate multi-target binding, strongest for unsaturated/oxygenated fatty acids, supporting a synergistic rather than single-target mode of action. In vitro assays further validated this pattern, revealing moderate antioxidant capacity and AChE/BChE inhibition compared with controls, aligning with the predicted mid-range affinities across several proteins. Overall, the findings indicate that *C. racemosa* extract may offer neuroprotective potential through combined cholinergic support, oxidative/nitrosative stress reduction, and anti-inflammatory lipid modulation appropriate for the multifactorial pathology of AD.

5.2. Recommendation

Future work should isolate and quantify the major bioactive lipids, confirm their mechanisms through enzyme-kinetic and target-validation assays (ACHE/BChE, NOS1/NOS2, and arachidonic-pathway enzymes), and evaluate efficacy in AD-relevant cellular and animal models while assessing BBB permeability, pharmacokinetics, safety, and synergistic interactions among metabolites to clarify therapeutic feasibility.

6. Patents

The authors disclose that the invention related to this work is covered by an Indonesian patent application S00202511597, filed by Universitas Islam Negeri Sunan Kalijaga Yogyakarta, with inventors Dr. Nita Handayani and Fahrul Nurkolis.

Author Contributions: Conceptualization, N.H. and F.N.; Methodology, F.N., N.H. and A.S.; Software, F.N. and A.F.H.; Validation, N.H., A.S., L.D.L., R.R. and F.N.; Formal Analysis, F.N., A.Y., N.H., R.R., A.S. and D.W.C.N.; Investigation, N.H., F.N., R.R. and A.S.; Resources, N.H. and F.N.; Data Curation, F.N., A.F.H. and D.W.C.N.; Writing—Original Draft Preparation, N.H. and F.N.; Writing—Review and Editing, F.N., A.Y., N.H., L.D.L., A.S. and R.R.; Visualization, A.F.H., and F.N.; Supervision, N.H., A.S., L.D.L., R.R. and F.N.; Project Administration, N.H.; Funding Acquisition, N.H. All authors have read and agreed to the published version of the manuscript.

Funding: This research was funded by the *Penelitian Inovasi Teknologi* Program of UIN Sunan Kalijaga Yogyakarta, grant number 3268.5.1/Un.02/PPK.3/TL/07/2025.

Institutional Review Board Statement: The study was approved by the Ethics Committee of the Faculty of Medicine, Islamic University of Indonesia (Universitas Islam Indonesia), under Ethical Approval Number 1/Ka.Kom.Et/70/KE/X/2025 (approved on 3 October 2025).

Data Availability Statement: All original data and materials supporting the findings of this study are provided within the article and additional information or clarifications can be obtained by contacting the corresponding authors.

Acknowledgments: We acknowledge the use of AI assistance, specifically ChatGPT (Version 5.1), for language refinement and improving the clarity and conciseness of the manuscript. No AI tools were used for data analysis, interpretation, or generating scientific content. All scientific concepts, results, and conclusions were developed and verified by the authors.

Conflicts of Interest: The authors declare no conflicts of interest. The funders had no role in the design of the study; in the collection, analyses, or interpretation of data; in the writing of the manuscript; or in the decision to publish the results.

References

1. Kumar, A.; Sidhu, J.; Lui, F.; Tsao, J.W. Alzheimer Disease. In *StatPearls*; StatPearls Publishing: Treasure Island, FL, USA, 2025.
2. Dhapola, R.; Beura, S.K.; Sharma, P.; Singh, S.K.; HariKrishnaReddy, D. Oxidative Stress in Alzheimer's Disease: Current Knowledge of Signaling Pathways and Therapeutics. *Mol. Biol. Rep.* **2024**, *51*, 48. [CrossRef]
3. Singh, B.; Day, C.M.; Abdella, S.; Garg, S. Alzheimer's Disease Current Therapies, Novel Drug Delivery Systems and Future Directions for Better Disease Management. *J. Control. Release* **2024**, *367*, 402–424. [CrossRef]
4. Matin, M.; Koszarska, M.; Atanasov, A.G.; Król-Szmajda, K.; Jóźwik, A.; Stelmasiak, A.; Hejna, M. Bioactive Potential of Algae and Algae-Derived Compounds: Focus on Anti-Inflammatory, Antimicrobial, and Antioxidant Effects. *Molecules* **2024**, *29*, 4695. [CrossRef]
5. López-Santamarina, A.; Roade-Pérez, P.; del Mondragón-Portocarrero, A.C.; Cardelle-Cobas, A.; Cepeda, A.; Miranda, J.M. Effects of a Green Seaweed from the Atlantic Coast (Ulva Lactuca) on Gut Microbiota, Using an in Vitro Colon Model. *Food Biosci.* **2025**, *63*, 105596. [CrossRef]
6. Nurkolis, F.; Taslim, N.A.; Hardinsyah; Radu, S.; Mayulu, N.; Tsopmo, A.; Kurniawan, R.; Tallei, T.E.; Herlina, T.; Maksum, I.P. Metabolomic Profiling, in Vitro Antioxidant and Cytotoxicity Properties of Caulerpa Racemosa: Functional Food of the Future from Algae. *Res. Sq.* **2024**. [CrossRef]
7. Nam, H.Y.; Na, E.J.; Lee, E.; Kwon, Y.; Kim, H.-J. Antiepileptic and Neuroprotective Effects of Oleamide in Rat Striatum on Kainate-Induced Behavioral Seizure and Excitotoxic Damage via Calpain Inhibition. *Front. Pharmacol.* **2017**, *8*, 817. [CrossRef] [PubMed]
8. Maleki, M.F.; Nadri, H.; Kianfar, M.; Edraki, N.; Eisvand, F.; Ghodsi, R.; Mohajeri, S.A.; Hadizadeh, F. Design and Synthesis of New Carbamates as Inhibitors for Fatty Acid Amide Hydrolase and Cholinesterases: Molecular Dynamic, in Vitro and in Vivo Studies. *Bioorg. Chem.* **2021**, *109*, 104684. [CrossRef] [PubMed]
9. Kita, M.; Ano, Y.; Inoue, A.; Aoki, J. Identification of P2Y Receptors Involved in Oleamide-Suppressing Inflammatory Responses in Murine Microglia and Human Dendritic Cells. *Sci. Rep.* **2019**, *9*, 3135. [CrossRef]
10. Wang, F.; Chen, H.; Hu, Y.; Chen, L.; Liu, Y. Integrated Comparative Metabolomics and Network Pharmacology Approach to Uncover the Key Active Ingredients of Polygonati Rhizoma and Their Therapeutic Potential for the Treatment of Alzheimer's Disease. *Front. Pharmacol.* **2022**, *13*, 934947. [CrossRef] [PubMed]
11. Kageyama, H.; Waditee-Sirisattha, R. Antioxidative, Anti-Inflammatory, and Anti-Aging Properties of Mycosporine-like Amino Acids: Molecular and Cellular Mechanisms in the Protection of Skin-Aging. *Mar. Drugs* **2019**, *17*, 222. [CrossRef]
12. Taslim, N.A.; Hardinsyah, H.; Radu, S.; Mayulu, N.; Tsopmo, A.; Kurniawan, R.; Tallei, T.E.; Herlina, T.; Maksum, I.P.; Nurkolis, F. Functional Food Candidate from Indonesian Green Algae Caulerpa Racemosa (Försskal) J. Agardh by Two Extraction Methods: Metabolite Profile, Antioxidant Activity, and Cytotoxic Properties. *J. Agric. Food Res.* **2024**, *18*, 101513. [CrossRef]
13. Palaniyappan, S.; Sridhar, A.; Kari, Z.A.; Téllez-Isaías, G.; Ramasamy, T. Evaluation of Phytochemical Screening, Pigment Content, in Vitro Antioxidant, Antibacterial Potential and GC-MS Metabolite Profiling of Green Seaweed Caulerpa Racemosa. *Mar. Drugs* **2023**, *21*, 278. [CrossRef] [PubMed]
14. Ghimire, A.; Rehman, S.A.; Subhani, A.; Khan, M.A.; Rahman, Z.; Iqubal, M.K.; Iqubal, A. Mechanism of Microglia-Mediated Neuroinflammation, Associated Cognitive Dysfunction, and Therapeutic Updates in Alzheimer's Disease. *Hlife* **2025**, *3*, 64–81. [CrossRef]
15. Tang, K.S. The Cellular and Molecular Processes Associated with Scopolamine-Induced Memory Deficit: A Model of Alzheimer's Biomarkers. *Life Sci.* **2019**, *233*, 116695. [CrossRef]
16. Amirahmadi, S.; Farimani, F.D.; Akbarian, M.; Mirzavi, F.; Eshaghi Ghalibaf, M.H.; Rajabian, A.; Hosseini, M. Minocycline Attenuates Cholinergic Dysfunction and Neuro-Inflammation-Mediated Cognitive Impairment in Scopolamine-Induced Alzheimer's Rat Model. *Inflammopharmacology* **2022**, *30*, 2385–2397. [CrossRef]
17. Xu, M.; Zhang, L.; Li, P.; Wang, C.; Shi, Y. Network Pharmacology Used to Decode Potential Active Ingredients in Ferula Assafoetida and Mechanisms for the Application to Alzheimer's Disease. *J. Tradit. Chin. Med. Sci.* **2020**, *7*, 199–209. [CrossRef]
18. Kim, M.; Snowden, S.; Suvitaival, T.; Ali, A.; Merkler, D.J.; Ahmad, T.; Westwood, S.; Baird, A.; Proitsi, P.; Nevado-Holgado, A.; et al. Primary Fatty Amides in Plasma Associated with Brain Amyloid Burden, Hippocampal Volume, and Memory in the European Medical Information Framework for Alzheimer's Disease Biomarker Discovery Cohort. *Alzheimers. Dement.* **2019**, *15*, 817–827. [CrossRef]
19. Bronzuoli, M.R.; Facchinetti, R.; Steardo, L., Jr.; Romano, A.; Stecca, C.; Passarella, S.; Steardo, L.; Cassano, T.; Scuderi, C. Palmitoylethanolamide Dampens Reactive Astrogliosis and Improves Neuronal Trophic Support in a Triple Transgenic Model of Alzheimer's Disease: In Vitro and in Vivo Evidence. *Oxid. Med. Cell. Longev.* **2018**, *2018*, 4720532. [CrossRef]

20. Colizzi, M.; Bortoletto, R.; Colli, C.; Bonomo, E.; Pagliaro, D.; Maso, E.; Di Gennaro, G.; Balestrieri, M. Therapeutic Effect of Palmitoylethanolamide in Cognitive Decline: A Systematic Review and Preliminary Meta-Analysis of Preclinical and Clinical Evidence. *Front. Psychiatry* **2022**, *13*, 1038122. [CrossRef]
21. Assogna, M.; Di Lorenzo, F.; Martorana, A.; Koch, G. Synaptic Effects of Palmitoylethanolamide in Neurodegenerative Disorders. *Biomolecules* **2022**, *12*, 1161. [CrossRef] [PubMed]
22. Lee, A.Y.; Lee, M.-H.; Lee, S.; Cho, E.J. Alpha-Linolenic Acid Regulates Amyloid Precursor Protein Processing by Mitogen-Activated Protein Kinase Pathway and Neuronal Apoptosis in Amyloid Beta-Induced SH-SY5Y Neuronal Cells. *Appl. Biol. Chem.* **2018**, *61*, 61–71. [CrossRef]
23. Tofighi, N.; Asle-Rousta, M.; Rahnema, M.; Amini, R. Protective Effect of Alpha-Linoleic Acid on Aβ-Induced Oxidative Stress, Neuroinflammation, and Memory Impairment by Alteration of A7 NAChR and NMDAR Gene Expression in the Hippocampus of Rats. *Neurotoxicology* **2021**, *85*, 245–253. [CrossRef]
24. Nurkolis, F.; Taslim, N.A.; Subali, D.; Kurniawan, R.; Hardinsyah, H.; Gunawan, W.B.; Kusuma, R.J.; Yusuf, V.M.; Pramono, A.; Kang, S.; et al. Dietary Supplementation of Caulerpa Racemosa Ameliorates Cardiometabolic Syndrome via Regulation of PRMT-1/DDAH/ADMA Pathway and Gut Microbiome in Mice. *Nutrients* **2023**, *15*, 909. [CrossRef]
25. Hardinsyah, H.; Gunawan, W.B.; Nurkolis, F.; Alisaputra, D.; Kurniawan, R.; Mayulu, N.; Taslim, N.A.; Tallei, T.E. Antiobesity Potential of Major Metabolites from Clitoria Ternatea Kombucha: Untargeted Metabolomic Profiling and Molecular Docking Simulations. *Curr. Res. Food Sci.* **2023**, *6*, 100464. [CrossRef]
26. Kim, S. Getting the Most out of PubChem for Virtual Screening. *Expert Opin. Drug Discov.* **2016**, *11*, 843–855. [CrossRef]
27. Williams, A.; Tkachenko, V. The Royal Society of Chemistry and the Delivery of Chemistry Data Repositories for the Community. *J. Comput. Aided Mol. Des.* **2014**, *28*, 1023–1030. [CrossRef]
28. Min, S.; Lee, B.; Yoon, S. TargetNet: Functional MicroRNA Target Prediction with Deep Neural Networks. *Bioinformatics* **2022**, *38*, 671–677. [CrossRef]
29. Brown, G.R.; Hem, V.; Katz, K.S.; Ovetsky, M.; Wallin, C.; Ermolaeva, O.; Tolstoy, I.; Tatusova, T.; Pruitt, K.D.; Maglott, D.R.; et al. Gene: A Gene-Centered Information Resource at NCBI. *Nucleic Acids Res.* **2015**, *43*, D36–D42. [CrossRef]
30. Liu, T.; Wang, J.; Tong, Y.; Wu, L.; Xie, Y.; He, P.; Lin, S.; Hu, X. Integrating Network Pharmacology and Animal Experimental Validation to Investigate the Action Mechanism of Oleanolic Acid in Obesity. *J. Transl. Med.* **2024**, *22*, 86. [CrossRef] [PubMed]
31. Szklarczyk, D.; Kirsch, R.; Koutrouli, M.; Nastou, K.; Mehryary, F.; Hachilif, R.; Gable, A.L.; Fang, T.; Doncheva, N.T.; Pyysalo, S.; et al. The STRING Database in 2023: Protein-Protein Association Networks and Functional Enrichment Analyses for Any Sequenced Genome of Interest. *Nucleic Acids Res.* **2023**, *51*, D638–D646. [CrossRef] [PubMed]
32. Kuleshov, M.V.; Jones, M.R.; Rouillard, A.D.; Fernandez, N.F.; Duan, Q.; Wang, Z.; Koplev, S.; Jenkins, S.L.; Jagodnik, K.M.; Lachmann, A.; et al. Enrichr: A Comprehensive Gene Set Enrichment Analysis Web Server 2016 Update. *Nucleic Acids Res.* **2016**, *44*, W90–W97. [CrossRef] [PubMed]
33. Qin, Y.; Yan, G.; Qiao, Y.; Wang, D.; Tang, C. Identification of Hub Genes Based on Integrated Analysis of Single-Cell and Microarray Transcriptome in Patients with Pulmonary Arterial Hypertension. *BMC Genom.* **2023**, *24*, 788. [CrossRef]
34. Kouranov, A. The RCSB PDB Information Portal for Structural Genomics. *Nucleic Acids Res.* **2006**, *34*, D302–D305. [CrossRef]
35. Liu, Y.; Yang, X.; Gan, J.; Chen, S.; Xiao, Z.-X.; Cao, Y. CB-Dock2: Improved Protein-Ligand Blind Docking by Integrating Cavity Detection, Docking and Homologous Template Fitting. *Nucleic Acids Res.* **2022**, *50*, W159–W164. [CrossRef] [PubMed]
36. Nurkolis, F.; Purnomo, A.F.; Alisaputra, D.; Gunawan, W.B.; Qhabibi, F.R.; Park, W.; Moon, M.; Taslim, N.A.; Park, M.N.; Kim, B. In Silico and in Vitro Studies Reveal a Synergistic Potential Source of Novel Anti-Ageing from Two Indonesian Green Algae. *J. Funct. Foods* **2023**, *104*, 105555. [CrossRef]
37. Ellman, G.L.; Courtney, K.D.; Andres, V., Jr.; Feather-Stone, R.M. A New and Rapid Colorimetric Determination of Acetylcholinesterase Activity. *Biochem. Pharmacol.* **1961**, *7*, 88–95. [CrossRef]
38. Bonesi, M.; Menichini, F.; Tundis, R.; Loizzo, M.R.; Conforti, F.; Passalacqua, N.G.; Statti, G.A.; Menichini, F. Acetylcholinesterase and Butyrylcholinesterase Inhibitory Activity of Pinus Species Essential Oils and Their Constituents. *J. Enzyme Inhib. Med. Chem.* **2010**, *25*, 622–628. [CrossRef] [PubMed]

marine drugs

MDPI

Article

A New Algal Friendly Extract from *Euglena cantabrica* with Potential Applications in Biomedical Field

Silvia Buonvino [1,*], Carolina Trinca [2], Stefan Leu [3], Silvia Licoccia [4,5] and Sonia Melino [2,5,*]

1 Departmental Faculty of Medicine, UniCamillus-Saint Camillus International University of Health and Medical Sciences, Via di Sant'Alessandro 8, 00131 Rome, Italy
2 Department of Experimental Medicine, University of Rome Tor Vergata, Via Montpellier, 00133 Rome, Italy
3 Microalgal Biotechnology Laboratory, French Associates Institute for Agriculture and Biotechnology of Drylands, The Jacob Blaustein Institutes for Desert Research, Ben-Gurion University of the Negev, Sede-Boqer Campus, Beersheba 84990, Israel; stefanleu3@gmail.com
4 Department of Chemical Science and Technologies, University of Rome "Tor Vergata", Via Della Ricerca Scientifica, 00133 Rome, Italy; licoccia@uniroma2.it
5 NAST Center, University of Rome Tor Vergata, 00133 Rome, Italy
* Correspondence: silvia.buonvino@unicamillus.org (S.B.); melinos@uniroma2.it (S.M.); Tel.: +39-0672596204 (S.M.)

Abstract: Microalgae, such as *Euglena cantabrica*, are rich in secondary metabolites, including polyphenols, which are valued for their antioxidant and therapeutic properties. Here a rapid, cost-effective and efficient protocol using a trichloroacetic acid (TCA) solution was developed for the production of an extract from *E. cantabrica* (EuPoly). The potential environmental and biomedical applications of this new extract were evaluated. The effects of EuPoly extract were tested on normal human dermal fibroblasts (NHDFs) and on breast cancer cells of the triple-negative MDA-MB-231 cell line. EuPoly was able to increase the NHDFs survival in oxidative -stress conditions and, on the contrary, to induce a decrease in cell viability of the breast cancer cells. EuPoly was also used to functionalize frustules (FEuPoly), mesoporous silica structures from diatoms. FEuPoly were investigated for the complexation of Cu^{2+} and Ni^{2+}, as new potential tools for metal-ion decontamination. Finally, the scaffolding properties of FEuPoly were here assessed in the bone marrow mesenchymal stem cells (BM-MSCs) growth and their osteo-differentiation. This study provides new insights into the sustainable valorization of algae extracts, showing that TCA *E. cantabrica* extract and functionalized frustules may serve as multifunctional, eco-friendly resources for biomedical applications, as antioxidants and cancer cell inhibitor, metal ions-trapping and tissue osteo-repair.

Keywords: *E. cantabrica*; polyphenols; frustules; breast cancer cells; osteo-differentiation; mesenchymal stem cells

1. Introduction

The current political priorities of the European Union (EU) are focused on promoting a sustainable economic model that balances economic growth with the preservation of natural resources. The EU's action plan supports the development and strengthening of bio-based sectors, highlighting the importance of advancing sustainable food systems and production processes, with the goal of transitioning to a circular economy [1]. Algae and microalgae, as crucial components of the marine environment, could play a significant role in addressing the EU's priorities of overcoming the current linear and open-loop fossil fuel-based economic model. In this context, the use of algae in an increasing variety of

 https://doi.org/10.3390/md23120453

commercial applications makes them particularly relevant to the aims of a circular bioeconomy [1], as they are capable of producing a wide range of bioactive compounds, from antioxidants and anti-inflammatory agents to antimicrobial and anticancer molecules. This ability has spurred their use in a variety of industrial applications, including pharmaceuticals, nutraceuticals, and biofuels [2–5]. Within this broad framework of high-value products, secondary metabolites derived from microalgae have garnered significant interest due to their roles in adapting to environmental stress and defending against external threats, presenting possibilities for the use of microalgae in biosensing devices [6,7]. Among microalgae, one particularly intriguing group is the euglenoids, a class of unicellular protists known for their metabolic versatility and adaptability to various environmental conditions. Euglenoids have been investigated for their potential in environmental bioremediation and bio-medical tools for the high presence of polyphenols. Polyphenols are well known for their antioxidant properties and for their chelating abilities, which are mainly thanks to their chemical structure, particularly the presence of hydroxyl groups. Among euglenoids, *E. cantabrica* has recently emerged due to its remarkable ability to shift between photosynthetic and heterotrophic modes of nutrition, allowing it to survive and thrive in diverse environments [8]. This metabolic flexibility and its resilience to environmental stressors such as fluctuating light, temperature, and nutrient availability, combined with its high intrinsic polyphenol content, make *E. cantabrica* a promising candidate for both biomedical and environmental applications [8]. Among the polyphenols identified in *E. cantabrica*, gallic acid (5.87 μg/g), protocatechuic acid (2.97 μg/g), and epicatechin have been shown to contribute significantly to its antioxidant capacity [9–11]. Moreover, a notable amount of caffeic acid, p-coumaric acid, and of the flavanone naringenin have been detected [12]. Polyphenols are potent scavengers of reactive oxygen species (ROS), mitigating oxidative stress, which is a major contributing factor in the pathogenesis of various chronic diseases, including neurodegenerative diseases, cardiovascular conditions, and cancer [13–16]. In recent years, various approaches for the extraction of polyphenols from algae, plants and other agri-food products have been explored [17,18]. Polyphenol-rich extracts from euglenoids have been reported to exhibit significant antioxidant activity, along with a broad range of bioactive effects, including antiviral, anti-inflammatory, anti-cancer, and wound-healing properties [19–22]. Live *Euglena gracilis* cells and their aqueous extracts were found to facilitate wound healing by enhancing re-epithelization and reducing fibroplasia, without stimulating an excessive inflammatory response [23]. Recently, it has been demonstrated that *E. gracilis*-derived extracellular vesicles enhance skin-regenerative wound healing, promoting the proliferation and migration of skin cells, thereby increasing both collagen synthesis and the expression of proliferation-associated proteins [24]. Anti-inflammatory studies on *Euglena tuba* methanolic extracts have also been performed, employing macrophage cell lines in lipopolysaccharide-induced inflammation mice models, where the extracts reduced free radical generation [25]. In recent years, interest has grown in the use of algae- and plant-derived polyphenols for cancer treatment [26,27], as these compounds, either alone or in combination, target distinct molecular pathways and exhibit enhanced therapeutic efficacy [28–30]. A methanolic extract of E. tuba was found to inhibit the growth of human lung (A549) and breast cancer (MCF-7) cells in vitro through ROS-mediated regulation of MAPKs (Mitogen-activated protein kinases) [31]. Finally, it was recently reported that aqueous *E. gracilis* extract can protect against tobacco smoke carcinogen-induced lung cancer by altering the gut microbiota metabolome [32].

Herein, we aimed to obtain and characterize a new polyphenol-rich extract from *E. cantabrica* and evaluate its biological activity. In particular, the extract was investigated for its potential to protect normal human dermal fibroblasts (NHDFs) from oxidative stress induced by oxygen radicals. Furthermore, the ability of the extract to affect the viability of MDA-MB-231 triple-negative breast cancer cells was also investigated.

Beyond their therapeutic properties, algal-derived polyphenols have also been investigated for their ability to bind metal ions. Indeed, the hydroxy groups in polyphenols can form strong bonds with metal ions; therefore, polyphenols could potentially be employed in the treatment of pathological conditions, such as metal overload, or heavy metal contamination, including arsenic, cadmium, chromium, lead, mercury, nickel, and copper. Heavy metal contamination in wastewater is identified as a risk to public health and the environment, and has been since the late 19th century [33], as repeated exposure to these metals leads to bioaccumulation in tissues and organs [34], consequently causing adverse effects on human health [35]. *E. gracilis* has demonstrated significant tolerance to a wide range of heavy metals, making it a promising candidate for bioremediation in environments contaminated by multiple metals [22,36–38]. Nickel and copper are widely distributed pollutants with both industrial and consumer-related sources. In particular, nickel is one of the most prevalent contact allergens and skin exposure to nickel ions leads to allergic dermatitis and eczema. Moreover, Ni-containing compounds have also been linked to carcinogenic effects depending on the dose, duration, and route of exposure, and are also frequently detected in ground-water, raising concerns for both environmental and human health [39]. Regarding copper ions, although they are essential in trace amounts in cells, they can become toxic when accumulated in excess. Chronic copper ion overload is implicated in several pathological conditions, most notably in Wilson's disease, a rare genetic disorder characterized by impaired copper metabolism and accumulation in the liver, brain, and other organs, leading to hepatic and neurological symptoms [40]. In addition, elevated copper levels have been associated with oxidative stress and cellular damage, and are potentially involved in neurodegenerative diseases such as Alzheimer's [40].

In this context, we sought to functionalize frustules of diatoms, natural three-dimensional silica structures with micro- and nano-meter-sized pores, with the algal extract, and to evaluate its ability to scavenge biologically relevant divalent met-al ions (Cu^{2+} and Ni^{2+}). These ions were specifically selected due to their involvement in biological systems: Cu^{2+} can act as a pro-oxidant agent, with elevated levels contributing to oxidative stress, neurodegeneration, and inflammatory responses, while Ni^{2+} is recognized for its cytotoxic and genotoxic effects, with involvement in allergic contact dermatitis, lung fibrosis, and carcinogenesis. Given these effects, the ability to bind and remove Cu^{2+} and Ni^{2+} is of particular relevance for applications in health protection and biomedical contexts, and could enable the development of new tools to mitigate metal-induced toxicity and enhance therapeutic strategies. Moreover, we aimed to investigate the potential applications of these functionalized structures in tissue repair. In a recent study, *E. gracilis* cells and their aqueous extracts mixed with chitosan–hyaluronic acid were used to create new bioactive hydrogels, and the efficacy of these mixtures in accelerating the wound healing process was demonstrated using a mouse model with deep skin burns [23]. However, the use of euglenoids and/or their derived bioactive compounds in combination with biomaterials for tissue regeneration represents an unexplored area of research. In this context, the ability of the *E. cantabrica* extract–functionalized frustules to act as a scaffold for human mesenchymal stem cells was assessed, paving the way for investigating these new systems as natural bioactive scaffolds with potential applications in stem cell-based tissue regeneration.

In this study, a new algal friendly extract has been characterized and investigated for its effects on the cancer and stem cells and to functionalize natural silica mesoporous structures for metal-ion trapping and improving their scaffolding properties.

2. Results and Discussion

2.1. Production and Characterization of the E. cantabrica Extract

Herein, a new protocol was developed for the production of a non-protein extract from *E. cantabrica* (EuPoly) using 50% trichloroacetic acid solution (TCA). The TCA extraction process was also compared with those using other classical solvents for polyphenol extraction (see Supplementary Information, Figure S1A) with the same incubation times and temperatures. Only the extract obtained through treating *E. cantabrica* with TCA showed a green color, demonstrating better pigment extraction. The extracts were then analyzed using the Folin–Ciocalteu assay (see Supplementary Information, Figure S1B), demonstrating the TCA solution's major ability to extract polyphenols compared to that of the other solvents used under the same experimental conditions.

Figure 1A shows the scheme of the algal extract production protocol. The absence of proteins in the extract was also demonstrated by the SDS-PAGE analysis, as shown in Figure 1B. SPE chromatography of the EuPoly was performed following the elution at 280 nm, demonstrating the high presence of hydrophobic compounds, eluted by methanol (see Figure 1C(a)). The eluted peaks were analyzed by Folin–Ciocalteu assay, further demonstrating the presence of phenolic species in the EuPoly (see Figure 1C(b)). Figure 1D shows the RP-HPLC profile of EuPoly recorded at 280 nm, where the peaks in the blue box, recorded through three RP-HPLC analyses and subsequent lyophilization, were positive to Folin–Ciocalteu assay. Their retention times are consistent with those previously reported for polyphenols [41]. The quantitative determination of polyphenols in EuPoly was performed using the Folin–Ciocalteu assay. A total poly-phenolic content of 1.097 mg/mL (S.D. ± 0.058) expressed as gallic acid equivalents (GAE) (mg/mL of extract) (Figure 1E) was determined by measuring the absorbance at 750 nm and using a calibration curve obtained with solutions at different gallic acid concentrations (0–50 μg) (see Supplementary Information, Figure S2).

In this study, the protocol for obtaining EuPoly requires the use of TCA and represents a rapid, efficient, and low-cost extraction process, which we have previously used for polyphenol extraction by vegetable-waste derived bioplastic (BPLH) [42]. The use of TCA for polyphenolic compound extraction offers advantages over other extraction methods. For instance, extraction with organic solvents, such as ethanol, methanol, acetone, or isopropanol, mixed with water is commonly used to obtain polyphenolic ex-tracts from microalgae, plants, and food industry by-products [43,44], but it often requires long incubation durations and several subsequent purification steps. Additionally, water-based or microwave-assisted extraction methods may be less selective and lead to the degradation of heat-sensitive compounds [44]. Another common technique generally used with organic solvents is ultrasound-assisted extraction, which, despite being a fast and efficient method, requires the strict selection of extraction parameters depending on the sample, which involves the frequency, ultrasound power, time, temperature, and quantity and preparation of the sample, and the type, volume, and con-centration of solvent [43]. Moreover, although TCA is classified as a toxic solvent, its use at concentrations up to 50–80% (*w*/*v*) has recently been investigated for biomedical applications, including the treatment of chronic venous ulcers and dermatological procedures for photoaging, further supporting its suitability in biomedicine and in clinical settings [45,46]. The protocol presented here provides advantages over other extraction procedures since it is rapid, cost-effective, and enables easy and efficient polyphenol extraction from *E. cantabrica*, reducing the processing time and lowering the risk of thermal degradation. Moreover, the protocol's short incubation time (1 h) could allow for on-site extraction, providing possibilities for analysis device production. Furthermore, TCA acts as an effective protein precipitant, allowing for the ex-traction of an enriched polyphenolic fraction while minimizing the protein content. Although full characterization of the polyphenols in the extract is still needed, this innovative approach could represent a smart strategy to produce polyphenol-rich, bio-active, high-value extracts from microalgae.

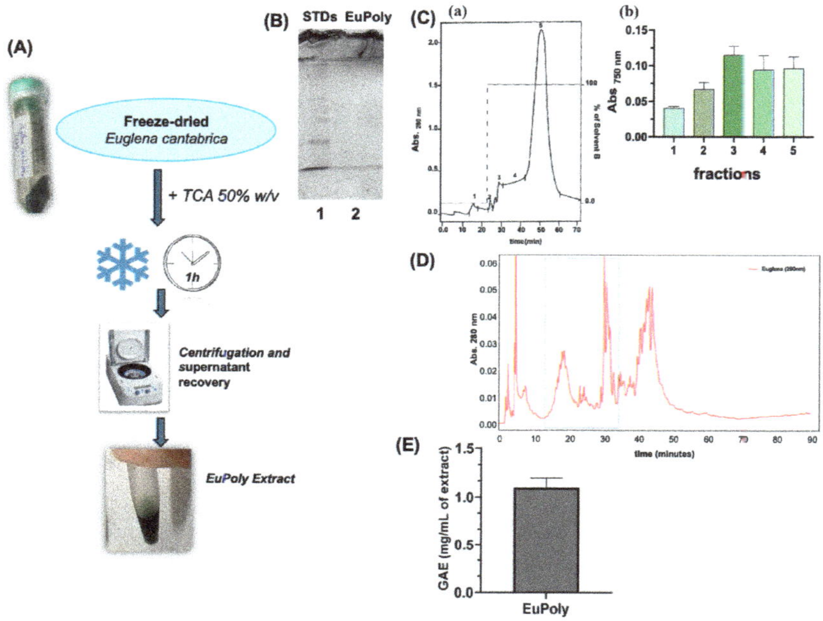

Figure 1. Production and Characterization of the Extract from *E. cantabrica*. (**A**) Schematic representation of *E. cantabrica* extract (EuPoly) production; (**B**) SDS-PAGE of the EuPoly extract (8 μL) (Lane 2) and molecular weight markers (Lane 1) using a 12% (*w*/*v*) polyacrylamide gel; (**C**) (a) SPE chromatogram of 40 μL of EuPoly obtained using an octadecyl column and H_2O_{dd} as solvent A (0–22 min) and methanol as solvent B (22–70 min), the elution was recorded at 280 nm; (b) absorbance at 750 nm after Folin–Ciocalteu assay of the collected peaks (30 μL) after freeze-drying and resuspension in 100 μL of buffer; (**D**) RP-HPLC chromatogram of EuPoly obtained with the following solvent B gradient: 0–5 min 0%; 5–65 min 60%; 65–90 min 90%. The absorbance at 280 nm was monitored; (**E**) the total polyphenolic content in the extract equal to 1.097 mg/mL (S.D. ± 0.058) of polyphenols expressed as Gallic Acid Equivalents (GAE) (mg/mL of extract). Error bar indicates S.D.

2.2. Effects of EuPoly on Human Dermal Fibroblasts (NHDFs)

Due to the role of oxidative stress in the development of various diseases, including neurodegenerative conditions, cardiovascular disorders, and, particularly, skin pathologies (i.e., photoaging, psoriasis, and dermatitis), there is a pressing need to identify new, effective natural antioxidants with therapeutic potential. Several studies have highlighted the antioxidant characteristics of various microalgae and of many micro-algae-derived metabolites such as polyphenols, polysaccharides, and carotenoids, suggesting their potential for treating skin diseases characterized by pro-oxidative and inflammatory conditions and UV light-induced damage [47,48].

The antioxidant properties of polyphenols have been extensively documented, with their mechanisms of action largely attributed to their ability to scavenge ROS, chelate metal ions, and modulate antioxidant enzyme activity [49]. Herein, the effects of EuPoly on normal human dermal fibroblasts (NHDFs) were evaluated in terms of cell viability and protection against oxidative stress. Figure 2A shows the brightfield micrographs and the results of the cell viability assay of the NHDFs after 24 h of treatment with and without

EuPoly (0.5 µL/mL). No significant effects on cell viability were observed in the samples treated with EuPoly with respect to the control samples. Subsequently, the ability of EuPoly to protect NHDFs from oxidative stress induced by H_2O_2 treatment was investigated. NHDFs were pre-treated for 3 h with EuPoly (0.5 µL/mL), followed by treatment with 100 µM H_2O_2 for 48 h. As shown in Figure 2B, a 20.65 % (S.D. ± 3.44) increase in cell viability compared to cells treated with H_2O_2 alone was observed, demonstrating that EuPoly provides significant protection to fibroblasts against H_2O_2-induced oxidative stress. This effect may result from both direct ROS scavenging and an induced increase in the oxidative damage resistance of cells enabled by EuPoly.

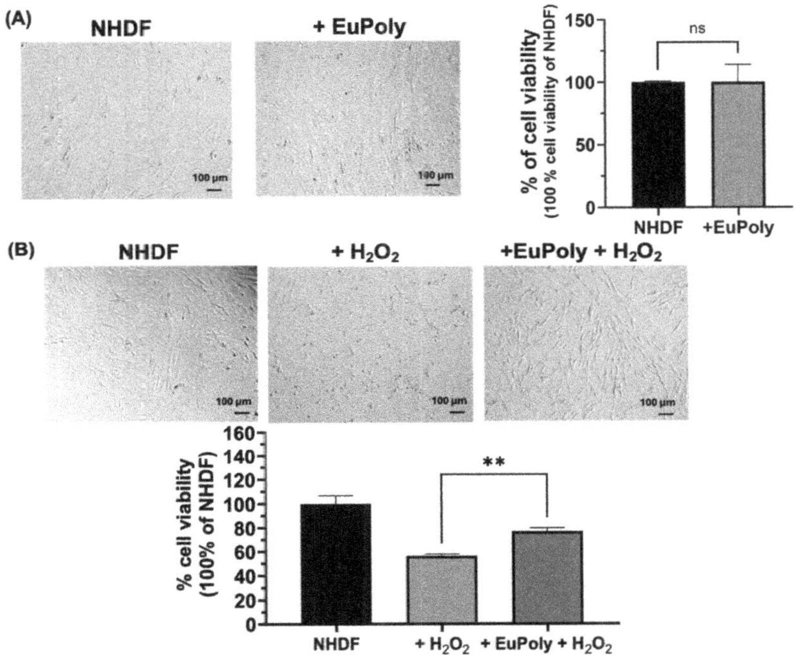

Figure 2. Effects of EuPoly on NHDFs' cell viability and protection against H_2O_2-induced oxidative stress. (**A**) Brightfield micrographs and the cell viability assay of NHDFs treated for 24 h with EuPoly (0.5 µL/mL) added in the cell culture medium (+EuPoly) or with the same concentration of 50% TCA (NHDF); (**B**) brightfield micrographs and the cell viability assay of untreated NHDFs (NHDF), of NHDFs treated for 48 h with 100 µM of H_2O_2 (+H_2O_2) and NHDFs first treated for 3 h with EuPoly (0.5 µL/mL) and then with 100 µM of H_2O_2 (+EuPoly + H_2O_2). The results were obtained by 3 experimental replicates. Error bars indicate S.D. ns: non-significant, ** p value ≤ 0.01. Scale bars are of 100 µm.

Our results are in agreement with recent studies that have reported polyphenol-rich extracts from microalgae, including euglenoids, to significantly reduce ROS levels in vitro and suppress oxidative damage markers [50,51]. For instance, a 70% methanol *E. tuba* extract was found to have scavenging abilities against superoxide, hydroxyl, and hypochlorous acid radicals [52]. Furthermore *E. gracilis* extract has been reported to promote the cellular reducing potential and prevent lipid peroxidation in the HT-29 human intestinal epithelial cell line, promoting conditions that counteract bacterial lipopolysaccharide-induced oxidative burst [19]. Moreover, algal polyphenols and other algal molecules, such as astaxanthin and fucoidans, have been shown to activate the Nrf2/ARE signaling pathway, enhancing the expression of antioxidant enzymes like HO-1 and NQO1, thereby providing protection against oxidative stress-induced cellular damage [53,54]. Our findings show EuPoly's antioxidant properties, highlighting its potential for further investigation as a therapeutic agent in skin disease treatment or in preventing oxidative stress-induced skin damage. Furthermore, TCA is widely used in dermatology from cosmetic peels to the treatment of actinic keratoses acne scars, warts, and at concentrations of from 40% to 60% it can stimulate the re-epithelialization process by activation of growth factors, such as TGF-α and PDGF-β [45,46]. Moreover, it is also reported to have a regulatory action on cytokines, including IL-1 and IL-10, which may also have a beneficial effect on wound healing [45]. In a dermatological study the topical application of 50% TCA on leg ulcers in 19 patients led to an evident reduction in the surface area of diabetic ulcers [45]. Therefore, EuPoly extract could combine the effect of 50% of TCA with the algal antioxidant molecules and our studies open the way for its medical application also in the treatment of diabetic ulcers.

2.3. Effects of EuPoly on MDA-MB-231 Breast Cancer Cells

Natural polyphenols at relatively high concentrations are known to have inhibitory effects on cancer cell proliferation, tumor growth, angiogenesis, metastasis, and inflammation, and also induce programmed cell death in different types of cancer including breast, colorectal, head, lung, ovarian, melanoma, and leukemia [55]. Polyphenolic compounds, and particularly those derived from microalgae, are able to sensitize cancer cells to various therapies and, therefore, their use in combination with chemotherapy and radiotherapy has recently gathered attention [28,56]. First, the effects of EuPoly on the cell viability and proliferation of triple-negative MDA-MB-231 breast cancer cells were evaluated. Figure 3A shows the brightfield micrographs and the cell viability results as assessed using Trypan Blue after 24 h of treatment with EuPoly (0.5 μL/mL). A statistically significant decrease in cell viability of 28.21% (S.D. ± 1.56) was observed as compared to the untreated samples. Moreover, the WST-1 cell viability assay performed after 48 h of cell growth in the presence or absence of EuPoly showed that the cells treated with EuPoly at a concentration of 0.5 μL/mL exhibited a 10.82% (S.D. ± 1.86) lower viability compared to the controls, while at a concentration of 1 μL/mL, the decrease was 22.96% (S.D. ± 1.88), indicating that EuPoly was able to affect the viability of the MDA-MB-231 cancer cells in a dose-dependent manner (Figure 3B). The observed decrease in cell viability and proliferation could likely be due to cell cycle arrest induced by EuPoly, rather than programmed cell death induction, as suggested by the Western blotting analysis, which shows a reduction in Cyclin D1 expression in the EuPoly-treated samples compared to the controls and the absence of cleaved forms of Caspase 3 protein (Figure 3C). Furthermore, no significant changes in MAP kinase ERK 1/2 phosphorylation were found.

Cyclin D1 is a cell cycle protein that plays a relevant role in regulating the progression from G1 phase to the S phase of the cell cycle. Increased expression levels of this protein have been positively correlated with increased aggressiveness, invasion, and metastasis of various types of tumors, particularly triple-negative breast cancer [57–60]. Studies on different cancer cell lines have reported the role of polyphenols as growth inhibitors, either by induction of G1 cell cycle arrest, G2/M arrest, or cell death [27]. Our findings are also consistent with evidence demonstrating the ability of euglenoid extracts to exert anticancer properties. It has been observed that methanolic *E. tuba* extract is able to inhibit the in vitro growth of human lung (A549) and breast cancer (MCF-7) cells [31] and shows anticancer activity in Dalton's lymphoma cells via reduction in mitochondrial potential and the induction of apoptosis [61]. Furthermore, an ethanol fractionated extract of *E. viridis* exerted cytotoxic activity in vitro against two prostate cancer cell lines, PC3 and Du145, and the colon cancer cell line HCT-116 [62]. Although further investigations are needed to elucidate the underlying molecular mechanisms, these findings demonstrate EuPoly's anticancer effects on triple-negative MDA-MB-231 breast cancer cells, highlighting its potential as a safe sensitizing agent in combination with other antitumor drugs, particularly given its lack of cytotoxicity toward normal fibroblasts (Figure 2A).

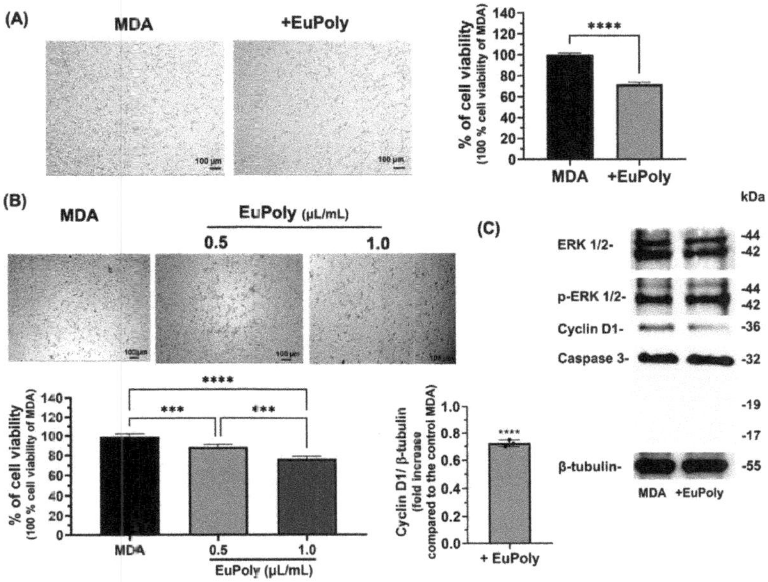

Figure 3. Effects of EuPoly on cell viability, proliferation and protein expression of MDA-MB-231 breast cancer cells. (**A**) Brightfield micrographs and cell counting trypan blue assay performed on MDA cells with 0.5 µL/mL of 50% TCA (MDA) and with EuPoly treatment (0.5 µL/mL) for 24 h (+EuPoly); (**B**) brightfield micrographs and WST-1 cell viability assay of MDA cells treated with 0.5 µL/mL of EuPoly (+EuPoly) added in the cell culture medium or with 0.5 µL/mL of 50% TCA (MDA) for 48 h and with 1 µL/mL of EuPoly or 50% TCA; (**C**) Western blotting analysis of Cyclin D1, p-ERK1/2, ERK1/2 and Caspase 3 protein expression of MDA cells treated with 0.5 µL/mL of EuPoly (+EuPoly) added in the cell culture medium or with 0.5 µL/mL of 50% TCA (MDA) for 48 h. The results were obtained by 3 experimental replicates. Error bars indicate S.D. *** p value ≤ 0.005, **** p value ≤ 0.0001. Scale bars are of 100 µm.

2.4. Diatoms Frustule Functionalization with EuPoly

Diatom frustules, composed of biogenic silica, have been extensively studied for their adsorption properties and potential applications in drug delivery, biosensing, and functional material development [63–65]. Their unique mesoporous structure provides a high surface area and chemical versatility for functionalization. In this study, S. pinnata frustules were functionalized with the EuPoly extract, with the aim of enhancing their bioactivity and potential applications in biomedicine. After the functionalization, performed by incubating frustules overnight with EuPoly extract (FEuPoly) (Figure 4A), the samples were centrifuged and the ability of the functionalized frustules to trap polyphenols was evaluated using the Folin–Ciocalteu assay on the supernatant fraction (superEuPoly + F). A statistically significant polyphenol trapping rate of 34.84% (S.D. ± 7.38) was found (Figure 4B). FEuPoly frustules were next characterized by brightfield microscopy and confocal fluorescence microscopy (Figure 4C). Figure 4C and Video S1 show confocal micrographs of the non-functionalized frustules (F) compared to the FEuPoly frustules.

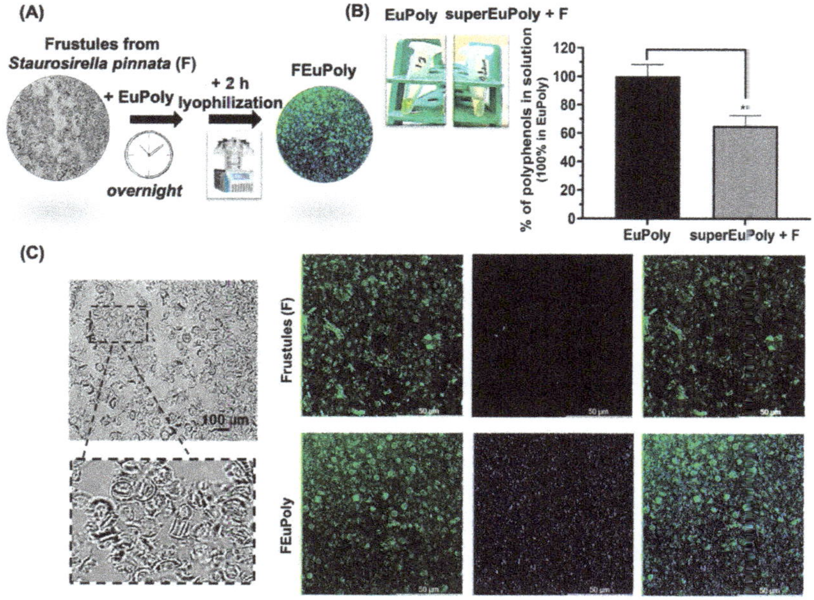

Figure 4. Functionalization and characterization of Frustules with EuPoly. (**A**) Schematic representation of the frustules functionalization with EuPoly to produce FEuPoly; (**B**) quantification of polyphenols by Folin–Ciocalteu assay with digital image of EuPoly and superEuPoly after incubation with frustules and centrifugation (superEuPoly + F); (**C**) brightfield micrographs of FEuPoly and confocal fluorescence micrographs of frustules with (FEuPoly) and without EuPoly functionalization (F). The green fluorescence signal (emission: 495–570 nm) was recorded using an excitation wavelength of 500 nm, while the blue fluorescence signal (emission 475–495 nm) with an excitation wavelength of 405 nm. Z-stacks were obtained with a 63× magnification and 1.5× zoom. The results were obtained by 3 experimental replicates. Error bars indicate S.D. ** p value $\leq$ 0.01. Scale bars are of 100 and 50 µm.

Notable autofluorescence in the green range (495–570 nm; excitation wavelength 500 nm) of the frustules was observed without and with functionalization, due to the intrinsic fluorescent property of these porous structures. The intrinsic photoluminescence of the diatom frustules in the green portion of the spectrum has been reported in the literature and specifically associated with their structural porous pattern, which resembles artificial photonic crystals and confers to frustules an active role in manipulation and exploitation of light [66,67]. However, as deduced from the confocal microscopy analysis, only the frustules functionalized with the polyphenolic extract emitted a strong fluorescence signal in the blue range of 475–495 nm when excited at 405 nm, indicating the strong presence of compounds that can be excited in the UV range and emit blue fluorescence, a characteristic typical of polyphenolic compounds that is attributed to their conjugated π-electron systems [68]. Therefore, these results represent further evidence of frustule functionalization with the EuPoly extract. The combination of frustules' distinctive features, such as their low cost and natural availability, as well as their large specific surface area, thermal stability, biocompatibility, and customizable surface chemistry, make them highly promising for environmental applications and biomedical tools [69]. Various strategies for frustule functionalization, including metal deposition and biomolecule adsorption, have been reported [68]. In line with these approaches, our results demonstrate that the rapid functionalization of frustules using a TCA polyphenol extract is feasible, enabling the simple production of novel bioactive silica-based materials.

2.5. Metal Ion Trapping by FEuPoly

Heavy metals are among the most common pollutants; they are not biodegradable and tend to accumulate in the environment, including in water, soil, and living organisms, leading to various illnesses and health disorders [70]. Among heavy metals, both cop-per (Cu^{2+}) and nickel (Ni^{2+}) ions are widely used across the domestic, industrial, medicinal, and agricultural sectors [71]. Polyphenols are well known for their ability to bind metal ions, primarily due to their multiple hydroxyl (-OH) groups and catechol or galloyl structures, which can chelate metal cations [72]; for this reason, polyphenol- rich extracts from algae have recently garnered attention in the field of environ-mental remediation. Herein, we investigated the potential trapping of the divalent metal ions Cu^{2+} and Ni^{2+} by frustules functionalized with polyphenolic extract. Figure 5A shows the schematic representation of FEuPoly's metal ion-binding property evaluation. The frustules were also functionalized with gallic acid (FGA) (Figure 5B) in order to compare its metal-binding ability with that of FEuPoly. Figure 5C shows that FEuPoly exhibited a 26.38% (S.D. $\pm$ 6.58) $\pm$ 6.59 higher Cu^{2+} binding capability com-pared to FGA, likely due to the presence of other molecules and further polyphenols with multiple functional groups (–OH, –COOH, –C=O, etc.) such as flavonoids, tannins, and floro-tannins present in the extract that are able to bind divalent metal cat-ions, enhancing the overall metal chelation rate. Interestingly, FEuPoly was found to bind Ni^{2+} more efficiently than Cu^{2+}, with a 25.03 % (S.D. $\pm$ 6.58) higher binding capability, as shown in Figure 5D. The preferential Ni^{2+} binding/coordination of FEuPoly in respect to Cu^{2+} ions could be advantageous in aquaculture or water remediation, considering the higher toxicity/allergenic properties of nickel ions than copper ions [73]. In light of the potential toxicity of these metal ions, the World Health Organization has set recommended maximum concentrations for these ions in drinking water: 31.5 μM for Cu^{2+} and 0.34 μM for Ni^{2+} [73]. Indeed, although these metals play essential roles in various biological and technological processes, excessive exposure can lead to serious health issues, including neurodegenerative diseases such as Parkinson's and Alzheimer's, as well as Wilson's disease, asthma, pneumonitis, lung cancer, and disorders of the central nervous system [71].

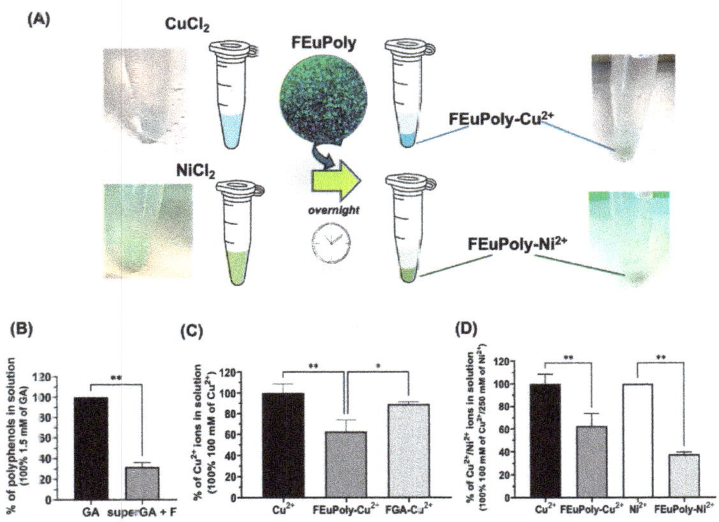

Figure 5. Evaluation of metal ions complexation by FEuPoly. (**A**) Schematic representation of FEuPoly's metal-ions binding property evaluation; (**B**) quantification of polyphenols by Folin–Ciocalteu assay of GA and superGA after incubation with frustules and centrifugation (superGA + F); (**C**) quantification

of Cu^{2+} ions left in solution after FEuPoly and FGA incubation with $CuCl_2$ (FEuPoly-Cu^{2+} and FGA-Cu^{2+}) determined measuring the absorbance at 750 nm; (**D**) quantification of Ni^{2+} ions left in solution after FEuPoly incubation with $NiCl_2$ (FEuPoly-Ni^{2+}) determined measuring the absorbance at 415 nm, compared to quantification of Cu^{2+} ions in solution. The results were obtained by 3 experimental replicates. Error bars indicate S.D. * p value ≤ 0.05, ** p value ≤ 0.01.

Recently, the development of polyphenol-functionalized platforms, such as porous particles, hydrogels, capsules, and films, mainly based on synthetic polymers (i.e., PEG, PVA, and PAAM) or nanomaterials able to exploit the metal chelation properties of polyphenols, has attracted significant interest in biomedicine (i.e., drug delivery, bioimaging, materials for bio-interfacial engineering) [74,75] and environmental remediation [76,77]. In this context, the preliminary data presented here may suggest that FEuPoly represents a natural, green, and sustainable platforms potentially useful for sensing applications, or reducing the metal overload in pathological conditions associated with abnormal metal ion accumulation [78,79].

2.6. Evaluation of Stem Cell Scaffolding Properties of FEuPoly

EuPoly's effects on the cell growth and differentiation of mesenchymal stem cells were also assessed in this study. Specifically, the potential use of EuPoly to produce new functionalized cellular scaffolds was investigated by assessing the ability of FEuPoly to support stem cell growth. Bone marrow mesenchymal stem cells (BM-MSCs) were seeded on F and FEuPoly and cultured for 7 days. Alizarin Red S staining was performed to detect the presence of calcium-rich deposits produced by the cells (Figure 6A). Our results revealed the strong presence of red-stained calcium deposits in the BM-MSC samples grown on F, and even greater presence was observed when the cells were grown on FEuPoly (Figure 6B). In contrast, no calcium deposits were detected in the cells grown on the plates without frustules.

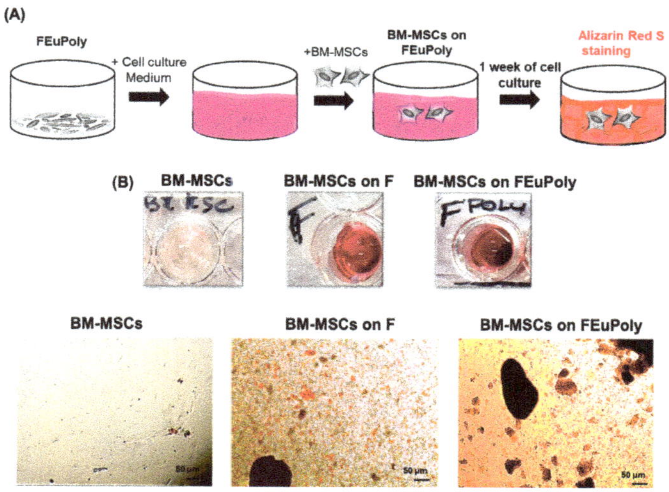

Figure 6. Evaluation of cell scaffolding properties of FEuPoly for cell growth and osteo-differentiation of BM-MSCs. (**A**) Schematic representation of the experimental set up to assess the osteo-differentiation of BM-MSCs grown on FEuPoly by Alizarin Red S assay; (**B**) digital images and brightfield micrographs after Alizarin Red S staining of BM-MSCs grown for 7 days on plates (BM-MSCs), on frustules (BM-MSCs on F) or on FEuPoly (BM-MSCs on FEuPoly). The results were obtained by 3 experimental replicates. Scale bars are of 50 μm.

The strong presence of Alizarin Red-positive deposits in the BM-MSCs grown on FEuPoly could be due to the combination of the silica frustules' mechanical properties and the Euglena polyphenols' biochemical activity, which creates a synergistic environment that promotes osteogenic differentiation. The use of polyphenols in tissue engineering applications has recently been investigated due to their potential ability to enhance the bioactivity and biocompatibility of scaffolds and promote cell adhesion, proliferation, and differentiation while showing anti-inflammatory, antioxidant, and antimicrobial properties, thus facilitating the tissue regeneration process. Certain polyphenols, including flavonoids, have also been reported to influence signaling path-ways relevant to wound healing and bone regeneration, suggesting a beneficial role in regenerative medicine applications [80–82].

Diatom silica frustules show a highly porous architecture and significant stiffness, closely resembling the structure of bone tissue. This structural mimicry provides mechanical cues that are critical for directing stem cell fate and promoting their osteo-genic differentiation by activating mechano-transduction pathways, such as the Wnt/β-catenin and TGF-β/BMP signaling cascades [83,84]. Furthermore, silica frustules' porosity can enhance cell adhesion, infiltration, and proliferation, also addressing the limit of oxygen deprivation and facilitating bone-specific extracellular matrix component deposition. Recently, diatoms were 3D bio-printed with stem cells in a gelatin methacryloyl (GelMA) bio-ink for bone repair in animal models, and the frustules present in the diatoms were able to reduce hypoxia damage and promote bone regeneration [85]. Therefore, frustule functionalization with the algal extract proposed in our study could be a novel approach for enhancing the osteogenic–regenerative properties of these natural mesoporous structures. Moreover, polyphenols alone have also been found to contribute to osteogenic differentiation by modulating key signaling pathways involved in bone formation [86–88]. For instance, flavonoids have been shown to modulate the ability of MSCs to self-renew and their osteogenic differentiation potential by targeting multiple signaling pathways such as the Wnt/β-catenin pathway, ERK pathway, and PI3K/Akt pathway, and regulating bone-specific markers and transcription factors including ALP, Runx2, BMP-2, Cbfa1, and Osx [86–88]. In recent years, polyphenol-functionalized scaffolds including hydrogels, films, and nano-fibers, mainly based on synthetic polymers, have emerged [80]. For instance, Lee et al. developed functionalized scaffolds based on different polymers, such as polystyrene and polydimethylsiloxane, for improving osteo-regeneration abilities of human adipose-derived stem cells through surface modification via catechin coating [89]. Although these emerging synthetic polyphenol-functionalized platforms have shown promise, our FEuPoly cell scaffold, as a fully natural, microalgae-derived system, potentially offers a more sustainable and biomimetic alternative, thus representing an innovative system with promising applications in biomedicine and bone tissue regeneration.

3. Materials and Methods

3.1. Preparation of Dried Algal Biomass

E. cantabrica (https://utex.org/products/utex-lb-1320, accessed on 20 May 2025) was obtained from the University of Texas's culture collection. The alga was cultured under photoautotrophic conditions in BG11 medium at 80 microeinstein light intensity in 4 cm glass bubble columns or at 200 microceinstein light intensity in 8 cm glass bubble columns placed in a water bath at a temperature of 25 °C. The first inoculum had to be prepared at a 5-fold lower light intensity until the green mobile Euglena cells emerged into the liquid medium. Cells were grown to about 2 g/L and harvested in a Sorvall tabletop centrifuge. Pellets were rinsed with deionized water, quick-frozen and stored at −80 °C, and lyophilized using a VirTis Benchtop 2K ES Freeze Dry System (Steroglass, Perugia, Italy).

3.2. Production of the E. cantabrica Extract (EuPoly) and Its Characterization by SPE, RP-HPLC and SDS-PAGE Analyses

The extract (EuPoly) was obtained from freeze-dried *E. cantabrica*. Approximately 12 mg of the lyophilized algae were resuspended in 500 μL of a 50% trichloroacetic acid (TCA) (*w*/*v*) solution and incubated on ice for 1 h. Subsequently, the samples were centrifuged at 8000× *g* for 15 min at 4 °C, and the supernatants were recovered for analysis. The obtained extract was stored at −20 °C. SPE chromatography of the extract was performed using a Bakerbond SPE oc-tadecyl column (J.T.Baker, Deventer, The Netherlands) [90]; the solvents used were H_2O_{dd} as solvent A and HPLC-grade methanol (Sigma-Aldrich, Milan, Italy) as solvent B. The chromatography was performed through isocratic elution 0–22 min at 0% of solv. B and then at 100% of solv. B (22–70 min) using a peristaltic pump, the elution was detected using an UV detector at 280 nm (Pharmacia LKB, Varese, Italy). The eluted fractions by SPE chromatography were collected, lyophilized, and then analyzed using the Folin–Ciocalteu assay. The extract was also characterized via reversed-phase high-performance liquid chromatography (RP-HPLC). RP-HPLC analysis of EuPoly was performed using mod. LC-10AVP (Shimadzu, Milan, Italy), equipped with a UV detector (Shimadzu, Milan, Italy) and a C_{18} column (150 mm × 4.6 mm, 5 μm, CPS Analitica, Rome, Italy), a loop of 20 μL, and a rate flow 0.8 mL/min. The solvents used were solvent A (0.1% (*v*/*v*) TFA) and solvent B (70% (*v*/*v*) CH_3CN, 0.1% (*v*/*v*) TFA in H_2O_{dd}). The solvent B gradient was 0–5 min 0%; 5–65 min 60%; 65–90 min 90%. The elution was monitored at 280 nm. The eluted peaks of three RP-HPLC analyses were collected, lyophilized, and then analyzed using the Folin–Ciocalteu assay. An SDS-PAGE analysis of the EuPoly extract was performed using a 12% *w*/*v* of polyacrylamide gel, and using a sample buffer with 2 μL of 1.5 M Tris-HCl, pH 8.8, for increasing the pH of the samples.

3.3. Quantitative UV Spectrophotometric Analysis for Polyphenolic Content Determination

Polyphenol quantification was performed using a modified Folin–Ciocalteu assay [91]: 250 μL of Folin–Ciocalteu reagent (diluted 1:10 *v*/*v*) was added to 30 μL of TCA extract for 4 min at room temperature in dark conditions. After that, 20 μL of 1 M KOH and 200 μL of 1 M $NaHCO_3$ were added and the samples were incubated in the dark for 2 h at room temperature. The absorbance at 750 nm of 200 μL of each sample was then recorded using an iMark™ Microplate Absorbance Reader (Bio-Rad, Milan, Italy). A calibration curve (see Supplementary Materials Figure S2) using gallic acid (GA) was created in order to assess the total polyphenol content in GA equivalents (GAE) (mg/mL of extract).

3.4. Cell Cultures and WST-1 Cell Viability Assay

Cell studies were performed on MDA-MB-231 cells, NHDFs (Lonza, Basel, Switzerland), and BM-MSCs (Gibco, StemPro®, Life Technologies, Monza, Italy). The cell lines were cultured at 37 °C, under 5% CO_2, in high-glucose Dulbecco's Modified Eagle's Medium (DMEM) (Gibco, Monza, Italy), containing 10% Fetal Bovine Serum (FBS) (*v*/*v*) (Gibco, Monza, Italy), 1% penicillin–streptomycin (*w*/*v*) (Sigma-Aldrich, Milan, Italy), and 2 mM of L-Glutamine solution (Gibco, Italy). The brightfield microscopy of the cell cultures was performed using a Zeiss microscope (Primovert, Zeiss, Milan, Italy). Cell viability was assessed by counting MDA-MB-231 breast cancer cells with Trypan Blue staining after 24 h of cell growth.

The cell viability of NHDFs and of MDA-MB-231 cells was assessed using a WST-1(4-[3-(4-lodophenyl)-2-(4-nitrophenyl)-2H-5-tetrazolium]-1,3-benzene disulfonate (Cell Proliferation Reagent WST-1, Roche, Mannheim, Germany) assay [92]. NHDFs were seeded at a density of 2×10^4 cells/cm^2. After 24 h of cell growth, the medium was changed, and cells were treated with 100 μM H_2O_2 for 48 h with and without a previous incubation with

EuPoly 0.5 μL/mL (0.55 μg/mL of GAE) for 3 h. After, the medium was replaced with fresh high-glucose DMEM without phenol red (GIBCO, Italy) containing tetrazolium salt WST-1 (5% *v*/*v*); the cells were incubated for 2 h at 37 °C, under 5% CO_2, and the absorbance of the medium was evaluated at 450 nm using a microplate reader (iMark^{TM} Microplate Absorbance Reader, Bio-Rad, Milan, Italy). MDA-MB-231 breast cancer cells were seeded at a cell density of 2 × 10^4 cells/cm^2, and the next day, the cells were treated at different EuPoly extract concentrations (0.5 and 1 μL/mL of EuPoly, corresponding to 0.55 μg/mL and 1.1 μg/mL of GAE). Cell viability was then assessed using the WST-1 assay at 48 h of cell growth, as described above. For each cell treatment with EuPoly, control samples with the same TCA concentration (50% *w*/*v*) were included in all experiments.

250 μL of Folin–Ciocalteu reagent (diluted 1:10 *v*/*v*) was added to 30 μL of TCA extract for 4 min at room temperature in dark conditions. After that, 20 μL of 1 M KOH and 200 μL of 1 M $NaHCO_3$ were added and the samples were incubated in the dark for 2 h at room temperature. The absorbance at 750 nm of 200 μL of each sample was then recorded using an iMark^{TM} Microplate Absorbance Reader (Bio-Rad). A calibration curve (see Supplementary Materials Figure S2) using gallic acid (GA) was created in order to assess the total polyphenol content in GA equivalents (GAE) (mg/mL of extract).

3.5. Western Blotting Analysis of Protein Expression

Proteins were extracted from 2 × 10^6 MDA-MB-231 cells per sample using RIPA buffer (50 μL) containing a protease inhibitor cocktail (Sigma-Aldrich, Milan, Italy) and per-vanadate (Sigma-Aldrich, Milan, Italy) as a phosphatase inhibitor for the cell lysis. After incubation for 90 min on ice, lysates were centrifuged for 10 min at 8000× *g* at 4 °C. The bicinchoninic acid (BCA) protein assay (Sigma-Aldrich, Milan, Italy) was used to determine the protein content, and SDS-PAGE for cell extracts (30 μg of protein) was performed using 15% polyacrylamide gel. Electroblotting was performed on PVDF membranes using a semi-dry Trans-Blot Turbo Transfer System (Bio-Rad). After blot-ting, the membrane was blocked and probed with the following primary monoclonal antibodies: Ab-cyclin D1 rabbit (2922S, Cell Signaling Technology, Danvers, MA, USA); Caspase 3 rabbit (D3R6Y, Cell Signaling Technology, USA); Ab-p-ERK1/2 rabbit (Anti-p-ERK1 (pThr202/pTyr204) and ERK2 (pThr185/pTyr187), ab136926 Abcam, Milan, Italy); and Ab-ERK1/2 rabbit (M5670, Sigma-Aldrich, Italy). Immunoblots were then incubated with the rabbit secondary antibody (dilution 1:3000) (7074S, Cell Signaling Technology, USA) for 4 h at room temperature. Immunoblots with Ab-β-tubulin–horseradish peroxidase conjugates (AB21058, Abcam, Milan, Italy) were also probed for controlling the protein loading. A SuperSignal West Pico kit (Thermo Scientific, Waltham, MA, USA) was used to visualize signals, followed by exposure to a FluorChem Imaging system (Alpha Innotech Corporation-Analitica De Mori, Milan, Italy).

3.6. Frustule Preparation, EuPoly Functionalization (FEuPoly), and Metal Ion Binding

Staurosirella pinnata biomass harvesting was carried out after 7 days of growth, and freeze-dried biomass was treated with a boiling acid mix (H_2SO_4:HNO_3:H_2O = 3:1:1), washed in bi-distilled water (H_2O_{dd}), and then freeze-dried according to a previously published protocol [93]. Frustules (2 mg) were functionalized by overnight incubation using 50 μL of EuPoly and 150 μL of H_2O_{dd}. The resulting pellet was resus-pended in 1 mL of 50 mM HEPES buffer, centrifuged at 2000 rpm for 5 min, and then lyophilized for 2 h. For the metal ion complexation analyses, samples of functionalized frustules (FEuPoly) were treated with 200 μL of either 100 mM $CuCl_2$ in 10 mM HEPES buffer, pH 5.5, or 100 mM $NiCl_2$, pH 5.5, and were left to oscillate in the dark overnight. The absorbances of the supernatants from the samples were measured at 750 nm and 415 nm, respectively, using the iMarkTM Microplate Reader (Bio-Rad). The brightfield microscopy analysis of frustules was performed using a BA310 Motic microscope (Motic, Hackensack, NJ, USA) Metal ion complexation was also assessed on frustules functionalized with gallic acid (FGA). Briefly, frustules were incubated overnight with 50 μL of a gallic acid (GA) solution (1 mg/mL) and 150 μL of H_2O_{dd}. After functionalization, the same protocol described for FEuPoly was used to perform Cu^{2+} ion complexation analyses.

3.7. Confocal Microscopy Analysis of FEuPoly

After frustule functionalization with EuPoly and centrifugation at 1342× g for 5 min, the pellet was washed with H_2O_{dd} and confocal fluorescence microscopy analysis of FEuPoly was performed using the Leica Stellaris platform. The excitation wavelength was set to 500 nm with an emission range of 495–570 nm (green), and to 405 nm with emission in the 475–495 nm range (blue).

3.8. FEuPoly Validation for BM-MSC Growth and Alizarin Red S Staining

FEuPoly was validated as a scaffold for BM-MSCs by seeding mesenchymal stem cells at a density of 6×10^3 cells/cm^2. After 7 days of cell culture, Alizarin Red S staining was performed to detect the presence of calcium-rich deposits. Alizarin Red S staining was performed as follows: the culture medium was removed, the well was washed twice with PBS, and cells were fixed with 4% PFA (paraformaldehyde) for 20 min in the dark. Then, after washing twice with H_2O_{dd}, the Alizarin Red S staining solution, at pH 4.1 (Sigma-Aldrich, Italy), was added for 3 min. Subsequently, the staining solution was removed, the samples were washed 3 times with H_2O_{dd}, and the red deposits were analyzed by optical microscopy using a BA310 Motic microscope (Motic, Hackensack, NJ, USA).

3.9. Statistical Analysis

GraphPad Prism version 8.0 for Windows (GraphPad Software, San Diego, CA, USA) was used for the statistical analysis. Data obtained from three or more experimental independent biological replicates were quantified and analyzed for each variable using a t-test or one-way ANOVA test followed by Tukey's multiple comparisons test. A p-value < 0.05 was considered statistically significant. Data are presented as mean ± standard deviation (S.D.).

4. Conclusions

Herein, we have described a new *E. cantabrica*-derived polyphenolic extract and investigated its potential use for biomedical applications. The successful development of a rapid and cost-effective extraction protocol highlights its scalability and applicability within a circular bioeconomy framework, offering advantages for analysis device production, which requires fast and efficient on-site ex-traction procedures. Furthermore, our results demonstrated that EuPoly was able to protect human fibroblasts from ROS-induced oxidative stress and to reduce the viability of MDA-MB-231 triple-negative breast cancer cells, suggesting its good potential for treating oxidative stress-related skin disorders and as an antitumor therapy. Although a full characterization of EuPoly is required and other bioactive compounds may contribute to the observed cellular effects described here, it is reasonable to attribute these effects primarily to the extract's polyphenolic content, also consistent with the extensive literature reporting polyphenols' antioxidant and anticancer properties. Herein, we have also functionalized diatom frustules with EuPoly, which showed good coordination of the heavy metal divalent ions Cu^{2+} and Ni^{2+}, suggesting promise for wastewater remediation and biomedical applications. Moreover, FEuPoly frustules were able to support the osteogenic differentiation of BM-MSCs, potentially offering a fully natural, microalgae-derived green scaffold for use in bone tissue re-generation. These findings highlight the innovative properties of the FEuPoly system, which combines the natural and unique mesoporous structure of diatom silica with the biochemical activity of a readily obtainable Euglena-derived polyphenolic extract for driving the osteo-differentiation of mesenchymal stem cells in bone tissue repair. In conclusion, our work contributes to the recent efforts directed towards harnessing the multifunctionality of algal bioproducts with the aim of providing new eco-sustainable tools for future applications in biomedicine.

Supplementary Materials: The following supporting information can be downloaded at: https://www.mdpi.com/article/10.3390/md23120453/s1, Figure S1: *E. cantabrica* extracts in different solvents; Figure S2: Folin–Ciocalteu assay of EuPoly and Gallic Acid calibration curve; Video S1: 3D confocal microscopy of FEuPoly.

Author Contributions: S.M., conceived the idea and designed the experiments; S.M., supervised the project and acquired the funding; S.B., C.T. and S.M. conducted the experiments; S.B. and S.M. analyzed the all data and interpreted the results and wrote the first draft; S.L. (Silvia Licoccia), writing—review and editing, and acquired the funding; S.L. (Stefan Leu), algae cultivation and production, methodology, data curation and writing—review and editing. All authors have read and agreed to the published version of the manuscript.

Funding: The research leading to these results has received funding from the European Union—Next Generation EU through the Italian Ministry of University and Research under PNRR-M4C2-I1.3 Project PE_00000019 "HEAL ITALIA". The views and opinions expressed are those of the authors only and do not necessarily reflect those of the European Union or the European Commission. Neither the European Union nor the European Commission can be held responsible for them. The research was also partially supported by the Italian network of excellence for advanced diagnosis (INNOVA) PNC-E3-2022-23683266, and by bi-national project BlueApp, funded by the Italian and Israeli Ministries of Science and Technology.

Institutional Review Board Statement: Not applicable.

Data Availability Statement: The authors declare that all data generated in this study are available within the article or the Supplementary Information. Other data related to this work are available from the corresponding authors upon request.

Acknowledgments: The authors thank Sammy Boussiba for his support and critical discussion of the project.

Conflicts of Interest: The authors declare no conflicts of interest.

Abbreviations

The following abbreviations are used in this manuscript:

ALP	Alkaline Phosphatase
BCA	Bicinchoninic acid
BM-MSCs	Bone marrow-mesenchymal stem cells
BMP	Bone morphogenetic protein
Cbfa1	Core Binding Factor 1
DMEM	Dulbecco's Modified Eagle Medium
ERK	Extracellular Signal-Regulated Kinase
EU	European Union
EuPoly	*Euglena cantabrica* extract
F	Frustules
FBS	Fetal Bovine Serum
FEuPoly	Frustules functionalized with *Euglena cantabrica* extract
GA	Gallic acid
GAE	Gallic acid equivalents
GelMA	Gelatin methacryloyl

HO-1	Heme Oxygenase-1
MAPKs	Mitogen-activated protein kinases
MSCs	Mesenchymal stem cells
NHDFs	Normal human dermal fibroblasts
NQO1	NAD(P)H:quinone oxidoreductase 1
Nrf2/ARE	Nuclear factor erythroid 2-related factor 2/ Antioxidant Response Element
Osx	Osterix
PAAM	Polyacrylamide
PBS	Phosphate Buffered Saline
PEG	Poly(ethylene glycol)
PFA	Paraformaldehyde
PI3K/Akt	Phosphatidylinositol 3-kinase/protein kinase B
PVA	Polyvinyl alcohol
PVDF	Polyvinylidene difluoride
ROS	Reactive oxygen species
RunX2	RUNT-related transcription factor 2
SDS-PAGE	Sodium dodecyl sulfate-polyacrylamide gel electrophoresis
TCA	Trichloroacetic acid
TFA	Trifluoroacetic acid
TGF-β	Transforming growth factor-beta
Wnt	Wingless-related integration site

References

1. Araújo, R.; Vázquez Calderón, F.; Sánchez López, J.; Azevedo, I.C.; Bruhn, A.; Fluch, S.; Garcia Tasende, M.; Ghaderiardakani, F.; Ilmjärv, T.; Laurans, M.; et al. Current Status of the Algae Production Industry in Europe: An Emerging Sector of the Blue Bioeconomy. *Front. Mar. Sci.* **2021**, *7*, 626389. [CrossRef]
2. Matin, M.; Koszarska, M.; Atanasov, A.G.; Król-Szmajda, K.; Jóźwik, A.; Stelmasiak, A.; Hejna, M. Bioactive Potential of Algae and Algae-Derived Compounds: Focus on Anti-Inflammatory, Antimicrobial, and Antioxidant Effects. *Molecules* **2024**, *29*, 4695. [CrossRef]
3. Guedes, A.C.; Amaro, H.M.; Malcata, F.X. Microalgae as Sources of High Added-Value Compounds—A Brief Review of Recent Work. *Biotechnol. Prog.* **2011**, *27*, 597–613. [CrossRef]
4. Bleakley, S.; Hayes, M. Algal Proteins: Extraction, Application, and Challenges Concerning Production. *Foods* **2017**, *6*, 33. [CrossRef] [PubMed]
5. Kumar, A.; Soratur, A.; Kumar, S.; Venmathi Maran, B.A. A Review of Marine Algae as a Sustainable Source of Antiviral and Anticancer Compounds. *Macromol* **2025**, *5*, 11. [CrossRef]
6. Antonacci, A.; Scognamiglio, V. Biotechnological Advances in the Design of Algae-Based Biosensors. *Trends Biotechnol.* **2020**, *38*, 334–347. [CrossRef]
7. Allouzi, M.M.A.; Allouzi, S.; Al-Salaheen, B.; Khoo, K.S.; Rajendran, S.; Sankaran, R.; Sy-Toan, N.; Show, P.L. Current Advances and Future Trend of Nanotechnology as Microalgae-Based Biosensor. *Biochem. Eng. J.* **2022**, *187*, 108653. [CrossRef]
8. Ciugulea, I.; Triemer, R.E. *A Color Atlas of Photosynthetic Euglenoids*; Michigan State University Press: East Lansing, MI, USA, 2010; ISBN 978-0-87013-879-9.
9. Jerez-Martel, I.; García-Poza, S.; Rodríguez-Martel, G.; Rico, M.; Afonso-Olivares, C.; Gómez-Pinchetti, J.L. Phenolic Profile and Antioxidant Activity of Crude Extracts from Microalgae and Cyanobacteria Strains. *J. Food Qual.* **2017**, *2017*, 2924508. [CrossRef]
10. Kapoor, S.; Singh, M.; Srivastava, A.; Chavali, M.; Chandrasekhar, K.; Verma, P. Extraction and Characterization of Microalgae-derived Phenolics for Pharmaceutical Applications: A Systematic Review. *J. Basic Microbiol.* **2022**, *62*, 1044–1063. [CrossRef]
11. Muñóz-Almagro, N.; Gilbert-López, B.; Carmen, P.-R.M.; García-Fernandez, Y.; Almeida, C.; Villamiel, M.; Mendiola, J.A.; Ibáñez, E. Exploring the Microalga Euglena Cantabrica by Pressurized Liquid Extraction to Obtain Bioactive Compounds. *Mar. Drugs* **2020**, *18*, 308. [CrossRef]
12. Cervantes-Garcia, D.; Troncoso-Rojas, R.; Sanchez-Estrada, A.; González-Mendoza, D.; Grimaldo-Juarez, O. Production of Phenolics and Flavonoids Compounds in Euglena Gracilis under Copper Stress. *J. Pure Appl. Microbiol.* **2013**, *7*, 93–100.
13. García-Lafuente, A.; Guillamón, E.; Villares, A.; Rostagno, M.A.; Martínez, J.A. Flavonoids as Anti-Inflammatory Agents: Implications in Cancer and Cardiovascular Disease. *Inflamm. Res.* **2009**, *58*, 537–552. [CrossRef]
14. Vauzour, D.; Rodriguez-Mateos, A.; Corona, G.; Oruna-Concha, M.J.; Spencer, J.P.E. Polyphenols and Human Health: Prevention of Disease and Mechanisms of Action. *Nutrients* **2010**, *2*, 1106–1131. [CrossRef] [PubMed]

15. Visioli, F.; De La Lastra, C.A.; Andres-Lacueva, C.; Aviram, M.; Calhau, C.; Cassano, A.; D'aRchivio, M.; Faria, A.; Favé, G.; Fogliano, V.; et al. Polyphenols and Human Health: A Prospectus. *Crit. Rev. Food Sci. Nutr.* **2011**, *51*, 524–546. [CrossRef]
16. Zhang, R.; Ren, Y.; Ren, T.; Yu, Y.; Li, B.; Zhou, X. Marine-Derived Antioxidants: A Comprehensive Review of Their Therapeutic Potential in Oxidative Stress-Associated Diseases. *Mar. Drugs* **2025**, *23*, 223. [CrossRef]
17. Vicente-Zurdo, D.; Gómez-Mejía, E.; Morante-Zarcero, S.; Rosales-Conrado, N.; Sierra, I. Analytical Strategies for Green Extraction, Characterization, and Bioactive Evaluation of Polyphenols, Tocopherols, Carotenoids, and Fatty Acids in Agri-Food Bio-Residues. *Molecules* **2025**, *30*, 1326. [CrossRef] [PubMed]
18. Bermudez, G.; Terenzi, C.; Medri, F.; Andrisano, V.; Montanari, S. Extraction and Analytical Methods for the Characterization of Polyphenols in Marine Microalgae: A Review. *Mar. Drugs* **2024**, *22*, 538. [CrossRef]
19. Brun, P.; Piovan, A.; Caniato, R.; Dalla Costa, V.; Pauletto, A.; Filippini, R. Anti-Inflammatory Activities of Euglena Gracilis Extracts. *Microorganisms* **2021**, *9*, 2058. [CrossRef] [PubMed]
20. Nakashima, A.; Horio, Y.; Suzuki, K.; Isegawa, Y. Antiviral Activity and Underlying Action Mechanism of Euglena Extract against Influenza Virus. *Nutrients* **2021**, *13*, 3911. [CrossRef]
21. Isegawa, Y. Activation of Immune and Antiviral Effects by Euglena Extracts: A Review. *Foods* **2023**, *12*, 4438. [CrossRef]
22. Bedard, S.; Roxborough, E.; O'Neill, E.; Mangal, V. The Biomolecules of Euglena Gracilis: Harnessing Biology for Natural Solutions to Future Problems. *Protist* **2024**, *175*, 126044. [CrossRef]
23. Li, J.; Zheng, Z.; Du, M.; Chen, J.; Zhu, H.; Hu, Z.; Zhu, Y.; Wang, J. Euglena Gracilis and Its Aqueous Extract Constructed With Chitosan-Hyaluronic Acid Hydrogel Facilitate Cutaneous Wound Healing in Mice Without Inducing Excessive Inflammatory Response. *Front. Bioeng. Biotechnol.* **2021**, *9*, 713840. [CrossRef]
24. Ko, Y.; Baek, H.; Hwang, J.-H.; Kim, Y.; Lim, K.-M.; Kim, J.; Kim, J.W. Nonanimal Euglena Gracilis-Derived Extracellular Vesicles Enhance Skin-Regenerative Wound Healing. *Adv. Mater. Interfaces* **2023**, *10*, 2202255. [CrossRef]
25. Kesherwani, R.; Kumar, R.; Minhas, U.; Rizvi, S.I. Euglena Tuba Extract Provides Protection against Lipopolysaccharide-Induced Inflammatory Response and Oxidative Stress in Mice. *Biologia* **2021**, *76*, 793–798. [CrossRef] [PubMed]
26. Ferdous, U.T.; Balia Yusof, Z.N. Insight into Potential Anticancer Activity of Algal Flavonoids: Current Status and Challenges. *Molecules* **2021**, *26*, 6844. [CrossRef] [PubMed]
27. Sharma, E.; Attri, D.C.; Sati, P.; Dhyani, P.; Szopa, A.; Sharifi-Rad, J.; Hano, C.; Calina, D.; Cho, W.C. Recent Updates on Anticancer Mechanisms of Polyphenols. *Front. Cell Dev. Biol.* **2022**, *10*, 1005910. [CrossRef]
28. Sharma, R.; Mondal, A.S.; Trivedi, N. Anticancer Potential of Algae-Derived Metabolites: Recent Updates and Breakthroughs. *Future J. Pharm. Sci.* **2023**, *9*, 44. [CrossRef]
29. Maleki Dana, P.; Sadoughi, F.; Asemi, Z.; Yousefi, B. The Role of Polyphenols in Overcoming Cancer Drug Resistance: A Comprehensive Review. *Cell. Mol. Biol. Lett.* **2022**, *27*, 1. [CrossRef] [PubMed]
30. Mileo, A.M.; Miccadei, S. Polyphenols as Modulator of Oxidative Stress in Cancer Disease: New Therapeutic Strategies. *Oxid. Med. Cell. Longev.* **2016**, *2016*, 6475624. [CrossRef]
31. Panja, S.; Ghate, N.B.; Mandal, N. A Microalga, Euglena Tuba Induces Apoptosis and Suppresses Metastasis in Human Lung and Breast Carcinoma Cells through ROS-Mediated Regulation of MAPKs. *Cancer Cell Int.* **2016**, *16*, 51. [CrossRef]
32. Upreti, D.; Ishiguro, S.; Phillips, M.; Nakashima, A.; Suzuki, K.; Comer, J.; Tamura, M. Euglena Gracilis Extract Protects From Tobacco Smoke Carcinogen-Induced Lung Cancer by Altering Gut Microbiota Metabolome. *Integr. Cancer Ther.* **2023**, *22*, 15347354231195323. [CrossRef] [PubMed]
33. Tchounwou, P.B.; Yedjou, C.G.; Patlolla, A.K.; Sutton, D.J. Heavy Metal Toxicity and the Environment. In *Molecular, Clinical and Environmental Toxicology*; Volume 3: Environmental Toxicology; Luch, A., Ed.; Springer Basel: Basel, Switzerland, 2012; pp. 133–164. ISBN 978-3-7643-8340-4.
34. Jaishankar, M.; Tseten, T.; Anbalagan, N.; Mathew, B.B.; Beeregowda, K.N. Toxicity, Mechanism and Health Effects of Some Heavy Metals. *Interdiscip. Toxicol.* **2014**, *7*, 60–72. [CrossRef] [PubMed]
35. Jomova, K.; Makova, M.; Alomar, S.Y.; Alwasel, S.H.; Nepovimova, E.; Kuca, K.; Rhodes, C.J.; Valko, M. Essential Metals in Health and Disease. *Chem. Biol. Interact.* **2022**, *367*, 110173. [CrossRef]
36. Jasso-Chávez, R.; Campos-García, M.L.; Vega-Segura, A.; Pichardo-Ramos, G.; Silva-Flores, M.; Santiago-Martínez, M.G.; Feregrino-Mondragón, R.D.; Sánchez-Thomas, R.; García-Contreras, R.; Torres-Márquez, M.E. Microaerophilia Enhances Heavy Metal Biosorption and Internal Binding by Polyphosphates in Photosynthetic Euglena Gracilis. *Algal Res.* **2021**, *58*, 102384. [CrossRef]
37. Rodríguez-Zavala, J.S.; García-García, J.D.; Ortiz-Cruz, M.A.; Moreno-Sánchez, R. Molecular Mechanisms of Resistance to Heavy Metals in the Protist Euglena Gracilis. *J. Environ. Sci. Health Part A* **2007**, *42*, 1365–1378. [CrossRef]
38. Khatiwada, B.; Hasan, M.T.; Sun, A.; Kamath, K.S.; Mirzaei, M.; Sunna, A.; Nevalainen, H. Proteomic Response of Euglena Gracilis to Heavy Metal Exposure—Identification of Key Proteins Involved in Heavy Metal Tolerance and Accumulation. *Algal Res.* **2020**, *45*, 101764. [CrossRef]

39. Ahlström, M.G.; Thyssen, J.P.; Wennervaldt, M.; Menné, T.; Johansen, J.D. Nickel Allergy and Allergic Contact Dermatitis: A Clinical Review of Immunology, Epidemiology, Exposure, and Treatment. *Contact Dermat.* **2019**, *81*, 227–241. [CrossRef]
40. Sailer, J.; Nagel, J.; Akdogan, B.; Jauch, A.T.; Engler, J.; Knolle, P.A.; Zischka, H. Deadly Excess Copper. *Redox Biol.* **2024**, *75*, 103256. [CrossRef]
41. Mizzi, L.; Chatzitzika, C.; Gatt, R.; Valdramidis, V. HPLC Analysis of Phenolic Compounds and Flavonoids with Overlapping Peaks. *Food Technol. Biotechnol.* **2020**, *58*, 12–19. [CrossRef]
42. Buonvino, S.; Ciocci, M.; Nanni, F.; Cacciotti, I.; Melino, S. New Vegetable-Waste Biomaterials by *Lupin albus* L. as Cellular Scaffolds for Applications in Biomedicine and Food. *Biomaterials* **2023**, *293*, 121984. [CrossRef]
43. Chaves, J.O.; de Souza, M.C.; da Silva, L.C.; Lachos-Perez, D.; Torres-Mayanga, P.C.; Machado, A.P.D.F.; Forster-Carneiro, T.; Vázquez-Espinosa, M.; González-de-Peredo, A.V.; Barbero, G.F.; et al. Extraction of Flavonoids From Natural Sources Using Modern Techniques. *Front. Chem.* **2020**, *8*, 507887. [CrossRef] [PubMed]
44. Gil-Martín, E.; Forbes-Hernández, T.; Romero, A.; Cianciosi, D.; Giampieri, F.; Battino, M. Influence of the Extraction Method on the Recovery of Bioactive Phenolic Compounds from Food Industry By-Products. *Food Chem.* **2022**, *378*, 131918. [CrossRef] [PubMed]
45. Zenjari, L.; Hali, F.; Chiheb, S. Trichloroacetic Acid (50%) in the Treatment of Venous Leg Ulcers. *JMV J. Médecine Vasc.* **2021**, *46*, 139–143. [CrossRef]
46. Sitohang, I.B.S.; Legiawati, L.; Suseno, L.S.; Safira, F.D. Trichloroacetic Acid Peeling for Treating Photoaging: A Systematic Review. *Dermatol. Res. Pract.* **2021**, *2021*, 3085670. [CrossRef]
47. Yu, Z.; Hong, Y.; Xie, K.; Fan, Q. Research Progresses on the Physiological and Pharmacological Benefits of Microalgae-Derived Biomolecules. *Foods* **2022**, *11*, 2806. [CrossRef] [PubMed]
48. Pereira, L.; Cotas, J.; Valado, A. Antioxidants from Microalgae and Their Potential Impact on Human Well-Being. *Explor. Drug Sci.* **2024**, *2*, 292–321. [CrossRef]
49. Belščak-Cvitanović, A.; Durgo, K.; Huđek, A.; Bačun-Družina, V.; Komes, D. 1—Overview of Polyphenols and Their Properties. In *Polyphenols: Properties, Recovery, and Applications*; Galanakis, C.M., Ed.; Woodhead Publishing: Sawston, UK, 2018; pp. 3–44. ISBN 978-0-12-813572-3.
50. Coulombier, N.; Jauffrais, T.; Lebouvier, N. Antioxidant Compounds from Microalgae: A Review. *Mar. Drugs* **2021**, *19*, 549. [CrossRef]
51. Del Mondo, A.; Smerilli, A.; Ambrosino, L.; Albini, A.; Noonan, D.M.; Sansone, C.; and Brunet, C. Insights into Phenolic Compounds from Microalgae: Structural Variety and Complex Beneficial Activities from Health to Nutraceutics. *Crit. Rev. Biotechnol.* **2021**, *41*, 155–171. [CrossRef]
52. Chaudhuri, D.; Ghate, N.B.; Deb, S.; Panja, S.; Sarkar, R.; Rout, J.; Mandal, N. Assessment of the Phytochemical Constituents and Antioxidant Activity of a Bloom Forming Microalgae Euglena Tuba. *Biol. Res.* **2014**, *47*, 24. [CrossRef]
53. Nisar, M.F.; Li, M.; Xu, J.; Wan, C. Anti-Diabetic Effects of Marine Natural Products through Redox Modulation via Nrf2/HO-1 Cytoprotective Pathways. *Front. Mar. Sci.* **2024**, *11*, 1438955. [CrossRef]
54. Chen, J.; Huang, Z.; Cao, X.; Chen, X.; Zou, T.; You, J. Plant-Derived Polyphenols as Nrf2 Activators to Counteract Oxidative Stress and Intestinal Toxicity Induced by Deoxynivalenol in Swine: An Emerging Research Direction. *Antioxidants* **2022**, *11*, 2379. [CrossRef]
55. Glasauer, A.; Chandel, N.S. Targeting Antioxidants for Cancer Therapy. *Biochem. Pharmacol.* **2014**, *92*, 90–101. [CrossRef]
56. Frazzini, S.; Rossi, L. Anticancer Properties of Macroalgae: A Comprehensive Review. *Mar. Drugs* **2025**, *23*, 70. [CrossRef]
57. Montalto, F.I.; De Amicis, F. Cyclin D1 in Cancer: A Molecular Connection for Cell Cycle Control, Adhesion and Invasion in Tumor and Stroma. *Cells* **2020**, *9*, 2648. [CrossRef]
58. Buonvino, S.; Arciero, I.; Martinelli, E.; Seliktar, D.; Melino, S. Modelling the Disease: H2S-Sensitivity and Drug-Resistance of Triple Negative Breast Cancer Cells Can Be Modulated by Embedding in Isotropic Micro-Environment. *Mater. Today Bio* **2023**, *23*, 100862. [CrossRef]
59. Buonvino, S.; Di Giuseppe, D.; Filippi, J.; Martinelli, E.; Seliktar, D.; Melino, S. 3D Cell Migration Chip (3DCM-Chip): A New Tool toward the Modeling of 3D Cellular Complex Systems. *Adv. Healthc. Mater.* **2024**, *13*, 2400040. [CrossRef] [PubMed]
60. Arciero, I.; Buonvino, S.; Palumbo, V.; Scimeca, M.; Melino, S. A 3D-Printable Cell Array for In Vitro Breast Cancer Modeling. *Int. J. Mol. Sci.* **2024**, *25*, 13068. [CrossRef]
61. Gupta, S.P.; Siddiqi, N.J.; Khan, H.A.; Alrokayan, S.H.; Alhomida, A.S.; Singh, R.K.; Verma, P.K.; Kumar, S.; Acharya, A.; Sharma, B. Phytochemical Profiling of Microalgae Euglena Tuba and Its Anticancer Activity in Dalton's Lymphoma Cells. *FBL* **2022**, *27*, 120. [CrossRef]
62. Das, B.; Pradhan, J.; Mahammad, S.; Nayak, K.K. In Vitro Cytotoxic and Antibacterial Activity of Ethanolic Extract of Euglena Viridis. *Int. J. Pharma. Bio Sci.* **2012**, *3*, 321–331.

63. Uthappa, U.T.; Brahmkhatri, V.; Sriram, G.; Jung, H.-Y.; Yu, J.; Kurkuri, N.; Aminabhavi, T.M.; Altalhi, T.; Neelgund, G.M.; Kurkuri, M.D. Nature Engineered Diatom Biosilica as Drug Delivery Systems. *J. Control. Release* **2018**, *281*, 70–83. [CrossRef] [PubMed]
64. Rabiee, N.; Khatami, M.; Jamalipour Soufi, G.; Fatahi, Y.; Iravani, S.; Varma, R.S. Diatoms with Invaluable Applications in Nanotechnology, Biotechnology, and Biomedicine: Recent Advances. *ACS Biomater. Sci. Eng.* **2021**, *7*, 3053–3068. [CrossRef]
65. Bhat, K.; Ajees, M.A.; Kumar, P.; Vibha, B.V.G.; Nayak, R.; Mazumder, N. Diatoms: Harnessing Nature's Microscopic Marvels for Biosensing and Multifaceted Applications. *Biophys. Rev.* **2025**, *17*, 103–125. [CrossRef]
66. Fuhrmann, T.; Landwehr, S.; El Rharbi-Kucki, M.; Sumper, M. Diatoms as Living Photonic Crystals. *Appl. Phys. B* **2004**, *78*, 257–260. [CrossRef]
67. De Tommasi, E.; Rea, I.; Mocella, V.; Moretti, L.; Stefano, M.D.; Rendina, I.; Stefano, L.D. Multi-Wavelength Study of Light Transmitted through a Single Marine Centric Diatom. *Opt. Express* **2010**, *18*, 12203–12212. [CrossRef]
68. Anouar, E.H.; Gierschner, J.; Duroux, J.-L.; Trouillas, P. UV/Visible Spectra of Natural Polyphenols: A Time-Dependent Density Functional Theory Study. *Food Chem.* **2012**, *131*, 79–89. [CrossRef]
69. Terracciano, M.; De Stefano, L.; Rea, I. Diatoms Green Nanotechnology for Biosilica-Based Drug Delivery Systems. *Pharmaceutics* **2018**, *10*, 242. [CrossRef]
70. Gupta, A.; Sharma, V.; Sharma, K.; Kumar, V.; Choudhary, S.; Mankotia, P.; Kumar, B.; Mishra, H.; Moulick, A.; Ekielski, A.; et al. A Review of Adsorbents for Heavy Metal Decontamination: Growing Approach to Wastewater Treatment. *Materials* **2021**, *14*, 4702. [CrossRef]
71. Loya, M.; Ghosh, S.; Atta, A.K. A Review on Dual Detection of Cu^{2+} and Ni^{2+} Ions by Using Single Fluorometric and Colorimetric Organic Molecular Probes. *J. Mol. Struct.* **2023**, *1278*, 134949. [CrossRef]
72. Chen, Z.; Świsłocka, R.; Choińska, R.; Marszałek, K.; Dąbrowska, A.; Lewandowski, W.; Lewandowska, H. Exploring the Correlation Between the Molecular Structure and Biological Activities of Metal–Phenolic Compound Complexes: Research and Description of the Role of Metal Ions in Improving the Antioxidant Activities of Phenolic Compounds. *Int. J. Mol. Sci.* **2024**, *25*, 11775. [CrossRef] [PubMed]
73. Available online: https://www.who.int/teams/environment-climate-change-and-health/water-sanitation-and-health/water-safety-and-quality/drinking-water-quality-guidelines (accessed on 24 May 2025).
74. Xu, L.Q.; Neoh, K.-G.; Kang, E.-T. Natural Polyphenols as Versatile Platforms for Material Engineering and Surface Functionalization. *Prog. Polym. Sci.* **2018**, *87*, 165–196. [CrossRef]
75. Cao, H.; Yang, L.; Tian, R.; Wu, H.; Gu, Z.; Li, Y. Versatile Polyphenolic Platforms in Regulating Cell Biology. *Chem. Soc. Rev.* **2022**, *51*, 4175–4198. [CrossRef]
76. Cheng, W.; Wen, J. Now and Future: Development and Perspectives of Using Polyphenol Nanomaterials in Environmental Pollution Control. *Coord. Chem. Rev.* **2022**, *473*, 214825. [CrossRef]
77. Lin, Z.; Liu, H.; Richardson, J.J.; Xu, W.; Chen, J.; Zhou, J.; Caruso, F. Metal–Phenolic Network Composites: From Fundamentals to Applications. *Chem. Soc. Rev.* **2024**, *53*, 10800–10826. [CrossRef]
78. Gerosa, C.; Fanni, D.; Congiu, T.; Piras, M.; Cau, F.; Moi, M.; Faa, G. Liver Pathology in Wilson's Disease: From Copper Overload to Cirrhosis. *J. Inorg. Biochem.* **2019**, *193*, 106–111. [CrossRef]
79. Jomova, K.; Alomar, S.Y.; Nepovimova, E.; Kuca, K.; Valko, M. Heavy Metals: Toxicity and Human Health Effects. *Arch. Toxicol.* **2025**, *99*, 153–209. [CrossRef]
80. Zhang, X.; Li, Z.; Yang, P.; Duan, G.; Liu, X.; Gu, Z.; Li, Y. Polyphenol Scaffolds in Tissue Engineering. *Mater. Horiz.* **2021**, *8*, 145–167. [CrossRef] [PubMed]
81. Zulkefli, N.; Che Zahari, C.N.; Sayuti, N.H.; Kamarudin, A.A.; Saad, N.; Hamezah, H.S.; Bunawan, H.; Baharum, S.N.; Mediani, A.; Ahmed, Q.U.; et al. Flavonoids as Potential Wound-Healing Molecules: Emphasis on Pathways Perspective. *Int. J. Mol. Sci.* **2023**, *24*, 4607. [CrossRef]
82. Liu, Y.; Shi, Y.; Zhang, M.; Han, F.; Liao, W.; Duan, X. Natural Polyphenols for Drug Delivery and Tissue Engineering Construction: A Review. *Eur. J. Med. Chem.* **2024**, *266*, 116141. [CrossRef] [PubMed]
83. Han, S.-B.; Kim, J.-K.; Lee, G.; Kim, D.-H. Mechanical Properties of Materials for Stem Cell Differentiation. *Adv. Biosyst.* **2020**, *4*, 2000247. [CrossRef] [PubMed]
84. Wang, L.; Ruan, M.; Bu, Q.; Zhao, C. Signaling Pathways Driving MSC Osteogenesis: Mechanisms, Regulation, and Translational Applications. *Int. J. Mol. Sci.* **2025**, *26*, 1311. [CrossRef]
85. Han, Y.; Du, L.; Wu, J.; Zhang, H.; Yang, G.; Zheng, Y.; Wu, C. Diatomaceous Cross-Species Constructs for Tendon-to-Bone Regeneration. *Mat. Today* **2025**, *83*, 64–84. [CrossRef]
86. An, J.; Yang, H.; Zhang, Q.; Liu, C.; Zhao, J.; Zhang, L.; Chen, B. Natural Products for Treatment of Osteoporosis: The Effects and Mechanisms on Promoting Osteoblast-Mediated Bone Formation. *Life Sci.* **2016**, *147*, 46–58. [CrossRef]
87. Zhang, Q.; Chang, B.; Zheng, G.; Du, S.; Li, X. Quercetin Stimulates Osteogenic Differentiation of Bone Marrow Stromal Cells through miRNA-206/Connexin 43 Pathway. *Am. J. Transl. Res.* **2020**, *12*, 2062. [PubMed]

88. Zhang, J.; Liu, Z.; Luo, Y.; Li, X.; Huang, G.; Chen, H.; Li, A.; Qin, S. The Role of Flavonoids in the Osteogenic Differentiation of Mesenchymal Stem Cells. *Front. Pharmacol.* **2022**, *13*, 2022. [CrossRef]
89. Lee, J.S.; Lee, J.S.; Lee, M.S.; An, S.; Yang, K.; Lee, K.; Yang, H.S.; Lee, H.; Cho, S.-W. Plant Flavonoid-Mediated Multifunctional Surface Modification Chemistry: Catechin Coating for Enhanced Osteogenesis of Human Stem Cells. *Chem. Mater.* **2017**, *29*, 4375–4384. [CrossRef]
90. López-Fernández, O.; Domínguez, R.; Pateiro, M.; Munekata, P.E.S.; Rocchetti, G.; Lorenzo, J.M. Determination of Polyphenols Using Liquid Chromatography–Tandem Mass Spectrometry Technique (LC–MS/MS): A Review. *Antioxidants* **2020**, *9*, 479. [CrossRef]
91. Singleton, V.L.; Rossi, J.A. Colorimetry of Total Phenolics with Phosphomolybdic-Phosphotungstic Acid Reagents. *Am. J. Enol. Vitic.* **1965**, *16*, 144–158. [CrossRef]
92. Koyanagi, M.; Kawakabe, S.; Arimura, Y. A Comparative Study of Colorimetric Cell Proliferation Assays in Immune Cells. *Cytotechnology* **2016**, *68*, 1489–1498. [CrossRef] [PubMed]
93. De Angelis, R.; Melino, S.; Prosposito, P.; Casalboni, M.; Lamastra, F.R.; Nanni, F.; Bruno, L.; Congestri, R. The Diatom Staurosirella Pinnata for Photoactive Material Production. *PLoS ONE* **2016**, *11*, e0165571. [CrossRef]

marine drugs

MDPI

Article

Botryocladia leptopoda Extracts Promote Wound Healing Ability via Antioxidant and Anti-Inflammatory Activities and Regulation of MMP/TIMP Expression

Shin-Ping Lin [1,2,3], Tsung-Kai Yi [4], Yi-Feng Kao [4], Ming-Chieh Tu [4], Chen-Che Hsieh [5], Yu-Chieh Chou [2], Jheng-Jhe Lu [6], Shella Permatasari Santoso [7,8,9], Huey-Jine Chai [4,*] and Kuan-Chen Cheng [6,10,11,12,13,*]

1 School of Food Safety, Taipei Medical University, Taipei 11031, Taiwan
2 Ph.D. Program in Drug Discovery and Development Industry, Taipei Medical University, Taipei 11031, Taiwan
3 Research Center of Biomedical Device, Taipei Medical University, Taipei 11031, Taiwan
4 Seafood Technology Division, Fisheries Research Institute, Ministry of Agriculture, Keelung 20246, Taiwan
5 Department of Seafood Science, College of Hydrosphere, National Kaohsiung University of Science and Technology, Kaohsiung 81157, Taiwan
6 Institute of Biotechnology, National Taiwan University, Taipei 10617, Taiwan
7 Department of Chemical Engineering, Faculty of Engineering, Widya Mandala Surabaya Catholic University, Surabaya 60114, Indonesia
8 Chemical Engineering Master Program, Widya Mandala Surabaya Catholic University, Surabaya 60114, Indonesia
9 Collaborative Research Center for Zero Waste and Sustainability, Widya Mandala Surabaya Catholic University, Surabaya 60114, Indonesia
10 Institute of Food Science and Technology, National Taiwan University, Taipei 10617, Taiwan
11 Department of Medical Research, China Medical University Hospital, China Medical University, Taichung 40402, Taiwan
12 Department of Optometry, Asia University, Taichung 41354, Taiwan
13 Department of Food Science, Fu Jen Catholic University, New Taipei City 242062, Taiwan
* Correspondence: hjchai@mail.tfrin.gov.tw (H.-J.C.); kccheng@ntu.edu.tw (K.-C.C.)

Abstract: Wound healing is a complex process involving coordinated actions of multiple cell types. Therefore, when developing therapeutics to promote wound healing, it is essential to consider the synergistic contributions of various cells at different stages of the healing process. In this study, we evaluated the potential of different extracts of *Botryocladia leptopoda* as wound-healing agents by examining their effects on antioxidant activity, cytotoxicity, cell migration, anti-inflammatory properties, and expressions of specific biomarkers associated with wound healing. Results indicated that the ethanol extract (FE) and hexane extract (HE) exhibited the highest DPPH radical scavenging activity, reaching up to 94%. The alkaline extract (AE) showed the strongest antioxidant ability in the FICA assay, with a maximum of 99%. In addition, the FE and AE provided anti-inflammatory actions that inhibited tumor necrosis factor (TNF)-α and interleukin (IL)-6 in lipopolysaccharide (LPS)-treated RAW 264.7 cells. Further analyses suggested that the FE and AE enhanced cell proliferation (210% and 112%) and migration (442.2% and 535.6%) and regulated wound healing-related genes, including matrix metalloproteinase 2, *MMP9*, and tissue inhibitor of metalloproteinase 2 (*TIMP2*) to avoid scar formation and accelerate wound healing. Lastly, the identification of potential compounds within the extract using the UHPLC system further supports its prospective medical applications. Taken together, these findings indicated that the FE and AE from *B. leptopoda* exhibited remarkable in vitro wound-healing properties, highlighting their potential for applications in pharmaceutical industries and health food development.

https://doi.org/10.3390/md23110444

Keywords: emphBotryocladia leptopoda; cell proliferation; antioxidant; anti-inflammation; wound healing

1. Introduction

Wound healing is an intricate process with interactions among various cells, extracellular compositions, and structures [1,2]. Different types of wounds require different care needs, such as accelerating wound healing, preventing pathogen infections, decreasing pain, and avoiding excessive tissue fluid leakage from the wound [3]. Although medications have been combined with dressings for wound care for many years, these medications often have side effects [4]. Natural compounds from marine or plant sources generally show better biocompatibility and lower cytotoxicity than synthetic drugs. They promote wound healing through mild antioxidant and anti-inflammatory actions, thereby reducing the risk of irritation or allergic reactions [5]. Therefore, developing novel wound-healing agents from natural sources has become a popular focus in recent years.

Marine algae are an unexploited reservoir of biologically active substances due to their abundant biodiversity [6]. Numerous studies have investigated their chemical constituents and bioactivities; however, further exploration of specific species and targeted applications remains highly valuable for future research.

Recent studies demonstrated that extracts from algae provide specific biological functions such as antioxidation [7], antimicrobial properties [8], and antiviral abilities [9], and could be helpful for issues such as high blood pressure [10], obesity problems [11], cardiac diseases [12], and specific cancers [13]. These biofunctions may arise from various types of bioactive molecules, such as proteins, compounds, polysaccharides, and peptides [14,15]. Therefore, it is essential to evaluate the functions and health benefits of different crude extracts within specific disease models, with the ultimate goal of isolating a purified bioactive molecule in alga-related research.

When applying marine algae for wound healing, most studies focused on developing wet wound dressings using algal polysaccharides [16,17], which form the structure of dressing materials and provide a surface for cell adhesion or attachment to promote wound healing. In addition, bioactive compounds from marine algae also participate in the wound-healing process and skin tissue regeneration by regulating cellular signaling pathways [18]. Given the high potential for the use of marine algae to promote wound healing, a number of ongoing studies are attempting to identify and isolate ideal materials for wound healing, especially through various types and rare macroalgae as research targets [16,19,20].

Botryocladia leptopoda (*B. leptopoda*) is a kind of marine red alga that has been used as feed, fertilizer, and in food manufacturing at an industrial level [21]. However, its biomedical potential, especially in skin repair and wound healing, remains largely unexplored. To the best of our knowledge, this is the first study to investigate the wound- healing potential of *B. leptopoda* extracts, providing novel insights into the therapeutic applications of marine red algae and expanding their value beyond conventional uses.

In our previous study [22], we focused on the effects of *B. leptopoda* extracts on the repair of skin cells under photo-damage conditions and found that the extracts exhibited strong protective activity. Therefore, the antioxidant and anti-inflammatory properties were further investigated. The cell-based experiments were conducted to assess cytotoxicity, cell adhesion, and cell proliferation for evaluating their potential for wound-care applications. Finally, the potential compounds present in the *B. leptopoda* extract were also analyzed using the negative ion mode of the ultra-high performance liquid chromatography (UHPLC) system to identify key bioactive constituents.

2. Results

2.1. Total Phenolic Content (TPC) and Antioxidant Capacity of B. leptopoda Extracts

In the past, many plants have been used for wound care and were later found to be rich in polyphenolic compounds [23]. These polyphenols exhibit strong anti-inflammatory effects [24], reduce oxidative stress [25], promote collagen regeneration [26], enhance re-epithelialization [27], and effectively accelerate wound healing [28]. Therefore, analyzing the TPC can aid in evaluating the potential of extracts from *B. leptopoda* as wound-care agents. *B. leptopoda* was extracted using four different methods: alkaline extraction with NaOH at 25 °C, ethanol extraction at 25 °C, ethanol extraction at 70 °C, and hot water extraction at 100 °C. The resulting products were designated as AE, FE, HE, and HW, respectively, according to their extraction processes.

Results (Figure 1a) indicated that phenolic compounds from *B. leptopoda* extracts were much more soluble in alkaline solvents than in water or weak polar organic solvents. The AE presented the highest TPC of 6.4 mg GA/g, compared to FE, HE, and HW (at 3.1, 2.7, and 1.7 mg/GA/g, respectively). Sun et al. [29] compared water, acidic, and alkaline solvent extracts and found the highest bioactive components were achieved in an alkaline environment. This may have been due to alkaline extraction helping break down algal cell walls composed of cellulose leading to release of components out of the algae [30]. Results from Peasura et al. [31] also showed a similar trend of alkaline extraction yielding higher sulfated polysaccharides compared to water and acidic extraction, which provided higher antioxidation abilities. Additionally, AE exhibited the highest polyphenol content, suggesting its potential as a promising wound-healing agent. Utpal et al. [32] have emphasized that polyphenols can modulate multiple stages of the wound-healing cascade, including antioxidation, inflammation control, angiogenesis, and tissue remodeling. Their bioactivities are primarily attributed to their strong radical-scavenging ability, regulation of cytokines (e.g., TNF-α, IL-6, VEGF, TGF-β1), and promotion of fibroblast and keratinocyte proliferation.

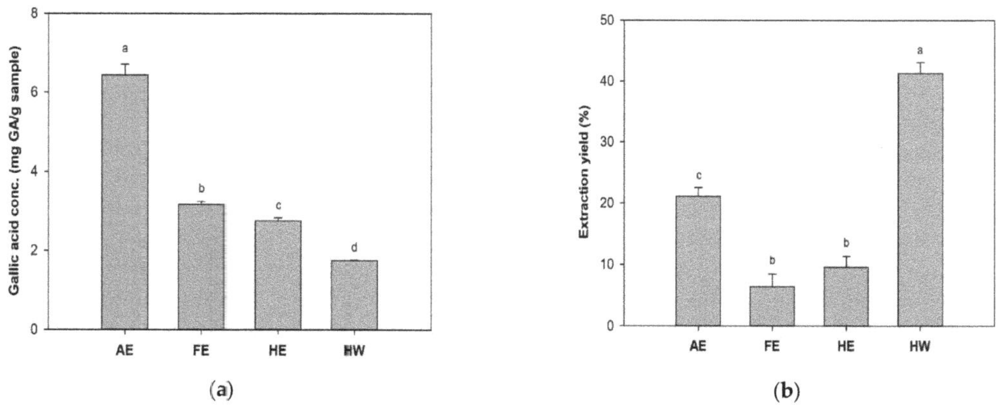

Figure 1. Effects of different solvent extracts on total phenolic contents of *Botryocladia leptopoda* (**a**, **b**) extraction yields. Different letters on the error bars indicate significant differences among the extraction groups and treatments ($p < 0.05$). AE: alkaline extract obtained at 25 °C; FE: ethanol extract obtained at 25 °C; HE: ethanol extract obtained at 70 °C; HW: hot water extract obtained at 100 °C.

In results of the extraction efficiency (Figure 1b), the HW group showed the highest yield, reaching 41.3%. Concentrations in descending order were the AE group (21.1%), HE group (9.5%), and FE group (6.4%). Harb et al. [33] found that water extraction showed 3–13-fold higher yields compared to methanolic extraction, which was similar to our results.

Owing to high polysaccharide contents in algae, the water extraction method was used to facilitate polysaccharide extraction, which may explain the results.

Free radical-scavenging properties were proven to promote wound-healing processes [34]. Therefore, evaluating the antioxidative abilities is crucial for biological ingredients applied to wound care, especially specific wounds such as diabetic wounds [35]. Results for DPPH (Figure 2a) showed that both the FE and HE groups exhibited strong antioxidation at 73.8~94.8% and 45.7~94.7%, respectively. These results suggested that the FE and HE samples contained significantly higher amounts of lipophilic antioxidants due to extraction with ethanol. In the AE and HW groups, hydrophilic solvents proved inadequate to extract lipophilic antioxidants, thereby resulting in reduced DPPH radical-scavenging activities (of 21.1~25.4% and 26.3~43.3%, respectively).

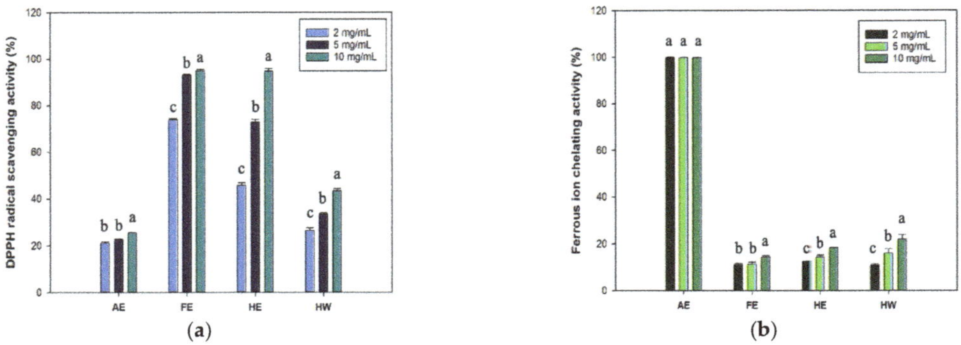

Figure 2. Antioxidant effects of various extracts (**a**) against DPPH radicals and (**b**) in a FICA assay. Different letters on the error bars indicate significant differences among the extraction groups and treatments ($p < 0.05$). AE: alkaline extract obtained at 25 °C; FE: ethanol extract obtained at 25 °C; HE: ethanol extract obtained at 70 °C; HW: hot water extract obtained at 100 °C.

In the results of ferrous iron-chelating activity (Figure 2b), the AE group exhibited the highest ferrous iron-chelating capacity compared to the other groups. Interestingly, the iron-chelating activity followed a trend similar to that observed for TPC. This suggested that phenolic compounds in the AE may contribute to its high metal-chelating capacity. Previous studies showed that specific polyphenols derived from macroalgae possess ferrous iron-chelating properties [36,37]. Although the AE group demonstrated saturated ferrous iron-chelating activity, this finding confirmed its strong antioxidant potential. Subsequent experiments further assessed its wound-healing efficacy using different extract doses in cellular assays. Based on the potential of AE and FE in demonstrating antioxidant properties, these two groups were selected as the primary experimental groups for subsequent experiments.

2.2. Anti-Inflammatory Activity of *B. leptopoda* Extracts in Macrophages

In the non LPS-induced inflammation of TNF-α expression (Figure 3a), the TNF-α RNA level was found to have slightly increased or remained unchanged with increasing FE and AE treatment concentrations. Compared to the untreated group (92%), the highest treatment concentrations (1 mg/mL) reached 136% (in the FE group) and 81.75% (in the AE group). However, in the LPS-induced inflammation group, expression levels of TNF-α decreased from 13,376% to 6006.5% and 9072.2%, respectively.

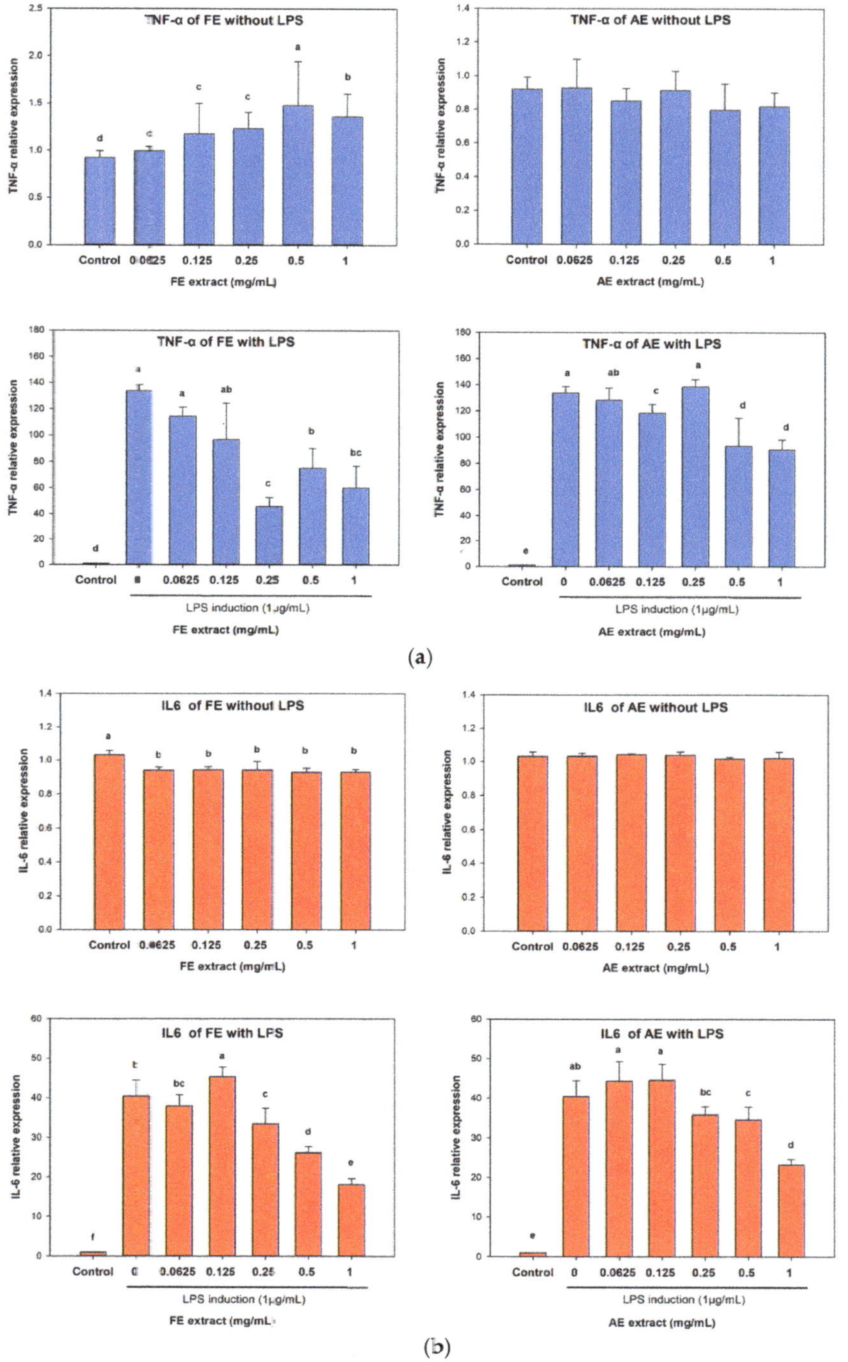

Figure 3. Effects of *Botryocladia leptopoda* extracts on expression levels of proinflammatory-associated genes in LPS-stimulated RAW 264.7 macrophages. (**a**) *TNF-α* and (**b**) *IL-6*. Different letters on the error bars indicate significant differences among the different concentrations of the extract ($p < 0.05$). AE: alkaline extract obtained at 25 °C; FE: ethanol extract obtained at 25 °C.

Interestingly, a similar trend was also observed in the analysis of IL-6 (Figure 3b). In the LPS-induced inflammation group, the highest treatment concentrations of FE and AE (1 mg/mL) suppressed IL-6 expression from 4042.9% to 1811.5% and 2327%, respectively. These results indicated that both the FE and AE exhibited anti-inflammatory effects by inhibiting TNF-α and IL-6 expressions. These proinflammatory cytokines are involved in different types of inflammation, which lead to apoptosis and cell death at the wound. Apoptosis of dermal keratinocytes was considered to have delayed the wound-healing process [38]. Furthermore, the over-inflammation of a wound also causes release of reactive oxygen species (ROS) resulting in the formation of granulation tissues [39]. Therefore, the anti-inflammatory properties of an extract can help the wound-healing processes of proliferation and remodeling.

2.3. Cell Cytotoxicity, Proliferation, and Migration of Fibroblast Cells

In the cytotoxicity results (Figure 4), the FE and AE groups both maintained at least 80% cell viability at treatment concentrations below 1.5 mg/mL. However, at 2 mg/mL, cell viability significantly decreased to 70.59% and 80.3%, respectively. Therefore, test concentrations of <2 mg/mL were utilized in subsequent cell-based experiments.

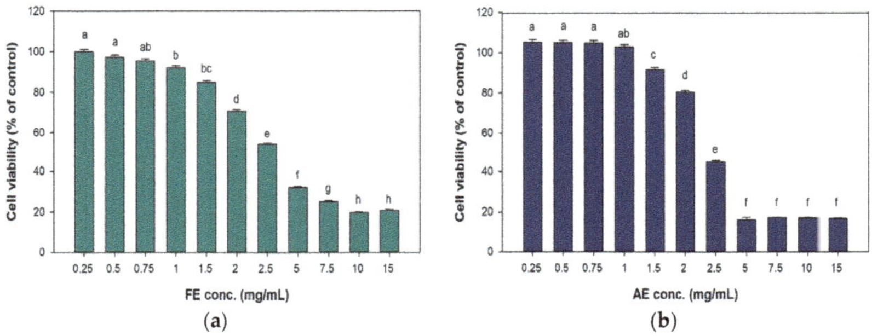

Figure 4. Cytotoxic effects on L929 fibroblast cells under different concentrations of (**a**) FE and (**b**) AE treatment. Different letters on the error bars indicate significant differences among the different concentrations of the extract ($p < 0.05$). FE: ethanol extract obtained at 25 °C; AE: alkaline extract obtained at 25 °C.

In the late stage of wound healing such as proliferation and remodeling, fibroblasts will adhere and migrate to the wound to release various signaling factors to enhance angiogenesis and granulation tissue formation [40]. Hence, proliferation and migration abilities are crucial to evaluate the potential of wound-healing agents and dressings [41].

In Figure 5a, the FE group demonstrated a similar increase in proliferation effects following treatment with concentrations ranging from 0.25 to 1.5 mg/mL; however, a significant reduction in proliferation was observed at a concentration of 2 mg/mL. With AE treatment (Figure 5b), although treatment with concentrations exceeding 1.5 mg/mL showed a slight reduction in their ability to enhance the proliferation ability, the overall treatment effects still promoted cell proliferation, ranging from approximately 112.3% to 87.7%. The observed results may be associated with cytotoxicity. By comparing cytotoxicity results with proliferation outcomes, it was evident that treatment groups showing a decline in the differentiation capacity exhibited a significant upward trend in cytotoxicity. Therefore, lower treatment concentrations of extracts (0.25 and 0.5 mg/mL) were used in the migration experiment. In addition, the observation that lower concentrations of the extract promoted cell migration may also have resulted from other potential mechanisms such as the involvement of bioactive compounds exhibiting biphasic effects. For instance, endostatin is known to enhance cell migration at specific concentrations, yet inhibits this process at higher concentrations, reflecting its dual functional characteristics [42]. To confirm these effects, it is essential to isolate and characterize the active compounds for targeted validation through subsequent studies.

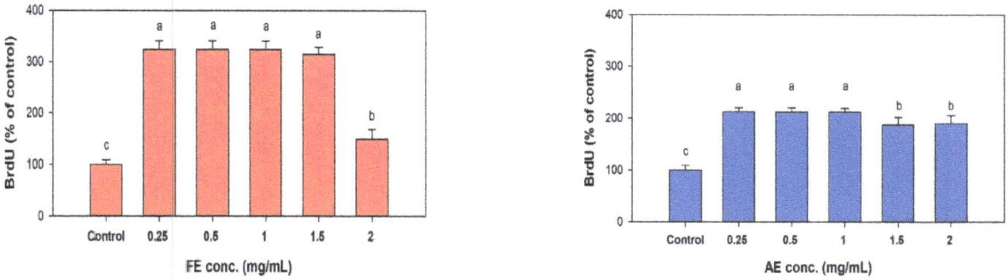

(a) (b)

Figure 5. Cell proliferation on L929 fibroblast cells under different concentrations of (**a**) FE and (**b**) AE treatment. Different letters on the error bars indicate significant differences among the different concentrations of the extract ($p < 0.05$). FE: ethanol extract obtained at 25 °C; AE: alkaline extract obtained at 25 °C.

In Figure 6a, all treatment groups exhibited significant cell migration, with cells moving from the seeding area to the central void within 24 h. Interestingly, in both the FE and AE groups, 0.25 mg/mL treatment (442.2% and 535.6%, respectively) demonstrated superior migration performance compared to 0.5 mg/mL treatment (398.7% and 387.8%, respectively) (Figure 6b).

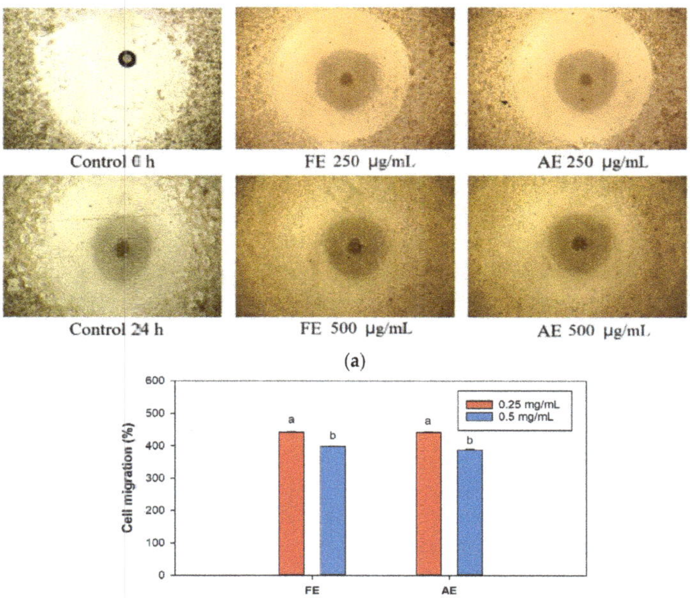

(a) (b)

Figure 6. Cell migration of L929 cells under different concentrations of *Botryocladia leptopoda* extracts. (**a**) In vitro scratch assay of cell diffusion and (**b**) quantitative analysis of cell diffusion. Original magnification ×40. Different letters on the error bars indicate significant differences among the different concentrations of the extract ($p < 0.05$). AE: alkaline extract obtained at 25 °C; FE: ethanol extract obtained at 25 °C.

2.4. Evaluation of Scar Inhibition In Vitro

To evaluate the effect of *B. leptopoda* extracts on scar inhibition in vitro, a PMA-induced L929 cell model was utilized to investigate the RNA-level overexpression of MMPs, specifically *MMP2*, and *MMP9* (Figure 7a–c).

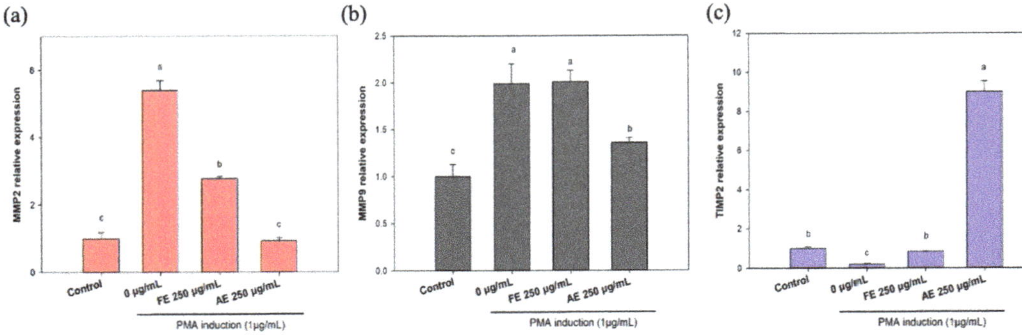

Figure 7. Effects of different *Botryocladia leptopoda* extracts on H_2O_2-induced changes in an intracellular reduced ratio of (**a**) *MMP-2*, (**b**) *MMP-9* and (**c**) *TIMP-2*, mRNA expressions. Different letters on the error bars indicate significant differences among the different concentrations of the extract ($p < 0.05$). AE: alkaline extract obtained at 25 °C; FE: ethanol extract obtained at 25 °C.

MMP2 is a kind of gelatinase which is involved in matrix remodeling, but its overexpression was implicated in delayed wound healing and tissue degradation [43]. MMP9 is essential for maintaining the dynamic equilibrium of the extracellular matrix (ECM) and is a key participant in wound-healing processes, serving as an important biomarker for anti-aging and skin regeneration [44]. Nevertheless, aberrant upregulation of MMP9 was associated with excessive granulation tissue formation [39], impaired healing, and the potential development of keloids [45].

In results of *MMP9* RNA expression (Figure 7c), the AE group exhibited a decrease in RNA expression from 199% to 136%. Interestingly, results for MMP2 (Figure 7a) showed that both the FE and AE inhibited *MMP2* RNA expression from 540% to 277% and 93%, respectively. These results suggested that the FE can inhibit MMP2 overexpression to avoid skin elasticity decrease and wrinkle formation. Jung et al. [46] reported that matrine can inhibit PMA-induced *MMP-1* mRNA expression by utilizing inhibition of activating protein (AP)-1 promoter activation, which may be helpful for anti-inflammation of dermatitis. Results also showed that the AE greatly repressed MMP2 and MM9, which may lead to acceleration of wound healing and wrinkle formation caused by collagen degradation.

However, this still needs to be further proven utilizing animal experiments. In addition, *TIMP-2* (the repressor gene of MMP2) RNA expression was also investigated (Figure 7c). Results indicated that AE treatment strongly enhanced TIMP-2 expression, which suggests that the AE can downregulate expression levels of MMP2 by modulating TIMP-2 activity. A previous study also demonstrated similar results that the *Davallia bilabiate* water extract decreased PMA-induced MMP2 expression by upregulating the *TIMP-2* RNA level, which provided a potential anti-angiogenic effect [47]. It should be noted that the current study evaluated MMP and TIMP expression only at the mRNA level, and it may still occur in the correlation of error with protein expression; therefore, future studies will therefore include protein-level validation and enzymatic assays to confirm the regulatory effects of the extracts on the MMP/TIMP pathway.

In this study, based on the high TPC of AE and FE, the negative ion mode of ultra-high-performance liquid chromatography (UHPLC) was used to characterize these two extracts

(Table 1 and Figure S1). Both were found to primarily exhibit functions associated with anti-inflammatory, antioxidant, and immunomodulatory activities. However, variations in the proportional distribution of these components were observed, which may account for the comparable effects of AE and FE in these functional domains. These findings provide additional evidence supporting their potential to promote wound healing. In addition, although UHPLC-MS was employed in this study for preliminary component identification, this analysis was insufficient to confirm the active constituents. Therefore, further studies will perform advanced characterization to determine the key bioactive compounds and elucidate their structures.

Table 1. Composition analysis of *B. leptopoda* extracts in negative ion mode. AE: alkaline extract obtained at 25 °C, FE: ethanol extract obtained at 25 °C.

Proportion (%)	Compound	Potential Skin Care Related Function
FE		
31.25	Quinolin-3-ol	Preservatives, disinfectants and pesticides
10.8	8-Hydroxyquinoline-5-carboxylic acid	Antioxidant
10.05	6-Methylnicotinic acid	Anti-inflammatory
8.61	4-Hydroxybenzaldehyde	Preservatives, skin whitening
5.64	1H-Indole-3-carboxylic acid	Antimicrobial property
3.84	4-Hydroxyquinoline	Dehydrogenase inhibition
AE		
37.2	Indoleacetic acid	Skin moisturizing, anti-oxidation
21.23	Quinolin-3-ol	Preservatives, disinfectants and pesticides
8.17	1H-Indole-3-carboxylic acid	Antimicrobial property, anti-inflammatory
3.6	2-(Formylamino)benzoic acid	Preservatives

3. Discussion

The present study demonstrated that AE and FE from *B. leptopoda* exhibit significant antioxidant, anti-inflammatory, and wound-healing properties. These biological activities can be attributed to the nitrogen-containing heterocycles and phenolic derivatives identified in the extracts. In agreement with previous studies also showing that phenolic and benzoic acid derivatives from marine algae exert potent anti-inflammatory and antioxidant effects that promote tissue regeneration [23,48,49], the high TPC observed in the AE supports its strong bioactive potential. AE group not only yielded higher TPC but also enhanced the solubilization of cell wall-bound phenolics by partially disrupting the cellulose structure of algal cell walls, consistent with prior findings by Sun et al. [29]. Although most of the compounds identified in the AE and FE fractions were not polyphenolic in nature, the TPC assay used in this study still exhibited high apparent TPC values due to the strong reducing capacity of these compounds. For instance, indole derivatives possess mild reducing power, whereas 4-hydroxybenzaldehyde contains a phenolic hydroxyl group contributing to the reaction.

The antioxidant assay results revealed that FE exhibited higher free radical scavenging activity, indicating the presence of lipophilic antioxidant compounds effectively extracted by ethanol. In contrast, AE showed a stronger ferrous ion-chelating capacity, consistent with its higher TPC value, suggesting a strong correlation between the concentration of extracted compounds and their metal-chelating activity. These findings are consistent with previous evidence that marine-derived indole and phenolic compounds can scavenge free radicals and bind transition metals, thereby alleviating oxidative stress and facilitating the wound-healing process [50,51].

The anti-inflammatory activity of the AE and FE were found to suppress TNF-α and IL-6 mRNA expression in LPS-induced macrophages. Overexpression of these proinflammatory cytokines is known to delay cellular regeneration by promoting apoptosis and excessive ROS generation. Therefore, the downregulation of TNF-α and IL-6 suggested that the extracts decreased the inflammatory cascades and restore redox balance to enhance the cell proliferation and remodeling [38,39].

In vitro scar inhibition assays revealed that both AE and FE could inhibit PMA-induced overexpression of MMP2, and MMP9 gene. These genes were related to the degradation of collagen and extracellular matrix components, leading to delayed healing and wrinkle formation [43]. Especially, AE significantly reduced MMP2 and MMP9 expression while enhancing TIMP-2 level, implying its regulatory effect on the MMP/TIMP. This balance is essential for maintaining extracellular matrix homeostasis and preventing excessive tissue remodeling [45]. This regulation may explain the superior wound-healing observed for AE in cell model.

UHPLC analysis identified quinolin-3-ol as the predominant compound in FE group, whereas indoleacetic acid was the major constituent in the AE group. Quinolin-derivatives have been reported to possess strong antioxidant and anti-inflammatory activities [52], which could explain the superior ROS-scavenging capacity and cytokine inhibition observed in FE-treated groups. In contrast, the study of indoleacetic acid and wound healing remains limited. Some studies have explored its use as a hydrogel component to enhance wound repair [53]; however, its underlying mechanism of action has not yet been clearly elucidated. Therefore, it still requires further identification and isolation to confirm the actual active components present in the extract.

In addition, the biochemical composition of macroalgae varies with species, season, and environmental conditions, which can influence their bioactivities. Although a detailed composition analysis of *B. leptopoda* was not performed in this study, previous reports indicate that *Botryocladia* species are rich in phenolic compounds with antioxidant and anti-inflammatory potential [21]. Future work will focus on correlating these constituents with the observed wound-healing effects.

In summary, these findings suggest that AE and FE from *B. leptopoda* exhibit multiple therapeutic functions—combining antioxidant and anti-inflammatory activities, as well as promoting cell proliferation and cell adhesion. These functions may contribute to skin regeneration and scar inhibition. The identification of key compounds not only reveals their biological mechanisms but also highlights the potential of *B. leptopoda* extracts for pharmaceutical and cosmeceutical applications. In future work, in vivo studies are necessary to further validate their potential for developing wound-healing formulations.

4. Materials and Methods

4.1. Materials and Chemicals

RAW 264.7 macrophage and L929 fibroblast cell lines were obtained from American Type Culture Collection (ATCC; Manassas, VA, USA). EDTA, trypsin, and antibiotics (penicillin/streptomycin) were obtained from GE Healthcare Life Science (Logan, UT, USA). Vivaspin 15R and Vivaspin Turbo 15 were obtained from Sartorius Stedim Biotech (Goettingen, Germany). Cell culture media (Dulbecco's modified Eagle medium (DMEM), supplemented with high glucose, phenol red, sodium pyruvate, and L-glutamine) and fetal bovine serum (FBS) were procured from Hyclone Laboratories (Logan, UT, USA). All chemicals used in this study were of analytical grade and purchased from Merck (Burlington, MA, USA). The Cell Proliferation ELISA (enzyme-linked immunosorbent assay) BrdU kit was purchased from Roche Applied Science (Mannheim, Germany). MTS reagent powder (G1111) and phenazine methosulfate were purchased from GeneLabs Life Science Corp. (Taipei, Taiwan).

4.2. Extraction of *B. leptopoda*

Raw material of *B. leptopoda* was obtained from the Eastern Marine Fishery Research Center of the Ministry of Agriculture (Taitung, Taiwan). After being thoroughly washed, the alga was dried and pulverized. The powder was sieved through a 40-mesh screen. *B. leptopoda* powder was then extracted at 25 °C using sodium hydroxide (alkaline extract, AE), at 25 °C using ethanol (FE), at 70 °C using ethanol (HE), and at 100 °C using deionization and distilled (dd)H_2O (HW extract). Extraction was performed using different solvents and temperatures under ultrasonic treatment at 20 kHz in an ice bath for 30 min. The mixtures were then centrifuged at 13,000× *g*, and the supernatants were collected and stored in light-protected tubes at −20 °C for further experiments. All experiments were conducted as repeated measurements using the same extraction sample, while independently re-extracted samples were also examined to verify the reproducibility and consistency of the results.

4.3. Identification of *B. leptopoda* Extracts Using Ultra-High-Performance Liquid Chromatograph (UHPLC)

In this study, 10 mg of freeze-dried microalgal biomass was suspended in 1 mL of chromatography-grade methanol containing 1% BHT, vortexed for 5 min, and then stored at 4 °C for 1 h. The mixture was subsequently subjected to ultrasonic extraction at 20 kHz in an ice bath for 30 min, followed by centrifugation at 12,000× *g* for 5 min at 4 °C. The resulting supernatant was filtered through a 0.22 µm PTFE membrane and used for further analysis. The chemical composition of the extract was analyzed using an UHPLC system (Vanquish Horizon, Thermo Scientific, Milan, Italy) coupled with a quadrupole-Orbitrap high-resolution mass spectrometer (Q-Orbitrap-HRMS) (Thermo Scientific). Separation was achieved on a Syncronis C18 column under chromatographic conditions, with a flow rate of 0.3 $mL\cdot min^{-1}$ and an injection volume of 5.0 µL. Full-scan mass spectrometric data were acquired in negative ion modes at a resolving power of 70,000 FWHM, covering an m/z range of 100–1200. The automatic gain control (AGC) target was set to 5×10^5 ions, with a maximum injection time of 200 ms. Data-dependent acquisition (DDA) was applied to obtain product ion spectra using collision energies of 45–60 eV and a resolution of 35,000 FWHM. A mass inclusion list containing precursor ion m/z values of target compounds and acquisition windows was employed.

4.4. Total Phenolic Content (TPC)

The TPC was used according to a method described by Pérez et al. [54] with slight modification: 0.25 mL of Folin–Ciocalteu reagent was mixed with 0.25 mL of an extract (volume ratio of 1:1), and the mixture was thoroughly mixed for 3 min at room temperature. Fifty milliliters of a 20% Na_2CO_3 solution was slowly added and incubated at 40 °C for 20 min. The absorbance of the mixture was determined at 755 nm. The TPC was calculated using a gallic acid standard curve, and results are expressed as milligrams of gallic acid equivalents per milliliter (mg GAE/mL).

4.5. Antioxidation Ability

Different concentrations of extracts (2, 5 and 10 mg/mL) were prepared using 80% methanol, and were shaken and extracted at 150 rpm and 25 °C for 30 min, followed by centrifugation at 8000× *g* and 4 °C for 20 min, and the supernatant was collected and used in the following experiment. L-Ascorbic acid (2, 5, and 10 mg/mL) was used as the positive control in the antioxidation ability assays.

In the diphenyl-1-picrylhydrazyl (DPPH) free radical-scavenging activity assay [55], 0.1 mM methanolic DPPH as a reaction solution was mixed with an extract (volume ratio of 1:1) at 25 °C in the dark for 30 min, and the absorbance value at 517 nm was measured.

The DPPH assay is based on the reduction in the stable purple DPPH radical to a yellow-colored diphenylpicrylhydrazine upon reaction with an antioxidant, which donates hydrogen or electrons. The decrease in absorbance at 517 nm indicates the free radical-scavenging ability of the sample.

Results were expressed as the scavenging activity (%) using Equation (1):

$$Scavenging\ activity\ (\%) = \frac{A_{nc} - \left(A_{sample} - A_{blank}\right)}{A_{nc}} \times 100\%; \quad (1)$$

where A_{nc}, A_{sample}, and A_{blank} are the absorbance at 517 nm for the negative control (0.1 mM methanolic DPPH, without the addition of sample), sample (0.1 mM methanolic DPPH, with the addition of extract at a specific concentration), and blank (sample with ddH_2O), respectively. Trolox (6-hydroxy-2,5,7,8-tetramethyl chroman-2-carboxylic acid) was used as the standard antioxidant for the assay.

In the ferrous ion-chelating activity (FICA) assay [56], 1 mL of extract was mixed with 0.1 mL of a 2 mM $FeCl_2$ solution for 30 s, and reacted with 0.2 mL of 5 mM ferrous hydrazine at room temperature for 10 min. The absorbance value at 562 nm was measured.

The FICA assay is based on the ability of antioxidants to compete with ferrozine for ferrous ions (Fe^{2+}). When chelating agents are present, they form complexes with Fe^{2+}, reducing the formation of the red-colored ferrozine–Fe^{2+} complex, which results in a lower absorbance at 562 nm.

Results are expressed as ferrous ion-chelating activity (%) using Equation (2):

$$\text{Ferrous ion} - \text{chelating activity}(\%) = \frac{A_{nc} - \left(A_{sample} - A_{blank}\right)}{A_{nc}} \times 100\%; \quad (2)$$

where A_{nc}, A_{sample}, and A_{blank} are the absorbance at 562 nm for the negative control (2 mM $FeCl_2$ solution, with ddH_2O), sample (2 mM $FeCl_2$ solution, with the addition of extract at specific concentration), and blank (sample with ddH_2O), respectively.

4.6. Detection of Anti-Inflammatory Ability

To confirm the ability of inflammatory inhibition by *B. leptopod* extracts, lipopolysaccharide (LPS)-treated RAW 264.7 macrophages were used as the detection cell model.

The anti-inflammatory was evaluated using ELISA kits to analyze levels of interleukin (IL)-6 (DY 406, R&D Systems Inc., Minneapolis, MN, USA), and tumor necrosis factor (TNF)-α (DY 410, R&D Systems Inc., Minneapolis, MN, USA). A 96-well plate coated with capture antibodies of IL-6 and TNF-α was washed with washing buffer, and 1× assay diluent (200 μL/well) was added at room temperature for 1 h. The assay diluent, AE or FE (62.5, 125, 250, 500, and 1000 μg/mL), and RAW 264.7 macrophage cells (10^6 cells/mL) with or without LPS treatment (1 μg/mL) were mixed at room temperature for 1 h. After washing buffer treatment, avidin-horseradish peroxidase (HRP) (100 μL/well) was added, and incubated for 30 min. After washing buffer treatment, the 3,3,5,5′-tetramethylbenzidine

(TMB) substrate (100 μL/well) was added and incubated for 15 min in a dark room. The reaction was stopped by adding a stop solution (50 μL/well), and the OD value at 450 nm was detected.

4.7. Cell Cytotoxicity, Proliferation, and Migration

For the cell cytotoxicity assay, L929 fibroblast cells were cultured in 90% DMEM and 10% FBS for 3 days in an incubator at 37 °C with 5% CO_2 airflow. L929 fibroblasts at a concentration of 10^6 cell/mL were plated in a 96-well plate with culture medium containing different concentrations of *B. leptopoda* extracts for 4 h of incubation. Treated cells were washed twice with phosphate-buffered saline (PBS), then 120 μL of 10-fold diluted MTS reagent was added to each well. Cells were left for 1 h in an incubator at 37 °C in the dark. The number of viable cells was measured at a wavelength of 490 nm. The diluted MTS reagent was used as a blank, and wells containing cells without extract addition were used as a negative control. Cell viability was calculated by comparing absorbance values of treated groups to that of the control group, which was set to 100%.

In the cell proliferation assay, L929 fibroblasts at a concentration of 2×10^5 cells/mL were plated in a 96-well plate with culture medium containing different concentrations of *B. leptopoda* extracts for 24 h of incubation and mixed with a BrdU solution (10 μL/well, 10 μM) for 4 h at 37 °C. After the medium was removed, cells were fixed and incubated for 30 min at room temperature. A solution of a BrdU antibody conjugated with peroxidase was added (100 μL/well) for 90 min of treatment. Wells were washed with washing solution (200 μL/well), and a substrate solution (100 μL/well) was added. The absorbance was monitored at 370 nm. The proliferation ability was calculated by comparing absorbance values of treated groups to that of the control group, which was set to 100%.

In the cell-migration assay, L929 cells were inoculated in a culture dish with a central void and incubated until 80~90% cell confluency was reached. Cells migrated directly from the surroundings into the central void, and cell fragments were cleaned with PBS. Different concentrations of extracts were added to the serum-free medium. The central void was measured under an inverted microscope at 24 h. ImageJ software (1.53 k, National Institutes of Health, Bethesda, MD, USA) was used to calculate the area of the void area, and the migration rate was calculated using Equation (3):

$$\text{Migration rate}(\%) = \frac{A_0 - A_{24}}{A_0} \times 100\%; \quad (3)$$

where A_0 and A_{24} are areas of the void area at 0 and 24 h, respectively, after treatment with the extract.

4.8. Quantitative Real-Time Polymerase Chain Reaction (qRT-PCR)

To detect the anti-scarring effects of different *B. leptopoda* extracts, messenger (m)RNA expressions of genes including matrix metalloproteinase genes (*MMP-1*, *MMP-2*, and *MMP-9*) and tissue inhibitor of metalloproteinase 2 (*TIMP-2*) were investigated. L929 cells (6×10^5 cell/mL) were seeded inT25 flasks for 4 h. Medium with extract was added and incubated at 37 °C for 24 h. Phorbol-12-myristate 13-acetate (PMA) (1 μg/mL) was also added to the medium before incubation to induce MMP-related gene activation.

Total RNA extracted from cell samples was converted to complementary (c)DNA using an iScript cDNA Synthesis Kit (Bio-Rad, Hercules, CA, USA). A reverse-transcription quantitative polymerase chain reaction (RT-qPCR) analysis was carried out using iScript RT-qPCR Sample Preparation Reagent (Bio-Rad).

The qPCR conditions were 2 min at 50 °C and then 10 min at 95 °C. Afterward, conditions were set to 40 cycles of 15 s in which the temperature was kept at 95 °C and subsequently dropped to 60 °C for 60 s. The qPCR analysis involved the use of specific forward (F) and reverse (R) primers, namely MMP-2 RNA-F (5′-ATCGCAGACTCCTGGAATG-3′) and MMP-2 RNA-R (5′-CCAGCCAGTCTGATTTGATG-3′) for the *MMP-2* RNA gene, MMP-9 RNA-F (5′-GAGCCCTAGTTCAAGGGCAC-3′) and MMP-9 RNA-R (5′-TCCAGTACCAAGACAAAGC-3′) for the *MMP-9* RNA gene, and TIMP-2 RNA-F (5′-GGTAGCCTGTGAATGTTCCT-3′) and TIMP-2 RNA-R (5′-ACGAAAATGCCCTCAGAAG-3′) for the *TIMP-2* gene. Expression levels were standardized to those of the housekeeping gene, GAPDH RNA-F (5′-ACTCCACTCACGGCAAATTCA-3′) and GAPDH RNA-R (5′-CGCTCCTGGAAGATGGTGAT-3′) for the mouse *GAPDH* gene. Calculation formulas were as follows: Relative expression of gene = 2ΔΔCT.

$$\triangle CT = CT(target\ gene) - CT\ (reference\ gene)$$

$$\triangle \triangle CT = \triangle Ct(control\ target\ gene) - \triangle Ct\ (treatment\ target\ gene)$$

4.9. Statistical Analysis

All experiments were independently repeated at least three times, and the obtained data are expressed as the mean ± standard deviation (SD). Statistical data analyses were performed using SPSS Statistics 22 (IBM, Armonk, NY, USA). A one-way analysis of variance (ANOVA) with Tukey's honest significant difference (HSD) test was applied to determine significant differences ($p < 0.05$).

5. Conclusions

In summary, different *B. leptopoda* extracts were investigated for their in vitro antioxidation, proliferation, migration, and scar-inhibition activities. Result for the TPC showed that the AE had the highest phenolic compound contents. As to the antioxidative ability, the FE and HE presented the greatest DPPH-scavenging activities, and the AE exhibited an excellent FITA antioxidant ability. The FE and AE blocked LPS-induced inflammation in RAW 264.7 macrophages via suppressing proinflammatory cytokines such as TNF-α and IL-6 in concentration-dependent manners. As to proliferation, the FE and AE both presented an ability to enhance cell proliferation and migration at a low concentration of 0.25 mg/mL. Lastly, the FE and AE suppressed MMP2 overexpression, while further, respectively, inhibiting MMP9. This may help prevent wrinkle formation and the loss of skin elasticity and promote wound healing. In the future, further studies will focus on exploring the effects of specific compounds within the extracts on wound healing. Additionally, animal experiments will be conducted to validate the biological efficacy of these extracts in promoting wound healing.

Supplementary Materials: The following supporting information can be downloaded at: https://www.mdpi.com/article/10.3390/md23110444/s1, Figure S1: The profile of *B. leptopoda* extracts. (A) AE extraction and (B) FE extraction.

Author Contributions: Conceptualization, T.-K.Y., Y.-F.K. and H.-J.C.; methodology, T.-K.Y., Y.-F.K., M.-C.T. and H.-J.C.; validation, C.-C.H., Y.-C.C., S.P.S. and J.-J.L.; data curation, S.-P.L.; writing—original draft preparation, C.-C.H., J.-J.L., Y.-C.C. and S.-P.L.; writing—review and editing, S.-P.L., C.-C.H. and K.-C.C. All authors have read and agreed to the published version of the manuscript.

Funding: This research was funded by the National Science and Technology Council, Taiwan (NSTC 112-2221-E-002-040-MY3, NSTC 112-2320-B-002-013-MY3, NSTC 113-2321-B-002-037 and NSTC114-2221-E-038-004) and the Fisheries Research Institute, Ministry of Agriculture, Taiwan (111AS-6.3.1-A1 and 112AS-6.3.1-A1).

Institutional Review Board Statement: Not applicable.

Informed Consent Statement: Informed consent was obtained from all subjects involved in the study.

Data Availability Statement: The data presented in this study are available on request from the corresponding author.

Conflicts of Interest: The authors declare no conflicts of interest.

References

1. Gouripriya, D.; Adhikari, J.; Debnath, P.; Ghosh, S.; Ghosh, P.; Thomas, S.; Ghandilyan, E.; Gorbatov, P.; Kuchukyan, E.; Gasparyan, S. 3D printing of bacterial cellulose for potential wound healing applications: Current trends and prospects. *Int. J. Biol. Macromol.* **2024**, *279*, 135213. [CrossRef]
2. Gonzalez, A.C.d.O.; Costa, T.F.; Andrade, Z.d.A.; Medrado, A.R.A.P. Wound healing-A literature review. *An. Bras. Dermatol.* **2016**, *91*, 614–620.
3. Powers, J.G.; Higham, C.; Broussard, K.; Phillips, T.J. Wound healing and treating wounds: Chronic wound care and management. *J. Am. Acad. Dermatol.* **2016**, *74*, 607–625. [CrossRef]
4. Bennett, G.; Abbott, J.; Sussman, G. The negative impact of medications on wound healing. *Wound Pract. Res.* **2024**, *32*, 17–24. [CrossRef]
5. Menaa, F.; Wijesinghe, U.; Thiripuranathar, G.; Althobaiti, N.A.; Albalawi, A.E.; Khan, B.A.; Menaa, B. Marine algae-derived bioactive compounds: A new wave of nanodrugs? *Mar. Drugs* **2021**, *19*, 484. [CrossRef]
6. Chandrasekhar, T.; Riazunnisa, K.; Vijaya Lakshmi, D.; Anu Prasanna, V.; Veera Bramhachari, P. Exploration of Bioactive Functional Molecules from Marine Algae: Challenges and Applications in Nutraceuticals. *Mar. Bioact. Mol. Biomed. Pharmacother. Appl.* **2024**, *2024*, 187–196.
7. Pruteanu, L.L.; Bailey, D.S.; Grădinaru, A.C.; Jäntschi, L. The biochemistry and effectiveness of antioxidants in food, fruits, and marine algae. *Antioxidants* **2023**, *12*, 860. [CrossRef]
8. Imchen, T.; Singh, K.S. Marine algae colorants: Antioxidant, anti-diabetic properties and applications in food industry. *Algal Res.* **2023**, *69*, 102898. [CrossRef]
9. Pradhan, B.; Ki, J.-S. Biological activity of algal derived carrageenan: A comprehensive review in light of human health and disease. *Int. J. Biol. Macromol.* **2023**, *238*, 124085. [CrossRef]
10. Leong, Y.K.; Chang, J.-S. Proteins and bioactive peptides from algae: Insights into antioxidant, anti-hypertensive, anti-diabetic and anti-cancer activities. *Trends Food Sci. Technol.* **2024**, *145*, 104352.
11. Fernandes, F.; Martins, R.; Barbosa, M.; Valentão, P. Algae-based supplements claiming weight loss properties: Authenticity control and scientific-based evidence on their effectiveness. *Mar. Drugs* **2024**, *22*, 123. [CrossRef]
12. Yurika, N.; Montuori, E.; Lauritano, C. Marine microalgal products with activities against age-related cardiovascular diseases. *Mar. Drugs* **2024**, *22*, 229. [CrossRef] [PubMed]
13. Minhas, L.A.; Kaleem, M.; Farooqi, H.M.U.; Kausar, F.; Waqar, R.; Bhatti, T.; Aziz, S.; Jung, D.W.; Mumtaz, A.S. Algae-derived bioactive compounds as potential nutraceuticals for cancer therapy: A comprehensive review. *Algal Res.* **2024**, *78*, 103396. [CrossRef]
14. Chénais, B. Algae and microalgae and their bioactive molecules for human health. *Molecules* **2021**, *26*, 1185. [CrossRef] [PubMed]
15. Mimouni, V.; Ulmann, L.; Pasquet, V.; Mathieu, M.; Picot, L.; Bougaran, G.; Cadoret, J.-P.; Morant-Manceau, A.; Schoefs, B. The potential of microalgae for the production of bioactive molecules of pharmaceutical interest. *Curr. Pharm. Biotechnol.* **2012**, *13*, 2733–2750. [CrossRef] [PubMed]
16. Kuznetsova, T.A.; Andryukov, B.G.; Besednova, N.N.; Zaporozhets, T.S.; Kalinin, A.V. Marine algae polysaccharides as basis for wound dressings, drug delivery, and tissue engineering: A review. *J. Mar. Sci. Eng.* **2020**, *8*, 481. [CrossRef]
17. Kumar, M.; Kumar, D.; Garg, Y.; Mahmood, S.; Chopra, S.; Bhatia, A. Marine-derived polysaccharides and their therapeutic potential in wound healing application—A review. *Int. J. Biol. Macromol.* **2023**, *253*, 127331. [CrossRef] [PubMed]
18. Chandika, P.; Ko, S.-C.; Jung, W.-K. Marine-derived biological macromolecule-based biomaterials for wound healing and skin tissue regeneration. *Int. J. Biol. Macromol.* **2015**, *77*, 24–35. [CrossRef]
19. Ajayi, E.I.; Oladele, J.O.; Nkumah, A.O. Application of algae in wound healing. *Next-Gener. Algae* **2023**, *2*, 251–284.
20. Ma, J.; Fang, Y.; Yu, H.; Yi, J.; Ma, Y.; Lei, P.; Yang, Q.; Jin, L.; Wu, W.; Li, H. Recent advances in living algae seeding wound dressing: Focusing on diabetic chronic wound healing. *Adv. Funct. Mater.* **2024**, *34*, 2308387. [CrossRef]
21. Suthan, P. Secondary metabolites screening, in vitro antioxidant and antidiabetic activity of marine red alga *Botryocladia leptopoda* (J. Agardh) Kylin. *Orient. J. Chem.* **2022**, *38*, 16–27. [CrossRef]

22. Hsieh, C.-C.; Yi, T.-K.; Kao, Y.-F.; Lin, S.-P.; Tu, M.-C.; Chou, Y.-C.; Lu, J.-J.; Chai, H.-J.; Cheng, K.-C. Comparative efficacy of *Botryocladia leptopoda* extracts in scar Inhibition and skin regeneration: A study on UV protection, collagen synthesis, and fibroblast proliferation. *Molecules* **2024**, *29*, 5688. [CrossRef]
23. Mssillou, I.; Bakour, M.; Slighoua, M.; Laaroussi, H.; Saghrouchni, H.; Amrati, F.E.-Z.; Lyoussi, B.; Derwich, E. Investigation on wound healing effect of Mediterranean medicinal plants and some related phenolic compounds: A review. *J. Ethnopharmacol.* **2022**, *298*, 115663. [CrossRef] [PubMed]
24. Fu, J.; Huang, J.; Lin, M.; Xie, T.; You, T. Quercetin promotes diabetic wound healing via switching macrophages from M1 to M2 polarization. *J. Surg. Res.* **2020**, *246*, 213–223. [CrossRef]
25. Zhang, S.; Ou, Q.; Xin, P.; Yuan, Q.; Wang, Y.; Wu, J. Polydopamine/puerarin nanoparticle-incorporated hybrid hydrogels for enhanced wound healing. *Biomater. Sci.* **2019**, *7*, 4230–4236. [CrossRef]
26. Salehi, M.; Vaez, A.; Naseri-Nosar, M.; Farzamfar, S.; Ai, A.; Ai, J.; Tavakol, S.; Khakbiz, M.; Ebrahimi-Barough, S. Naringin-loaded poly (ε-caprolactone)/gelatin electrospun mat as a potential wound dressing: In vitro and in vivo evaluation. *Fibers Polym.* **2018**, *19*, 125–134. [CrossRef]
27. Ponrasu, T.; Veerasubramanian, P.K.; Kannan, R.; Gopika, S.; Suguna, L.; Muthuvijayan, V. Morin incorporated polysaccharide–protein (psyllium–keratin) hydrogel scaffolds accelerate diabetic wound healing in Wistar rats. *RSC Adv.* **2018**, *8*, 2305–2314. [CrossRef]
28. Liu, Y.-Y.; Wu, J.-Q.; Fan, R.-Y.; He, Z.-H.; Li, C.-Y.; He, M.-F. Isoliquiritin promote angiogenesis by recruiting macrophages to improve the healing of zebrafish wounds. *Fish Shellfish Immunol.* **2020**, *100*, 238–245. [CrossRef]
29. Sun, Y.; Hou, S.; Song, S.; Zhang, B.; Ai, C.; Chen, X.; Liu, N. Impact of acidic, water and alkaline extraction on structural features, antioxidant activities of Laminaria japonica polysaccharides. *Int. J. Biol. Macromol.* **2018**, *112*, 985–995. [CrossRef] [PubMed]
30. Li, R.; Xing, R.; Li, H.; Ren, J.; Chen, L.; Yu, Z.; Zhang, H.; Wu, W.; Li, C.; Zhu, L. From Terrestrial Plants to Marine Macroalgae: A Comprehensive Review of Cell Wall Component-Properties, Extraction, Modification, and Application of Algal Cellulose. *J. Agric. Food Chem.* **2025**, *73*, 23759–23782. [CrossRef]
31. Peasura, N.; Laohakunjit, N.; Kerdchoechuen, O.; Wanlapa, S. Characteristics and antioxidant of Ulva intestinalis sulphated polysaccharides extracted with different solvents. *Int. J. Biol. Macromol.* **2015**, *81*, 912–919. [CrossRef]
32. Utpal, B.K.; Sutradhar, B.; Zehravi, M.; Sweilam, S.H.; Panigrahy, U.P.; Urs, D.; Fatima, A.F.; Nallasivan, P.K.; Chhabra, G.S.; Sayeed, M. Polyphenols in wound healing: Unlocking prospects with clinical applications. *Naunyn-Schmiedeberg's Arch. Pharmacol.* **2025**, *398*, 2459–2485. [CrossRef]
33. Harb, T.B.; Pereira, M.S.; Cavalcanti, M.I.L.; Fujii, M.T.; Chow, F. Antioxidant activity and related chemical composition of extracts from Brazilian beach-cast marine algae: Opportunities of turning a waste into a resource. *J. Appl. Phycol.* **2021**, *33*, 3383–3395. [CrossRef]
34. Joorabloo, A.; Liu, T. Recent advances in reactive oxygen species scavenging nanomaterials for wound healing. *Exploration* **2024**, *4*, 20230066. [CrossRef]
35. Li, J.; Shen, Y.; Wang, X.; Wu, T.; Huang, Q.; Shen, M.; Xu, S.; Li, Y. A multilayer hydrogel incorporating urolithin B promotes diabetic wound healing via ROS scavenging and angiogenesis. *Chem. Eng. J.* **2024**, *496*, 153661. [CrossRef]
36. Chew, Y.L.; Lim, Y.Y.; Omar, M.; Khoo, K.S. Antioxidant activity of three edible seaweeds from two areas in South East Asia. *LWT-Food Sci. Technol.* **2008**, *41*, 1067–1072. [CrossRef]
37. Wang, T.; Jónsdóttir, R.; Ólafsdóttir, G. Total phenolic compounds, radical scavenging and metal chelation of extracts from Icelandic seaweeds. *Food Chem.* **2009**, *116*, 240–248. [CrossRef]
38. Secor, P.R.; James, G.A.; Fleckman, P.; Olerud, J.E.; McInnerney, K.; Stewart, P.S. Staphylococcus aureus Biofilm and Planktonic cultures differentially impact gene expression, mapk phosphorylation, and cytokine production in human keratinocytes. *BMC Microbiol.* **2011**, *11*, 143. [CrossRef] [PubMed]
39. Häkkinen, L.; Larjava, H.; Koivisto, L. Granulation tissue formation and remodeling. *Endod. Top.* **2011**, *24*, 94–129. [CrossRef]
40. Werner, S.; Grose, R. Regulation of wound healing by growth factors and cytokines. *Physiol. Rev.* **2003**, *83*, 835–870. [CrossRef]
41. Lin, S.-P.; Kung, H.-N.; Tsai, Y.-S.; Tseng, T.-N.; Hsu, K.-D.; Cheng, K.-C. Novel dextran modified bacterial cellulose hydrogel accelerating cutaneous wound healing. *Cellulose* **2017**, *24*, 4927–4937. [CrossRef]
42. Celik, I.; Sürücü, O.; Dietz, C.; Heymach, J.V.; Force, J.; Höschele, I.; Becker, C.M.; Folkman, J.; Kisker, O. Therapeutic efficacy of endostatin exhibits a biphasic dose-response curve. *Cancer Res.* **2005**, *65*, 11044–11050. [CrossRef]
43. Caley, M.P.; Martins, V.L.; O'Toole, E.A. Metalloproteinases and wound healing. *Adv. Wound Care* **2015**, *4*, 225–234. [CrossRef]
44. Mohan, R.; Chintala, S.K.; Jung, J.C.; Villar, W.V.; McCabe, F.; Russo, L.A.; Lee, Y.; McCarthy, B.E.; Wollenberg, K.R.; Jester, J.V. Matrix metalloproteinase gelatinase B (MMP-9) coordinates and effects epithelial regeneration. *J. Biol. Chem.* **2002**, *277*, 2065–2072. [CrossRef]
45. Tanriverdi-Akhisaroglu, S.; Menderes, A.; Oktay, G. Matrix metalloproteinase-2 and -9 activities in human keloids, hypertrophic and atrophic scars: A pilot study. *Cell Biochem. Funct.* **2009**, *27*, 81–87. [CrossRef] [PubMed]

46. Jung, E.; Lee, J.; Huh, S.; Lee, J.; Hwang, H.; Kim, Y.; Kim, Y.W.; Park, D.; Yo Byun, S. Matrine inhibits PMA-induced MMP-1 expression in human dermal fibroblasts. *Biofactors* **2008**, *33*, 121–128. [CrossRef] [PubMed]
47. Liu, C.-T.; Bi, K.-W.; Huang, C.-C.; Wu, H.-T.; Ho, H.-Y.; Pang, J.-H.S.; Huang, S.-T. Davallia bilabiata exhibits anti-angiogenic effect with modified MMP-2/TIMP-2 secretion and inhibited VEGF ligand/receptors expression in vascular endothelial cells. *J. Ethnopharmacol.* **2017**, *196*, 213–224. [CrossRef] [PubMed]
48. Pei, J.; Kanwal, S.; Sivaramakrishnan, R.; Katelakha, K. Therapeutic potential of microalgae-derived natural compounds in diabetic wound healing: A comprehensive review. *Heliyon* **2025**, *11*, e42723. [CrossRef]
49. Gager, L.; Lalegerie, F.; Connan, S.; Stiger-Pouvreau, V. Marine algal derived phenolic compounds and their biological activities for medicinal and cosmetic applications. In *Recent Advances in Micro and Macroalgal Processing: Food and Health Perspectives*; John Wiley & Sons, Inc: Hoboken, NJ, USA, 2021; pp. 278–334.
50. Fernández, S.; Arnáiz, V.; Rufo, D.; Arroyo, Y. Current status of indole-derived marine natural products: Synthetic approaches and therapeutic applications. *Mar. Drugs* **2024**, *22*, 126. [CrossRef]
51. Vasilakis, G.; Marka, S.; Ntzouvaras, A.; Zografaki, M.-E.; Kyriakopoulou, E.; Kalliampakou, K.I.; Bekiaris, G.; Korakidis, E.; Papageorgiou, N.; Christofi, S. Wound healing, antioxidant, and antiviral properties of bioactive polysaccharides of microalgae strains isolated from Greek Coastal Lagoons. *Mar. Drugs* **2025**, *23*, 77. [CrossRef]
52. Orhan Puskullu, M.; Tekiner, B.; Suzen, S. Recent studies of antioxidant quinoline derivatives. *Mini Rev. Med. Chem.* **2013**, *13*, 365–372.
53. Chitra, G.; Selvi, M.; Franklin, D.; Sudarsan, S.; Sakthivel, M.; Guhanathan, S. pH-sensitive biopolymeric hydrogel-based on indole-3-acetic acid for wound healing and anti-cancer applications. *SN Appl. Sci.* **2019**, *1*, 1641. [CrossRef]
54. Pérez, M.; Dominguez-López, I.; Lamuela-Raventós, R.M. The Chemistry Behind the Folin–Ciocalteu method for the estimation of (Poly)phenol content in food: Total phenolic intake in a mediterranean dietary pattern. *J. Agric. Food Chem.* **2023**, *71*, 17543–17553. [CrossRef] [PubMed]
55. Shimada, K.; Fujikawa, K.; Yahara, K.; Nakamura, T. Antioxidative properties of xanthan on the autoxidation of soybean oil in cyclodextrin emulsion. *J. Agric. Food Chem* **1992**, *40*, 945–948. [CrossRef]
56. Dinis, T.C.; Madeira, V.M.; Almeida, L.M. Action of phenolic derivatives (acetaminophen, salicylate, and 5-aminosalicylate) as inhibitors of membrane lipid peroxidation and as peroxyl radical scavengers. *Arch. Biochem. Biophys.* **1994**, *315*, 161–169. [CrossRef]

marine drugs

MDPI

Article

Comparative Evaluation of Dynamic Maceration and Ultrasonic Assisted Extraction of Fucoidan from Four Arctic Brown Algae on Its Antioxidant and Anticancer Properties

Ekaterina D. Obluchinskaya [1], Olga N. Pozharitskaya [1], Irina M. Lapina [2], Anna A. Kulminskaya [2], Elena V. Zhurishkina [2] and Alexander N. Shikov [1,3,*]

[1] Murmansk Marine Biological Institute of the Russian Academy of Sciences (MMBI RAS), 17 Vladimirskaya Str., Murmansk 183038, Russia; obluchinskaya@gmail.com (E.D.O.); olgapozhar@mail.ru (O.N.P.)
[2] Petersburg Nuclear Physics Institute Named by B.P.Konstantinov of NRC "Kurchatov Institute" (NRC "Kurchatov Institute"—PNPI), 1 Orlova Roshcha Str., Leningradskaya Region, Gatchina 188300, Russia; lapina_im@pnpi.nrcki.ru (I.M.L.); kulminskaya_aa@pnpi.nrcki.ru (A.A.K.); zhurishkina_ev@pnpi.nrcki.ru (E.V.Z.)
[3] Department of Technology of Pharmaceutical Formulations, St. Petersburg State Chemical Pharmaceutical University, 14a Prof. Popov Str., Saint Petersburg 197022, Russia
* Correspondence: spb.pharmacy@gmail.com

Abstract: The technology of fucoidan extraction significantly affects its properties. This study aimed to evaluate the impact of dynamic maceration (DM) and ultrasound-assisted extraction (UAE) on the antioxidant and anticancer properties of fucoidan from Arctic brown algae. *Fucus vesiculosus* (Fv), *Fucus serratus* (Fs), *Fucus distichus* (Fd), and *Ascophyllum nodosum* (An) were collected from the Barents Sea. The average yield of fucoidan and uronic acid was higher (by 43.2% and 22.0%, respectively) after UAE, while phlorotannin content decreased by 53.7% compared with DM. The fucose level for all algae increased after UAE, while the molecular weight of fucoidans was lower. The highest antioxidant activity was noted for the fucoidan from An and Fv, which were obtained by DM and can be associated with the high concentrations of phlorotannins. The treatment of HeLa G-63 cells with all studied fucoidans for 48 h increased concentration-dependently the number of dead cells. The most promising were Fv and Fs fucoidans with high phlorotannins, low sulfates, and uronic acid extracted by DM. The co-administration of paclitaxel and fucoidan caused cell cycle arrest in the G2/M phase. The calculated for the first time combinatory effect showed that the simultaneous use of paclitaxel and fucoidan exposure leads to a synergistic interaction. Our results support the rationality of fucoidan use in complex chemotherapy to improve survival, quality of life and immunity in patients with cervical carcinoma.

Keywords: fucoidan; phlorotannins; paclitaxel; brown algae; extraction; activity; synergy

1. Introduction

Life originated in the seas and oceans with a vibrant biodiversity, covering more than 70% of the Earth's surface. The marine environment contains several species of plants, animals, and microorganisms producing various natural products [1]. Arctic brown algae are a perspective source of unique compounds that can create various products with beneficial properties. In the Northern Hemisphere, the genera Fucus, Ascophyllum, and Pelvetia of the family Fucaceae predominate in the intertidal zones of many cold and warm temperate regions [2,3]. These algae are the best known and are of increasing importance due to their high content of various phytochemicals with industrial applications [4–6].

https://doi.org/10.3390/md23060230

Various species of brown algae have traditionally been used as food or dietary supplements in people's daily diets, typically in Far East Asian countries where seaweed consumption is part of their culture. In addition, although less frequently, some species of Fucus have also been consumed in coastal countries of Western Europe, the Arctic region, and Alaska [7]. Long-term scientific studies on patients have revealed correlations between a diet containing algae and a reduced risk of developing arterial hypertension, coronary heart disease, and cerebrovascular and oncological diseases [8–10]. It has been shown that including algae in the diets of patients with cardiovascular diseases reduces the risk of death from complications [11]. In the case of patients with oncological diseases, it helps to increase life expectancy [12]. Expanding interest in algae as a wealthy source of bioactive metabolites (primarily polysaccharides) and macro- and micro-elements has revealed promising applications in functional foods and nutraceutical manufacturing [13,14].

The major sulfated polysaccharide known as fucoidan is extracted from marine brown algae. The structure of fucoidan is heterogeneous and varies significantly in composition and chemical structure between species, depending on both regional and seasonal influences and the extraction method, enzymatic structural modifications, and purification [15–17]. Fucoidan consists mainly of *L*-fucose and sulfate [18–20]. It also comprises other monosaccharides like galactose, glucose, mannose, rhamnose, arabinose and xylose, and uronic acids [21,22].

Fucoidan has been reported to have antioxidant, antiviral, antibacterial, anti-inflammatory, anticoagulant, antiobesity activities, etc. [23–25]. Accumulated evidence supports the notion that the use of fucoidan as a supplement offers protection against various types of cancer. Some authors have reported that fucoidan has antiangiogenic and antiproliferative activity against cancer cells in vitro, as well as inhibitory activity against tumor growth in mice [26]. Fucoidan has been shown to exhibit antimetastatic activity by blocking the interaction between cancer cells and the basement membrane. Fucoidan inhibits cancer cells proliferation and cancer cells adhesion to various substrates. Several in vitro and in vivo studies have shown that fucoidan has strong antitumor activity [27,28]. Fucoidans have been shown to have low toxicity to normal cells [29,30]. Since fucoidan also has an immunomodulatory effect [31], it has been postulated that it may have a protective effect against the development of side effects when combined with chemotherapeutic agents and radiation [32]. These studies showed the potency of fucoidan as a chemopreventive agent and are the basis for the effort to develop fucoidan as a chemotherapeutic agent to increase the cytotoxic activity and reduce the side effects of paclitaxel.

Diverse methods have been described for fucoidan extraction, ranging from traditional maceration to modern and advanced. According to the data discussed in a recent review [33], the yield of fucoidan varied from 2.26% (hot water maceration from *Sargassum vulgare*) up to 19.5% (extraction by McIlvaine's buffer solution at 60 °C and pH 4.0 from Sargassum spp.). In some studies, microwave-assisted extraction was established as an effective method for the extraction yield [34], while other authors have advocated ultrasound-assisted extraction [35].

In some publications, polyphenolics coextracted with fucoidan are considered as contaminants [24]. The brown color of the algae and, consequently, of the crude fucoidan, is primarily due to polyphenols (e.g., phlorotannins) and fucoxanthin, which are closely coupled with fucoidans in the cell wall [22]. Breaking this bond requires significant purification expenses. However, some authors have shown that polyphenolic impurities in fucoidan contribute to antioxidant, anti-inflammatory, anticancer, and other activities [15, 34,36].

Scientific teams from various countries have attempted to link the activities with fucoidan's structural features, including molecular weight, monomer composition, sulfate content, and sulfation pattern. Nevertheless, this structure-activity relationship is still not well verified and varies depending on the extraction methods used [37–40].

However, the systematic comparison of the effects of extraction methods on the antioxidant and anticancer activities of fucoidans isolated from different brown algae species has not been performed yet. Although synergy for fucoidan with some anticancer drugs was claimed in the literature, the synergistic effect was not calculated.

The aim of this study was (a) to compare the efficacy of dynamic maceration (DM) and ultrasound-assisted extraction (UAE) of fucoidan from four Arctic brown alga species, (b) to evaluate the antioxidant activity and cytotoxicity of isolated fucoidans on HeLa G-63 cells, and (c) to study synergistic effect of fucoidan with paclitaxel (Ptx) on inhibition of HeLa G-63 cells.

2. Results and Discussion

2.1. The Impact of Extraction Methods on the Yield and of Fucoidans Composition

The fucoidans analyzed in this study are native, unfractionated polysaccharides, which contain other co-extracted substances such as polyphenols and uronic acids. Therefore, the term "fucoidan yield" is used rather than "sulfated polysaccharide yield" [24]. The effectiveness of two intensive methods (DM and UAE) for the extraction of fucoidan was compared in this study (Figure 1).

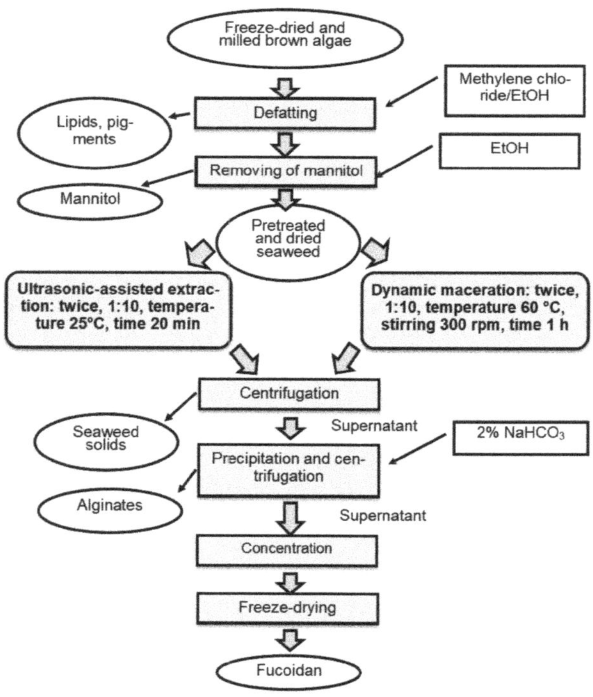

Figure 1. Scheme of extraction brown algae using dynamic maceration and ultrasound-assisted extraction.

The DM combines maceration with mechanical homogenization and temperature. In this case, a forced convection phenomenon allows a more efficient extraction in less time [41]. UAE was used to obtain polysaccharides from algae [42] and can be applied simultaneously to acid extraction [43] or as a previous pretreatment before acid extraction [44]. The effect of two different extraction methods on fucoidan yield is shown in Table 1.

Table 1. Yield and chemical composition of fucoidans isolated from Arctic brown algae.

Species	Extraction Method	Sample	Fucoidan Yield, %dw	Fucoidan, %dw	Mw, kDa	IC_{50}, µg/mL	TPC, %dw	FRAP, μM_{TE}
F. vesiculosus	DM	Fv1	9.4 ± 0.4 *	59.4 ± 0.2 *	244 ± 8 *	368 ± 13 *	5.4 ± 0.1 *	185 ± 4 *
	UAE	Fv2	17.4 ± 0.3	64.1 ± 0.4	195 ± 11	640 ± 12	3.3 ± 0.1	159 ± 5
F. distichus	DM	Fd1	11.2 ± 0.3 *	58.8 ± 0.3 *	273 ± 7 *	626 ± 20 *	4.2 ± 0.2 *	175 ± 5 *
	UAE	Fd2	14.9 ± 0.7	63.5 ± 0.2	229 ± 9	1212 ± 34	1.6 ± 0.1	96 ± 6
F. serratus	DM	Fs1	8.0 ± 0.3 *	53.1 ± 0.2 *	263 ± 8 *	301 ± 17 *	5.1 ± 0.3 *	176 ± 6 *
	UAE	Fs2	12.6 ± 0.5	57.7 ± 0.5	239 ± 6	1498 ± 54	1.4 ± 0.2	94 ± 4
A. nodosum	DM	An1	12.4 ± 0.4 *	58.8 ± 0.6 *	364 ± 10 *	667 ± 20 *	6.7 ± 0.3 *	194 ± 9 *
	UAE	An2	13.8 ± 0.3	60.7 ± 0.1	222 ± 7	1042 ± 30	3.6 ± 0.4	156 ± 6

Data is shown as a mean ± sd (n = 3). * Multiple comparison analyses show statistically significant differences ($p < 0.05$) between DM and UAE extraction methods. Mw—molecular weight; IC_{50}—anticancer activity; TPC—total phlorotannins content; FRAP—Ferric reducing antioxidant power.

It was found that the extraction method affects not only the yield of fucoidan and its composition, including sulfates, uronic acids, and total phlorotannins, but also the monosaccharide composition and molecular weight of the polysaccharide (Tables 1 and 2). When using UAE (mean for four algae species), a significant increase in fucoidan yield by 43.2% (Figure 2) and uronic acid levels by 22.0% (Figure 3) was observed. At the same time, the content of total phlorotannins was (on average) significantly lower by 53.7% than with DM (Figure 2). A two-way ANOVA analysis of the results revealed an extremely significant interaction between the extraction method and species of algae ($p < 0.0001$). The interaction of these factors was also statistically significant (Figure 2).

Table 2. Structural units of fucoidans vs. method extraction.

Sample	Monosaccharide Composition, mol.%					Uronic Acid, %	Sulfate, %
	Fucose	Xylose	Mannose	Glucose	Galactose		
Fv1	71.9 ± 0.9 *	9.4 ± 0.4	6.0 ± 0.2	8.3 ± 0.3	4.4 ± 0.1 *	5.3 ± 0.4 *	25.4 ± 0.3 *
Fv2	75.7 ± 1.1	7.6 ± 0.5	4.3 ± 0.1	5.8 ± 0.4	6.6 ± 0.1	6.4 ± 0.3	23.8 ± 0.2
Fd1	63.6 ± 1.2 *	4.2 ± 0.3	4.8 ± 0.2	21.6 ± 0.7	5.8 ± 0.2 *	5.9 ± 0.5 *	26.6 ± 0.5 *
Fd2	68.2 ± 0.8	5.8 ± 0.3	4.7 ± 0.2	17.9 ± 0.9	3.4 ± 0.1	7.0 ± 0.5	25.4 ± 0.3
Fs1	69.7 ± 0.7 *	5.9 ± 0.5	8.1 ± 0.3	3.0 ± 0.2	13.3 ± 0.3 *	4.1 ± 0.4 *	22.4 ± 0.4 *
Fs2	72.8 ± 1.0	4.5 ± 0.4	7.5 ± 0.2	4.4 ± 0.3	10.8 ± 0.4	4.8 ± 0.2	20.9 ± 0.2
An1	47.8 ± 1.2 *	12.4 ± 0.3	14.3 ± 0.4	13.3 ± 0.4	12.2 ± 0.5	3.3 ± 0.6 *	17.6 ± 0.2 *
An2	49.3 ± 0.9	11.7 ± 0.5	14.0 ± 0.5	13.4 ± 0.3	11.6 ± 0.4	4.5 ± 0.5	16.4 ± 0.4

Data is shown as a mean ± sd (n = 3). * Multiple comparison analyses show statistically significant differences ($p < 0.05$) between DM and UAE extraction methods.

It is known that fucoidan fractions with similar structural characteristics often exhibit identical biological activity [45]. All fucoidans obtained by two technologies from the studied algae contained fucose as the main monosaccharide, galactose, mannose, xylose, glucose, uronic acid residues, and sulfate and were, thus, heteropolysaccharides [46]. The changes in the monosaccharide composition of fucoidan were detected after the exposure of algae material to low-frequency ultrasound. The fucose level for all algae significantly increased (Table 2), while a tendency to decrease in other monosaccharides, such as xylose, mannose, and glucose, was observed. The content of uronic acid residues and sulfates also changed under the influence of ultrasound for each algae species (Table 2).

The influence of the extraction procedure conditions on the molecular weight of fucoidan is shown in Figure 4.

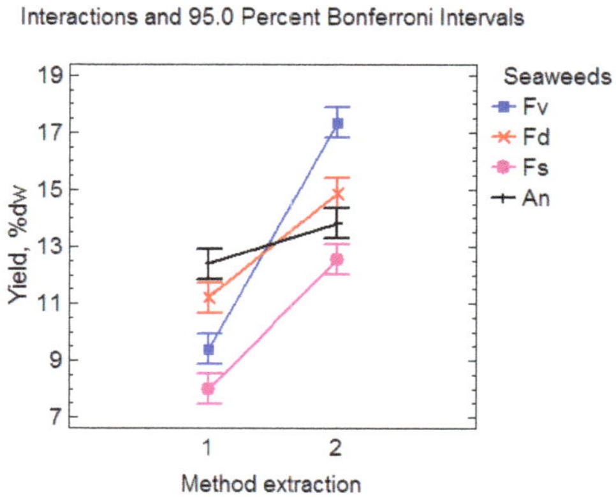

Figure 2. Effect of extraction method on fucoidan yield: 1—dynamic maceration and 2—ultrasound-assisted extraction.

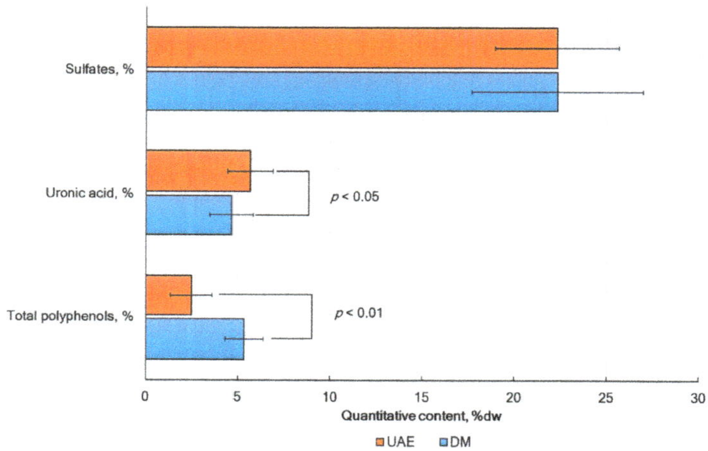

Figure 3. Impact of method extraction on biochemical composition of fucoidans. Data are shown as a mean ± sd (n = 3) for four types of algae. Multiple comparison analyses show statistically significant differences between DM and UAE extraction methods.

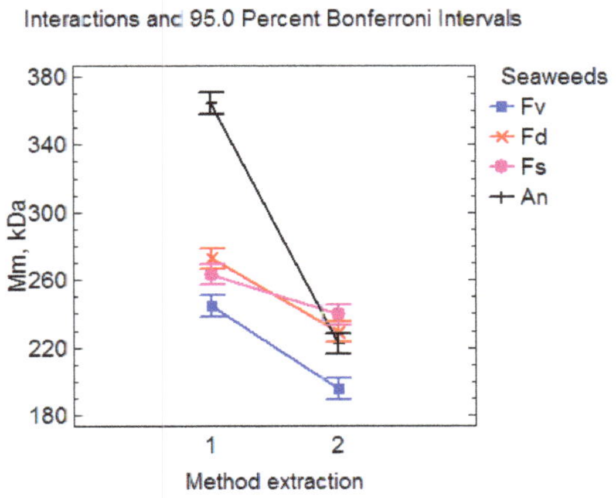

Figure 4. Effect of extraction method on the mean molecular weight of fucoidan. 1—dynamic maceration and 2—ultrasound-assisted extraction.

The molecular weight of all fucoidan samples after extraction in ultrasound was statistically lower than after extraction by the dynamic maceration method. It has been previously reported that high-molecular-weight polymers with long chains are preferentially destroyed under the action of shear forces arising from the rapid collapse of cavitation bubbles [47,48].

2.2. The Antioxidant Activities of Fucoidans

The antioxidant potential of algae makes them interesting candidates for pharmacological, food, and medicinal applications. The ferric reducing antioxidant power (FRAP) assay was conducted on the fucoidans to study the effect of the method intensification strategy. The antioxidant capacity of fucoidan fractions is presented in Table 1. The analysis of the FRAP values shown in Figure 5 shows significant differences between the species and between the extraction methods used. The highest FRAP activity was noted for the fucoidan An1 (193 ± 9 μM_{TE}) and Fv1 (185 ± 4 μM_{TE}) which can again be attributed to the presence of high TPC in the same samples (6.7 ± 0.3 %dw and 5.4 ± 0.1 %dw). The FRAP value of the fucoidan extracted with UAE was decreased by 31.1% (from 13.8% for Fv to 46.5% for Fs) for fucoidan obtained by DM. These results are in line with recent findings [48–51] and support the assumption that rather co-extracted phenolic compounds (e.g., phlorotannins) and terpenoids (e.g., fucoxanthin) than the fucoidan itself exhibit antioxidant effects. In the former studies, the radical scavenging potential of fucoidans correlated with their total phenolic content and fell after purification by ion exchange chromatography. A similar effect was achieved by simply incubating *F. vesiculosus* fucoidan with H_2O_2, which destroyed most of the brown-colored co-extracted polyphenols and terpenoids and, thus, also reduced its antioxidant activity [51]. It was noted that the fraction with the highest fucoidan content ($p < 0.05$) had the least antioxidant activity [52]. The influence of different extraction methods, including ultrasound, was discussed in [53]. The authors showed that the FRAP activity for fucoidan samples of brown macroalgae (*Padina tetrastromatica* and *Turbinaria conoides*) obtained using ultrasound was lower than the conventional approach. A strong positive correlation was observed between FRAP and TPC (Pearson correlation coefficient r = 0.95, $p < 0.05$). Our results are consistent with previous studies reporting a positive correlation between FRAP and polyphenolic compounds for seaweed extracts [15,54]. We observed a negative correlation between FRAP levels and sulfates (Pearson correlation coefficient r = −0.26, $p < 0.05$) and uronic acid (Pearson correlation coefficient r = −0.47, $p < 0.05$). It was suggested that this was associated with phlorotannins and sulfates.

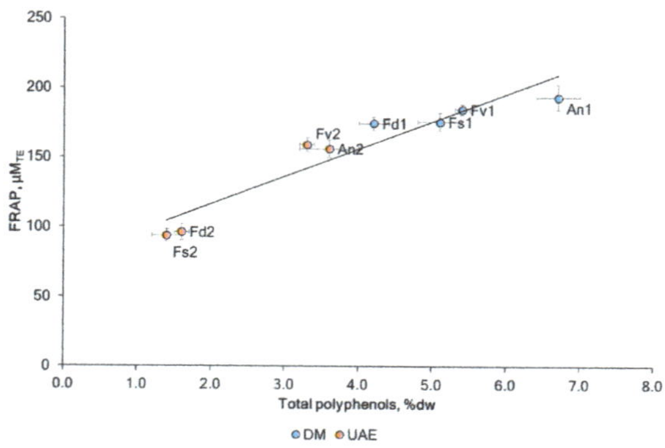

Figure 5. The antioxidant activity (FRAP) in Trolox equivalents and total phlorotannins content (TPC) in (phloroglucinol equivalents/g DW) for fucoidans extracted from the tested brown seaweeds extracted by DM and UAE: *F. vesiculosus* (Fv), *F. distichus* (Fd), *F. serratus* (Fs), and *A. nodosum* (An). Values are expressed as the mean ± sd.

2.3. Anticancer Properties of Fucoidans

In the present study, the anticancer activities of fucoidans extracted from *F. vesiculosus*, *F. distichus*, *F. serratus*, and *A. nodosum* via DM and UAE were tested at five concentrations ranging from 150 to 750 μg/mL. According to the MTT test, treatment of HeLa G-63 cells with all studied fucoidans for 48 h increased the number of dead cells depending on the concentration of sulfated polysaccharides (Figure 6). It was found that the extraction method significantly affected the anticancer activity. A decrease in activity was observed under the action of ultrasound. UAE had a less pronounced effect on *A. nodosum*. No difference in the anticancer activity was observed for the fucoidan from this alga.

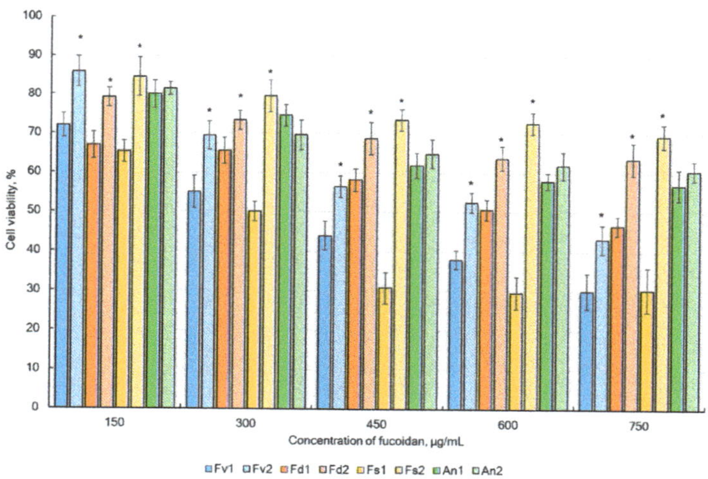

Figure 6. Dose-response of HeLa G-63 cell line treated with four different fucoidans extracted via DM and UAE in concentrations ranging from 150 μg/mL to 750 μg/mL: *F. vesiculosus* (Fv), *F. distichus* (Fd), *F. serratus* (Fs), and *A. nodosum* (An). The relative cell viability was calculated in comparison with the untreated negative control. * Multiple comparison analyses show statistically significant differences ($p < 0.05$) between DM and UAE extraction methods.

The anticancer properties of fucoidan have been studied since the 1980s. Further experiments have shown that these molecules can suppress cancer cell proliferation, induce apoptosis, suppress angiogenesis, etc., in vitro and in vivo studies [55,56]. According to literature data, fucoidan molecular weight has been considered one of the important factors that affect in vitro anticancer activities. Low molecular weight has been reported to have higher cytotoxicity due to its ability to increase solubility and penetration into the cell with a reduced toxic effect on normal cells [29,30]. An anticancer study using fucoidan fractions against the growth of U-251MG glioblastoma multiforme cancer cells demonstrated previously that the >300 kDa fraction had the lowest IC_{50} value against tumor cells compared to the other four fractions with a molecular weight of <300 kDa [57].

In the current study (Table 1, Figure 7), the most promising were fucoidans (<300 kDa) extracted via DM from *F. vesiculosus* and *F. serratus*. These two fucoidans presented the lowest IC_{50} value when compared with the other samples, especially those obtained using the UAE method.

The relationship between antioxidant activity and the anticancer efficacy of natural compounds has been the focus of numerous studies. In this work, we assessed the total antioxidant activity of fucoidan obtained from four various brown algae via two methods of extraction using the FRAP assay (Figure 7). Fucoidan from *F. vesiculosus* and *F. serratus*, obtained via DM showed the most prominent anticancer activity with an IC_{50} of 368 and 301 μg/mL, probably due to its high total phlorotannins content of about 5.4 and 5.1 %dw. The use of ultrasound resulted not only in a decrease in the level of TPC but also in a decrease in activity. Moreover, for the algae *F. vesiculosus*, *F. distichus*, and *A. nodosum*, the decrease in activity was 1.6–1.9 times, while for *F. serratus*, a decrease in activity by five times was observed. A significant reduction in TPC (by 73%) was also registered for *F. serratus* when DM was compared with UAE.

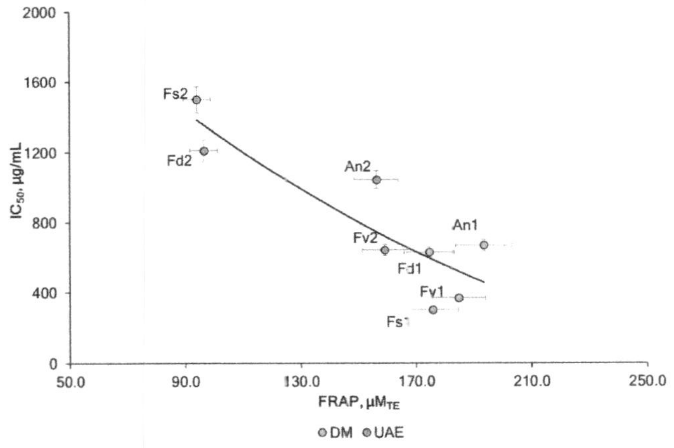

Figure 7. The antioxidant activity (FRAP) and anticancer activity (IC_{50}) for fucoidans from the tested brown algae extracted via DM and UAE: *F. vesiculosus* (Fv), *F. distichus* (Fd), *F. serratus* (Fs), and *A. nodosum* (An). Values are expressed as the mean ± sd.

The results showed that fucoidan containing higher amounts of phlorotannins and lower levels of sulfates and uronic acid obtained via DM exhibited the highest total antioxidant activity. The same samples Fv1 and Fs1 demonstrated higher cytotoxic activity against HeLa G-63 cells than the other samples. This finding is especially noteworthy as it indicates that both the algae species and the extraction method considerably influence the activity of fucoidan. A strong positive correlation was observed between IC_{50} and Mw (Pearson correlation coefficient r = 0.95, $p < 0.05$). The interaction between method and species continued to be extremely significant ($p < 0.0001$), also when the two-way ANOVA analysis was applied to the data of the antioxidant and anticancer activities.

2.4. Study of Synergism

Side effects restrain the application of chemotherapies in the clinic. Therefore, to improve drug efficacy, as well as reduce adverse effects, we tested whether fucoidan synergizes with Ptx in the treatment of cervical cancer. Based on the previously obtained IC_{50} values of fucoidan and Ptx, a dose-ranging experiment was designed and cell viability was determined in which fucoidan (25–750 µg/mL) and Ptx (0.001 and 0.05 µM) were added to HeLa G-63 cells at increasing doses either alone or in combination. The data are shown in Figure 8.

The exposition of HeLa G-63 cells to 0.001 µM Ptx together with fucoidan at 50–600 µg/mL for 24 h led to a significant ($p < 0.05$) increase in cell death (Figure 8A). When incubated for 48 h, significant increase in the anticancer effect was observed in the fucoidan concentrations from 50 to 150 µg/mL (Figure 8B).

Simultaneous application of Ptx at a concentration of 0.05 µM and fucoidan for 24 h on HeLa G-63 cells resulted in significant increase ($p < 0.05$) in dead cells at fucoidan concentrations of 50 and 150 µg/mL. Whereas, when incubated for 48 h, a statistically significant increase in the anticancer effect was observed in the fucoidan concentration range from 50 to 750 µg/mL (Figures 8C and 8D, respectively).

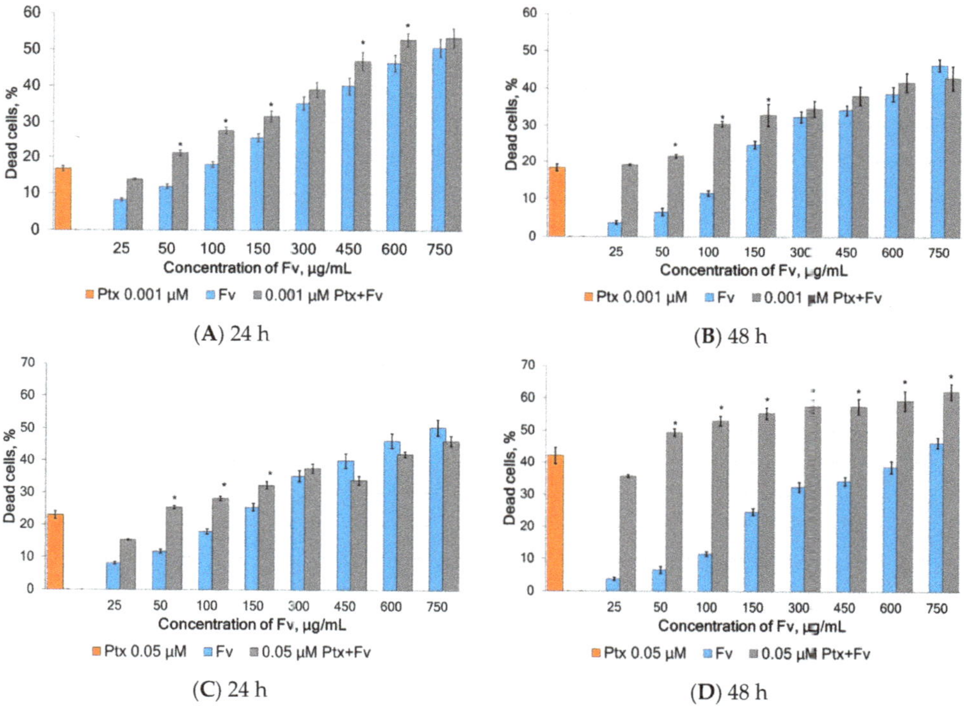

Figure 8. Inhibition of the viability of HeLa G-63 cells upon incubation with paclitaxel and different concentrations of fucoidan Fv alone or in combination for 24 and 48 h ($n = 5$). (**A**)—incubation with 0.001 µM Ptx and Fv for 24 h; (**B**)—incubation with 0.001 µM Ptx and Fv for 48 h; (**C**)—incubation with 0.05 µM Ptx and Fv for 24 h; (**D**)—incubation with 0.05 µM Ptx and Fv for 48 h. Results represent the mean ± sd from three independent experiments. * A significant difference from single treatments is indicated by $p < 0.05$.

To investigate the mechanisms of the synergistic effect of fucoidan in combination with Ptx on HeLa G-63 cells, a propidium iodide (PI) staining assay using flow cytometry was used to analyze the cell cycle distribution (Figure 9). Cell cycle assays were performed after

48 h exposure of HeLa G-63 cells to different concentrations of Ptx (0.001 and 0.05 μM) and Fv (25–750 μg/mL) both separately and combined to test the hypothesis that the growth suppression has stemmed from the disruption in the cell (Figure 9).

Ptx affects the cell cycle, causing a delay in the G2/M phase. It has a cytotoxic antimitotic effect. When HeLa G63 cells were incubated with 0.001 μM Ptx as well as with its combined action with various concentrations of fucoidan, no changes in the distribution of cells throughout the cycle were observed (Figure 9A). Whereas when cells were incubated with 0.05 μM Ptx as well as with its combined action with various concentrations of 25–100 μg/mL fucoidan, an accumulation of cells in the G2/M phase was observed (Figure 9B). The percentage of cells in the G1 and G2/M phases changed significantly as a result of the combination treatment, suggesting that the combination of the two drugs caused cell death more effectively than either of them alone. This experiment showed that co-administration of Ptx (0.05 μM) and fucoidan from *F. vesiculosus* at low concentrations (25–100 μg/mL) caused cell cycle arrest in the G2/M phase.

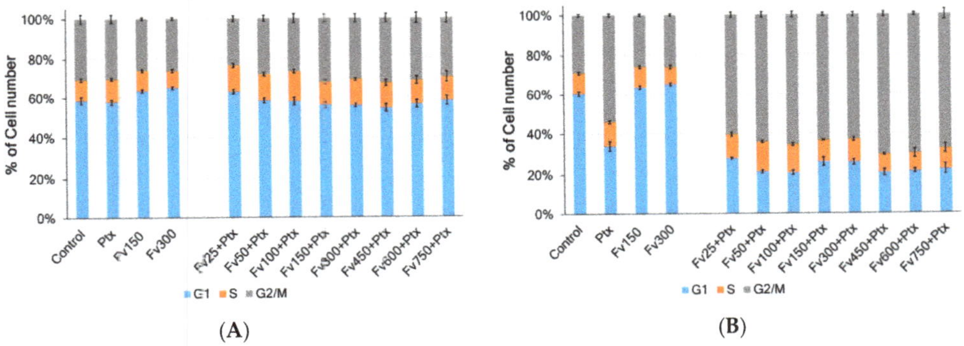

Figure 9. Distribution of HeLa G-63 cells by cell cycle phases under the combined action of paclitaxel (Ptx) (0.001 μM (**A**), 0.05 μM (**B**)) and different concentrations of fucoidan Fv after 48 h. The results are presented as mean ± sd from three separate experiments.

Mathew et al. (2017) performed combination growth inhibition assays using the IC_{50} concentration of the chemotherapeutic agents, which included paclitaxel and tamoxifen, as well as 0.3 mg/mL fucoidan UPF and 1.3 mg/mL fucoidan FVF [58]. It was demonstrated that both compounds appeared to have overall synergistic activity in inhibiting cancer cell growth when used in combination with paclitaxel or tamoxifen. Our results are consistent with the work [59], which showed that the semisynthetic alginate derivative polymannuroguluronate sulfate (2 mg/mL) in combination with Ptx (50 nM) blocked the cell cycle at the G2/M phase in HeLa G-63 cells, similar to Ptx treatment alone. Moreover, the sulfated polysaccharide itself did not show activity.

The calculation of the combinatory effect (CE) showed that the simultaneous use of Ptx at a concentration of 0.05 μM and fucoidan at a concentration of 25–600 μg/mL after 48 h exposure leads to a synergistic interaction (Figure 10). At the same time, the combined action of the same mixtures after 24 h exposure does not give a synergistic effect. A decrease in the concentration of Ptx at the same concentrations of fucoidan also does not form synergistic combinations. Thus, synergism depends not only on the concentrations of the components but also on the time of exposure. However, our fucoidan from *F. vesiculosus* led to increased activity Ptx at a much lower concentration (25–100 μg/mL), and the additivity effect was observed even when using a Ptx concentration lower than 50 times the IC_{50} (0.001 μM) (Figure 10).

The anticancer activity of the fucoidan (100–400 μg/mL) extracted from *Nizamuddinia zanardinii* by UAE was lower than that extracted via enzyme and enzyme-UAE [60]. A previous report [61] showed that the anticancer activity of bioactive polysaccharides is attributable to various factors such as sulfate content, monosaccharide composition, molecular weight and amount of impurity of protein, and total phenol. Yang et al. (2008) proposed that the anticancer activities of brown algae fucoidans depend on species and growing conditions of algae, extraction and purification methods, and the cancer cell lines used in the tests [37]. The effects of different extraction technologies on the extraction of phytochemicals (fucoidan, sulfates, uronic acid, and TPC) from the tested samples of brown algae are presented in Table 1. There was a significant variation in the extraction of each phytochemical depending on the macroalgal species and technological treatments. In general, extracts from *F. vesiculosus* contained the highest levels of fucoidan and TPC compared to others. The differences in the recovery of phytochemicals between species could be attributed to inter-species differences, while the effect of technological treatments on all species was similar (Figure 2). Harnedy & FitzGerald (2013) mentioned that strong cell walls containing variable types and amounts of polysaccharides, depending on the macroalgal species, were one of the main obstacles hindering an efficient extraction of compounds from macroalgae [62]. Thus, the type of polysaccharides and ionic interactions with other cell wall constituents will be strongly influenced by the macroalgal species studied [63], affecting the yields of compounds extracted depending on the macroalgal species.

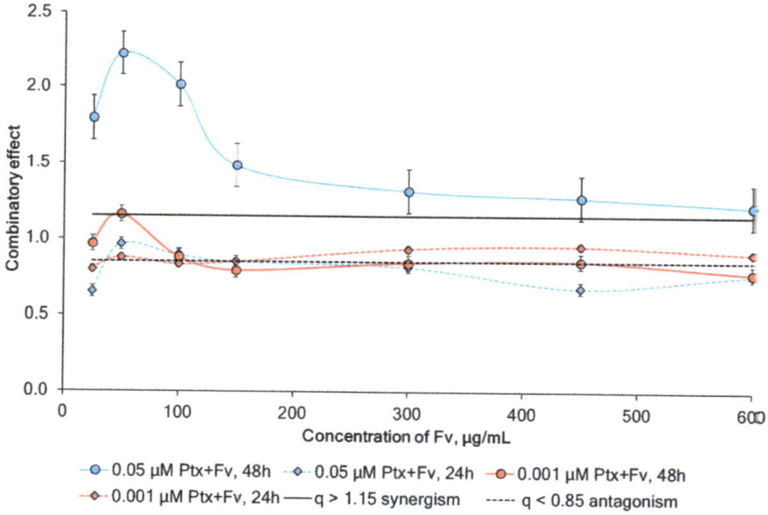

Figure 10. The combinatory effect (q) of paclitaxel (Ptx) and various concentrations of fucoidan (Fv) on HeLa G-63 cells.

The cell cycle is a sequence of synchronized activities that leads to cell division. When cellular control over this normal proliferation is compromised, a normal cell becomes cancerous. Consequently, chemotherapeutic drugs may aim to induce cell cycle arrest. The DNA synthesis (S phase), mitotic (M phase), and two gap phases (G1, G2) are among the phases of the cell cycle. The G0 segment is the resting length inside the molecular cycle, wherein the cells stay inactive. The sub-G1 segment represents the proportion of apoptotic cells, so the molecular cycle evaluation can offer apoptotic data. The G1 segment is, as a substitute, vital, considering the fact that arrest at this level affords a possibility for cells to both go through restore mechanisms or comply with the apoptotic pathway. Therefore, most of the anticancer drugs target this stage of the cell cycle [64]. Ptx + Fv showed a prominent cell cycle arrest at the G1 phase and accumulation of the cells in the S phase. The data indicate that the anticancer potential of ESPs-CP is mainly attributed to the induction of apoptosis and cell cycle arrest at the G1 phase. The anticancer activity of sulfated polysaccharides from brown alga *Ecklonia cava* [64], *Sargassum horneri* [65] and *Padina tetrastromatica* [66] also claimed the same pattern of cell cycle arrest.

The lack of selective targeting of chemotherapeutic agents such as Ptx leads to the high toxicity of therapy and the incidence of serious side effects, which not only reduces the quality of life but can also cause serious complications [67]. Consequently, there is an interest in agents that could either enhance the beneficial effects of conventional therapy or reduce the incidence of side effects. To date, several agents effective in enhancing the response to Ptx have emerged and include various flavonoids [68], green tea extract [69], etc. In the current study, we observed that co-administration of fucoidan to Ptx-treated cells enhanced the therapeutic effect in the tested cell line. In addition, subsequent analysis of the combined effect of the drug revealed synergy between fucoidan and Ptx. Similar results were obtained by Zhang et al. (2013), who investigated the effects of a common cytostatic combination with fucoidans [70]. The authors reported that the combined use of cytostatics and fucoidan provided a greater therapeutic effect compared to treatment with a single agent. They also showed that the combination of fucoidan and cisplatin was the most effective. Abudabbus et al. (2017) have suggested that co-incubation of cisplatin, doxorubicin, or Ptx with fucoidan enhanced the therapeutic effects compared to individual agents [71]; however, synergy was not calculated. The synergy between fucoidan and lapatinib [72] and fucoidan and cisplatin on HNSCC cell lines (H103, FaDu, and KB) was also reported [73].

This result may be explained by the multifactorial nature of the anticancer mechanisms of natural compounds. Although antioxidants can neutralize reactive oxygen species and decrease oxidative damage, which might also additionally save you from most cancers, the induction of apoptosis in most cancer cells regularly entails extra mechanisms inclusive of the modulation of molecular signaling pathways and induction of endoplasmic reticulum stress [74]. In this scenario, fucoidan derived from *F. vesiculosus*, exhibiting the most significant antioxidant properties and the highest level of cytotoxicity, could operate via several mechanisms to trigger cell death in HeLa G-63 cells. Studies of the synergistic effects of antioxidants with anticancer drugs may provide a promising basis for designing new agents for cancer therapy.

3. Materials and Methods

3.1. Sample Collection and Preparation of Alga

The brown alga, bladder wrack (*Fucus vesiculosus* L.) (Fv), toothed wrack (*Fucus serratus* L.) (Fs), rockweed (*Fucus distichus* L.) (Fd), and Icelandic kelp (*Ascophyllum nodosum* L.) Le Jolis) (An) were collected in August–September 2023 from the littoral of the Barents Sea (Zelentskaya Bay, Murmansk region, Russia) at low tide. Dr. E. Obluchinskaya identified the algae, and the voucher specimen (No. 9.2023) was deposited in the Collection of the Zoobentos Laboratory, Murmansk Marine Biological Institute. Collected algae were thoroughly washed in running tap water, followed by distilled water, to remove the adhering sand, epiphytes, extraneous matter, and necrotic parts, frozen within two hours of collection and subsequently freeze-dried for one week to ensure full lyophilization, and ground to a fine powder. Dried samples were stored in sealed containers at 4 °C until use.

3.2. Materials

Folin–Ciocalteu reagent, Trolox (6-hydroxy-2,5,7,8-tetramethylchroman-2-carboxylic acid), TPTZ (2,4,6-tripyridyl-s-triazine), ascorbic acid, phloroglucinol, L-cysteine, ammonium molybdate, analytical grade monosaccharides (fucose (Fuc), xylose (Xyl), mannose (Man), galactose (Gal), arabinose (Ara) and glucose (Glc), all purities > 99%), Shodex pullulan P-82 standard kit (Showa-Denko Co., Tokyo, Japan) and blue dextran-2000 (GE Healthcare, Chicago, IL, USA) were obtained from Sigma-Aldrich (St. Louis, MO, USA). Versene solution, phosphate-buffered saline (PBS), and Dulbecco's modified Eagle medium (DMEM) supplemented with 10% heat-inactivated fetal bovine serum (FBS) and 100 IU/mL penicillin and streptomycin were from BioloT Ltd., St. Petersburg, Russia. Propidium iodide (PI) and 3-(4,5-dimethylthiazole-2yl)-2,5-diphenyl tetrazolium bromide (MTT) were purchased from LLC Company Pushchino Laboratories, Pushchino, Russia. An aqueous solution of paclitaxel (Sandoz Pharmaceuticals d.d., Ljubljana, Slovenia) at a concentration of 6 mg/mL was stored at room temperature in the dark for future analysis. Ultrapure water was purified using a Milli-Q system (Millipore, Bedford, MA, USA). Other analytical grade chemicals and solvents for extraction and analysis were of analytical grade and purchased from local chemical suppliers.

3.3. Fucoidan Extraction

Fucoidans were prepared using a method modified from [49]. Briefly, samples of dried algae were pretreated sequentially with an azeotrope (methylene chloride/EtOH) and 80% EtOH in a Soxhlet apparatus to remove lipids, pigments, and mannitol. The defatted algae were extracted with 5% (*v*/*v*) EtOH at pH 4, and dry algae: liquid ratio of 1:10 (*w*/*v*). Fucoidan was isolated using UAE and DM. Residual supernatant and algae were separated. Alginate was removed by precipitation with 2% $NaHCO_3$ and centrifugation. The supernatant was concentrated using AR-3–100PS cassettes (NTP Biotest, Kirishi, Russia). After purification, the solution was lyophilized for 24 h on an Inei-4 freeze dryer (IBF RAS, Pushchino, Russia). The yield of fucoidan (g/100 g dw) was calculated using the following Equation (1):

$$\text{Yield Fucoidan} = [\text{dry wt. of fucoidan}/\text{dry wt. of algae}] \times 100 \quad (1)$$

3.3.1. Dynamic Maceration (DM)

Samples of defatted algae were twice macerated on a magnetic stirring apparatus equipped with a temperature-controlling system at 200 rpm with heating at 60 °C with the same solvent. All the other steps were equally performed in both UAE and DM (Fv1, Fd1, Fs1, and An1).

3.3.2. Ultrasonic-Assisted Extraction (UAE)

An ultrasonic processor (UZTA-0.4/22-OM, Biysk, Russia) with a 15 mm probe was used. Samples of defatted algae with a solvent were twice sonicated (22 kHz) at room temperature for 20 min (Fv2, Fd2, Fs2, and An2).

3.4. Analysis of Fucoidan Composition

The fucoidan content was determined using the method [75]. Fucoidan content was measured via the cysteine–sulfuric acid method using L-fucose as a reference [76] All measurements were done in duplicate, and results were expressed as the percentage of fucose in dry fucoidan. The sulfate residues were determined using the $BaCl_2$-gelatin method [77]. Uronic acid was determined following the Scott method (1979) with 3,5-dimethylphenol as the reagent [78] and alginic acid as a standard [79]. Impurities of polyphenols, as the total phlorotannin content (TPC), were quantified using Folin–Ciocalteau reagent with phloroglucinol as the standard [80], and the results were expressed as g of phloroglucinol equivalent per 100 g (%) of fucoidan DW.

The molecular weight (Mw) of fucoidan was analyzed using high-performance size-exclusion chromatography (HPSEC) [81], equipped with two TSKGel columns (Tosoh Bioscience, Stuttgart, Germany) and a PWX guard column. Water was used as the mobile phase at a rate of 0.4 mL/min at 70 °C. The monosaccharide compositions of fucoidans were analyzed using a high-performance liquid chromatography system (HPLC Model LC 20 AT Prominence, Shimadzu, Kyoto, Japan) with a refractive index detector (RID-10A, Shimadzu, Japan) after hydrolysis [82]. The samples were injected into a Shodex Asahipak NH2P-50 4E (4.6 × mm, 5 μm) column (Kanagawa, Japan) at 50 °C under isocratic conditions with a mobile phase consisting of 0.25 M H_3PO_4-acetonitrile (20:80, *v*/*v*) at a flow rate of 1.0 mL/min. Data are presented as relative mole percentages.

3.5. *In Vitro* Antioxidant Assays

Ferric reducing antioxidant power (FRAP) assay was performed following the method [83]. FRAP results were expressed as μM of Trolox equivalents (μM_{TE}).

3.6. Cell Culture

Human carcinoma HeLa G-63 cells were obtained from the shared research facility of Vertebrate Cell Culture Collection (Institute of Cytology RAS, St. Petersburg, Russia) and have been cultivated in the laboratory of PNPI since 1963.

After cryopreservation at −80 °C, thawed HeLa G-63 cells (1.5×10^6 cells/mL) were seeded in 60 mm culture dishes in 4 mL of culture medium. Cells were incubated at 37 °C in a humidified atmosphere with 5% CO_2, and the culture medium was changed every 24 h. For cell culture, cells were detached from the 60 mm culture dish using 0.25% trypsin: 0.02% Versene solution (1:3 *v*/*v*) and replated on a new culture dish. After 3–4 days, cells attached and spread on the 60 mm culture dishes and were subcultured to 80–90% confluence. Passages were repeated three to five times, the optimal density was 1.0–5.0 × 10^4 cells/cm^2. The HeLa G-63 was cultivated in monolayer culture in DMEM with L-glutamine and with 4.5 g/L glucose, and supplemented with 10% heat-inactivated FBS and 100 IU/mL penicillin and 100 μg/mL streptomycin in an incubator with 5% CO_2 at 37 °C.

3.6.1. Proliferation Assay and Cell Cycle Analysis

Cells were seeded at a density of 2×10^5 cells/well in 12-well plates and incubated for 24 h at 37 °C in a CO_2 incubator to form a monolayer. Then, the cells were treated with different concentrations of fucoidans and a reference drug for 24 h. After treatment, the cells were separated using Versene solution, washed with PBS, centrifuged (1000 rpm for 5 min), and the resulting suspension was stained with PI solution containing Rnase [84]. The antiproliferation activity and cell cycle analysis were carried out using a CytoFLEX B3-R2-V2 flow cytometer (Beckman Coulter, Brea, CA, USA; 20,000 cells per experiment) [85].

3.6.2. Cytotoxicity Assay

The cytotoxicity of the samples was determined via MTT assay [86]. In brief, HeLa G-63 cells were plated at 2×10^5 cells per well in 96-well microtiter plates (Cell+, Sarstedt, Germany) with 100 mL RPMI-1640 growth medium and incubated for 24 h at 37 °C, with 5% CO_2 in a humidified atmosphere. Thereafter, the medium was removed and fresh serum-free medium containing different concentrations (25, 50, 100, 150, 300, 450, 600 and 750 μg/mL) of the tested fucoidans and chemotherapeutic agents at a log range of concentrations (Ptx, 1 nM–800 μM) was added. After 44 h of incubation, the 10 μL MTT reagent (5 mg/mL) was added. After incubating at 37 °C for 2 h, the MTT reagent was removed, dimethyl sulphoxide (DMSO; 100 μL) was added to each well and thoroughly mixed by pipetting.

The absorbance was measured using a plate reader Multiskan FC (Thermo Scientific, Waltham, MA, USA) at 570 nm, and the percent cell death was calculated. Negative control cells were incubated without compounds. The percentage inhibition of proliferation was calculated using the formula below, and the half maximal inhibitory concentration of tested samples (IC_{50}) was calculated from the dose-response [87].

$$\text{Cell Viability (\%)} = 100\% \text{ (Test Concentration Reading} - \text{Blank Reading)/(Control Reading} - \text{Blank Reading)} \quad (2)$$

3.6.3. Analysis of Drug Combinatory Effect

The cytotoxicity of the combined use of fucoidan Fv and Ptx was assessed using flow cytometry in combinations of a constant concentration of Ptx with increasing concentrations of fucoidan. In the combined experiments, cells were incubated in 12-well plates and treated with Fv (500 μL) and Ptx (500 μL). After the incubation, the cells were removed with Versene solution, spun down, and the resulting suspension was stained with PI solution (50 μL/mL) for 20 min at 37 °C. The modified probability sum test [88] was applied to assess the mode of combinatory effect, according to the equation:

$$q = P[A + B]/(P[A] + P[B] - P[A] \times P[B]) \quad (3)$$

where P[A] represents the efficacy of drug A and P[B] the efficacy of drug B, while P[A + B] depicts the efficacy of a combination of both drugs at the same doses. Assessed value/expected value (sum of probability of independent events) ratios were defined: $q < 0.85$ as antagonism, while $q = 1.00 \pm 0.15$ indicates additivity, and $q > 1.15$ synergism.

3.7. Statistical Analysis

Each experiment was repeated three times. Data are represented by mean ± standard deviation (±sd). Statistical analysis was performed with STATGRAPHICS Centurion XV (StatPoint Technologies Inc., Warrenton, VA, USA).

4. Conclusions

The effect of the extraction method (dynamic maceration and ultrasound-assisted extraction) on the composition and properties of fucoidans from Arctic brown algae *F. vesiculosus*, *F. serratus*, *F. distichus*, and *A. nodosum* was explored. It was found that fucoidans containing higher TPC and lower levels of sulfates and uronic acid obtained via dynamic maceration exhibited the highest antioxidant and anticancer activity compared with fucoidans obtained via the UAE. For the first time, the synergy for a binary combination of 0.05 μM Ptx with 50–750 μg/mL Fv against HeLa G-63 cell growth was calculated. Thus, our results support the rationality of fucoidan use as a powerful antioxidant and in complex chemotherapy.

Our results open new perspectives and challenges. Future kinetic modeling of fucoidan degradation and more advanced characterization techniques could offer a deeper understanding of structural–function relationships. Our new data provide a reliable basis for the future validation of established synergy through additional mechanistic studies, such as apoptosis pathway analysis and gene expression profiling.

Author Contributions: Conceptualization, E.D.O. and O.N.P.; methodology, E.D.O. and O.N.P.; software, O.N.P.; validation, E.D.O. and E.V.Z.; formal analysis, O.N.P.; investigation, E.D.O., E.V.Z., I.M.L. and A.A.K.; resources, E.D.O.; data curation, A.N.S., O.N.P. and E.D.O.; writing—original draft preparation, O.N.P. and A.N.S.; writing—review and editing, A.N.S. and E.D.O.; visualization, O.N.P.; supervision, E.D.O.; project administration, E.D.O.; funding acquisition, E.D.O. All authors have read and agreed to the published version of the manuscript.

Funding: This study was funded by the Ministry of Science and Higher Education of the Russian Federation within the framework of the Government Assignment to the Murmansk Marine Biological Institute of the Russian Academy of Sciences (State Reg. No. 124013000732-7). The work with the cell line was performed at the Petersburg Nuclear Physics Institute named by B.P.Konstantinov of NRC «Kurchatov Institute» with the financial support of the Ministry of Science and Higher Education of the Russian Federation (Theme № 1023031500033-1-1.6.7;1.6.4;1.6.8).

Institutional Review Board Statement: Not applicable.

Data Availability Statement: Data are contained within the article.

Conflicts of Interest: The authors declare that they have no known competing financial interests or personal relationships that could be perceived as influencing the work reported in this study.

References

1. Costantino, V.; Fattorusso, E.; Menna, M.; Taglialatela-Scafati, O. Chemical diversity of bioactive marine natural products: An illustrative case study. *Curr. Med. Chem.* **2004**, *11*, 1671–1692. [CrossRef] [PubMed]
2. Guiry, M.D.; Guiry, G.M. *AlgaeBase*; World-Wide Electronic Publication, National University of Ireland: Galway, Ireland, 2025. Available online: https://www.algaebase.org (accessed on 9 April 2025).
3. WoRMS Editorial Board; World Register of Marine Species. 2025. Available online: https://www.marinespecies.org/aphia.php?p=taxdetails&id=145544 (accessed on 9 April 2025).
4. Varzugina, M.A.; Makarchuk, R.N.; Yavorsky, A.S.; Nikolaenko, O.A.; Kuranova, L.K. Fucus algae of the Arctic region—Characteristics, areas of use. News of higher educational institutions. *Arctic Region* **2015**, *1*, 48–53.
5. Leandro, A.; Pacheco, D.; Cotas, J.; Marques, J.C.; Pereira, L.; Gonçalves, A.M. Seaweed's bioactive candidate compounds to food industry and global food security. *Life* **2020**, *10*, 140. [CrossRef]
6. Shepeleva, O.A.; Degteva, G.N.; Novikova, I.I.; Shevkun, I.G.; Romanenko, S.P.; Semenikhina, M.V.; Popova, O.N.; Gudkov, A.B. Seaweed as an important functional ingredient and alimentary raw material for enriching the diet of the population in the Arctic Zone of the Russian Federation (Review). *J. Med. Biol. Res.* **2024**, *12*, 99–113. [CrossRef]
7. Pereira, L. *Edible Seaweeds of the World*, 1st ed.; CRC Press: Boca Raton, FL, USA, 2016. [CrossRef]
8. Cotas, J.; Pacheco, D.; Gonçalves, A.M.; Silva, P.; Carvalho, L.G.; Pereira, L. Seaweeds' Nutraceutical and Biomedical Potential in Cancer Therapy: A Concise Review. *J. Cancer Metastasis Treat.* **2021**, *7*, 13. Available online: https://www.oaepublish.com/articles/2394-4722.2020.134 (accessed on 2 May 2025). [CrossRef]
9. Park, G.H.; Cho, J.H.; Lee, D.; Kim, Y. Association between seafood intake and cardiovascular disease in South Korean adults: A community-based prospective cohort study. *Nutrients* **2022**, *14*, 4864. [CrossRef]
10. Ren, Y.; Feng, Y.; Qing, J.; Zhang, P.; Xiao, L.; Liang, X. The correlation between nuts and algae-less diet and children's blood pressure: From a cross-sectional study in Chongqing. *Clin. Exp. Hypertens.* **2023**, *45*, 2180024. [CrossRef]
11. Kishida, R.; Yamagishi, K.; Muraki, I.; Sata, M.; Tamakoshi, A.; Iso, H.; JACC Study Group. Frequency of seaweed intake and its association with cardiovascular disease mortality: The JACC study. *J. Atheroscl. Thromb.* **2020**, *27*, 1340–1347. [CrossRef]
12. Minami, Y.; Kanemura, S.; Oikawa, T.; Suzuki, S.; Hasegawa, Y.; Nishino, Y.; Fujiya, T.; Miura, K. Associations of Japanese food intake with survival of stomach and colorectal cancer: A prospective patient cohort study. *Cancer Sci.* **2020**, *111*, 2558–2569. [CrossRef]
13. Senthil, S.L. A comprehensive review to assess the potential, health benefits and complications of fucoidan for developing as functional ingredient and nutraceutical. *Int. J. Biol. Macromol.* **2024**, *277*, 134226. [CrossRef]
14. Lara-Hernández, G.; Ramos-Silva, J.A.; Pérez-Soto, E.; Figueroa, M.; Flores-Berrios, E.P.; Sánchez-Chapul, L.; Andrade-Cabrera, J.L.; Luna-Angulo, A.; Landa-Solís, C.; Avilés-Arnaut, H. Anticancer activity of plant tocotrienols, fucoxanthin, fucoidan, and polyphenols in dietary supplements. *Nutrients* **2024**, *16*, 4274. [CrossRef] [PubMed]
15. Obluchinskaya, E.D.; Pozharitskaya, O.N.; Shikov, A.N. In vitro anti-inflammatory activities of fucoidans from five species of brown seaweeds. *Mar. Drugs* **2022**, *20*, 606. [CrossRef] [PubMed]
16. Zayed, A.; Muffler, K.; Hahn, T.; Rupp, S.; Finkelmeier, D.; Burger-Kentischer, A.; Ulber, R. Physicochemical and biological characterization of fucoidan from *Fucus vesiculosus* purified by dye affinity chromatography. *Mar. Drugs* **2016**, *14*, 79. [CrossRef]
17. Zayed, A.; Cao, H.T.T.; Trang, V.T.D.; Ulber, R. Structural tailoring of fucoidan backbones for maximizing their benefits: Enzymatic, chemical, and physical strategies. *J. Appl. Phycol.* **2023**, *35*, 2445–2462. [CrossRef]
18. Cumashi, A.; Ushakova, N.A.; Preobrazhenskaya, M.E.; D'Incecco, A.; Piccoli, A.; Totani, L.; Tinari, N.; Morozevich, G.E.; Berman, A.E.; Bilan, M.I.; et al. A comparative study of the anti-inflammatory, anticoagulant, antiangiogenic, and antiadhesive activities of nine different fucoidans from brown seaweeds. *Glycobiology* **2007**, *17*, 541–552. [CrossRef]
19. Usov, A.I.; Bilan, M.I. Fucoidans—Sulfated polysaccharides of brown algae. *Russ. Chem. Rev.* **2009**, *78*, 785. [CrossRef]

20. Deghrigue, M.; Cherif, D.; Lajili, S.; ben Mesmia, H.; Muller, C.D.; Majdoub, H.; Bouraoui, A. Structural characterizations and bioactivities of fucoidans from *Dyctyopteris membranaceae* and *Padina pavonica* with in silico investigations. *Int. J. Biol. Macromol.* **2025**, *307*, 142133. [CrossRef]
21. Li, B.; Lu, F.; Wei, X.; Zhao, R. Fucoidan: Structure and bioactivity. *Molecules* **2008**, *13*, 1671–1695. [CrossRef]
22. Zayed, A.; Ulber, R. Fucoidan production: Approval key challenges and opportunities. *Carbohydr. Polym.* **2019**, *211*, 289–297. [CrossRef]
23. Fitton, J.H.; Stringer, D.N.; Park, A.Y.; Karpiniec, S.S. Therapies from fucoidan: New developments. *Mar. Drugs* **2019**, *17*, 571. [CrossRef]
24. Zayed, A.; El-Aasr, M.; Ibrahim, A.-R.S.; Ulber, R. Fucoidan characterization: Determination of purity and physicochemical and chemical properties. *Mar. Drugs* **2020**, *18*, 571. [CrossRef] [PubMed]
25. Zayed, A.; Al-Saedi, D.A.; Mensah, E.O.; Kanwugu, O.N.; Adadi, P.; Ulber, R. Fucoidan's molecular targets: A comprehensive review of its unique and multiple targets accounting for promising bioactivities supported by in silico studies. *Mar. Drugs* **2023**, *22*, 29. [CrossRef] [PubMed]
26. Oliveira, C.; Neves, N.M.; Reis, R.L.; Martins, A.; Silva, T.H. A review on fucoidan antitumor strategies: From a biological active agent to a structural component of fucoidan-based systems. *Carbohydr. Polym.* **2020**, *239*, 116131. [CrossRef]
27. Kwak, J.Y. Fucoidan as a marine anticancer agent in preclinical development. *Mar. Drugs* **2014**, *12*, 851–870. [CrossRef]
28. Alves, C.; Silva, J.; Pinteus, S.; Gaspar, H.; Alpoim, M.C.; Botana, L.M.; Pedrosa, R. From marine origin to therapeutics: The antitumor potential of marine algae-derived compounds. *Front. Pharmacol.* **2018**, *9*, 777. [CrossRef]
29. Yamasaki-Miyamoto, Y.; Yamasaki, M.; Tachibana, H.; Yamada, K. Fucoidan induces apoptosis through activation of caspase-8 on human breast cancer MCF-7 cells. *J. Agric. Food Chem.* **2009**, *57*, 8677–8682. [CrossRef]
30. Zhurishkina, E.V.; Lapina, I.M.; Ivanen, D.R.; Stepanov, S.I.; Shvetsova, S.V.; Shavarda, A.L.; Giliano, N.Y.; Kulminskaya, A.A. Effect of fucoidans isolated from seaweeds *Laminaria digitata* and *Fucus vesiculosus* on cell lines HeLa G-63, ECV 304 and PC 12. *Tsitologya* **2015**, *57*, 727–735. [PubMed]
31. Apostolova, E.; Lukova, P.; Baldzhieva, A.; Katsarov, P.; Nikolova, M.; Iliev, I.; Peychev, L.; Trica, B.; Oancea, F.; Delattre, C.; et al. Immunomodulatory and anti-inflammatory effects of fucoidan: A review. *Polymers* **2020**, *12*, 2338. [CrossRef]
32. Oh, B.; Kim, J.; Lu, W.; Rosenthal, D. Anticancer effect of fucoidan in combination with tyrosine kinase inhibitor lapatinib. *Evid. Based Complement. Altern. Med.* **2014**, *2014*, 865375. [CrossRef]
33. Anjana, K.; Arunkumar, K. Brown algae biomass for fucoxanthin, fucoidan and alginate; update review on structure, biosynthesis, biological activities and extraction valorisation. *Int. J. Biol. Macromol.* **2014**, *280*, 135632. [CrossRef]
34. Yuan, Y.; Macquarrie, D. Microwave assisted extraction of sulfated polysaccharides (fucoidan) from *Ascophyllum nodosum* and its antioxidant activity. *Carbohydr. Polym.* **2015**, *129*, 101–107. [CrossRef] [PubMed]
35. Hanjabam, M.D.; Kumar, A.; Tejpal, C.S.; Krishnamoorthy, E.; Kishore, P.; Kumar, K.A. Isolation of crude fucoidan from *Sargassum wightii* using conventional and ultra-sonication extraction methods. *Bioact. Carbohydr. Diet. Fibre* **2019**, *20*, 100200. [CrossRef]
36. Zayed, A.; Hahn, T.; Finkelmeier, D.; Burger-Kentischer, A.; Rupp, S.; Krämer, R.; Ulber, R. Phenomenological investigation of the cytotoxic activity of fucoidan isolated from *Fucus vesiculosus*. *Process Biochem.* **2019**, *81*, 182–187. [CrossRef]
37. Yang, C.; Chung, D.; Shin, I.S.; Lee, H.; Kim, J.; Lee, Y.; You, S. Effects of molecular weight and hydrolysis conditions on anticancer activity of fucoidans from sporophyll of *Undaria pinnatifida*. *Int. J. Biol. Macromol.* **2008**, *43*, 433–437. [CrossRef]
38. Ale, M.T.; Meyer, A.S. Fucoidans from brown seaweeds: An update on structures, extraction techniques and use of enzymes as tools for structural elucidation. *RSC Adv.* **2013**, *3*, 8131–8141. [CrossRef]
39. Obluchinsksaya, E.D.; Makarova, M.N.; Pozharitskaya, O.N.; Shikov, A.N. Effects of ultrasound treatment on the chemical composition and anticoagulant properties of dry fucus extract. *Pharm. Chem. J.* **2015**, *49*, 183–186. [CrossRef]
40. Zayed, A.; Finkelmeier, D.; Hahn, T.; Rebers, L.; Shanmugam, A.; Burger-Kentischer, A.; Ulber, R. Characterization and cytotoxic activity of microwave-assisted extracted crude fucoidans from different brown seaweeds. *Mar. Drugs* **2023**, *21*, 48. [CrossRef]
41. Manríquez-Zúñiga, A.N.; de la Torre, A.R.; Valdés-Santiago, L.; Hernández-Bustos, D.A.; Cuéllar-Sojo, S.; Hernández-Rayas, A.; Perez-Vega, S.; Molina-Guerrero, C.E. Broccoli leaves (*Brassica oleracea* var. *italica*) as a source of bioactive compounds and chemical building blocks: Optimal extraction using dynamic maceration and life cycle assessment. *Sustainability* **2023**, *15*, 16616. [CrossRef]
42. Flórez-Fernández, N.; Torres, M.D.; González-Muñoz, M.J.; Domínguez, H. Potential of intensification techniques for the extraction and depolymerization of fucoidan. *Algal Res.* **2018**, *30*, 128–148. [CrossRef]
43. Hmelkov, A.B.; Zvyagintseva, T.N.; Shevchenko, N.M.; Rasin, A.B.; Ermakova, S.P. Ultrasound-assisted extraction of polysaccharides from brown alga *Fucus evanescens*. Structure and biological activity of the new fucoidan fractions. *J. Appl. Phycol.* **2018**, *30*, 2039–2046. [CrossRef]
44. Dobrinčić, A.; Zorić, Z.; Pedisić, S.; Repajić, M.; Roje, M.; Herceg, Z.; Čož-Rakovac, R.; Dragović-Uzelac, V. Application of ultrasound-assisted extraction and non-thermal plasma for *Fucus virsoides* and *Cystoseira barbata* polysaccharides pre-treatment and extraction. *Processes* **2022**, *10*, 433. [CrossRef]

45. Jeong, S.; Lee, S.; Lee, G.; Hyun, J.; Ryu, B. Systematic characteristics of fucoidan: Intriguing features for new pharmacological interventions. *Int. J. Mol. Sci.* **2024**, *25*, 11771. [CrossRef]
46. Zvyagintseva, T.N.; Usoltseva, R.V.; Shevchenko, N.M.; Surits, V.V.; Imbs, T.I.; Malyarenko, O.S.; Besednova, N.N.; Ivanushko, L.A.; Ermakova, S.P. Structural diversity of fucoidans and their radioprotective effect. *Carbohydr. Polym.* **2021**, *273*, 118551. [CrossRef]
47. Jicsinszky, L.; Bucciol, F.; Chaji, S.; Cravotto, G. Mechanochemical degradation of biopolymers. *Molecules* **2023**, *28*, 8031. [CrossRef] [PubMed]
48. Obluchinskaya, E.D.; Pozharitskaya, O.N. Influence of ultrasound extraction of *Fucus vesiculosus* on the kinetics of fucoidan degradation and its properties. *Drug Dev. Regist.* **2025**, *14*, 54–63. [CrossRef]
49. Obluchinskaya, E.D.; Pozharitskaya, O.N. The efficacy of two methods for extracting fucoidan from frozen Arctic algae thalli: Chemical composition, kinetic study and process optimization. *J. Appl. Phycol.* **2024**, *36*, 1413–1432. [CrossRef]
50. Ivanova, J.G.; Toshkova-Yotova, T.S.; Toshkova, R.A.; Deleva, V.R.; Georgieva, A.K.; Gigova, L.G. Antioxidant and anticancer potential of extracellular polysaccharide from *Porphyridium aerugineum* (Rhodophyta). *Fermentation* **2024**, *10*, 259. [CrossRef]
51. Lahrsen, E.; Schoenfeld, A.K.; Alban, S. Size-dependent pharmacological activities of differently degraded fucoidan fractions from *Fucus vesiculosus*. *Carbohydr. Polym.* **2018**, *189*, 162–168. [CrossRef]
52. Rajauria, G.; Ravindran, R.; Garcia-Vaquero, M.; Rai, D.K.; Sweeney, T.; O'Doherty, J. Purification and molecular characterization of fucoidan isolated from *Ascophyllum nodosum* brown seaweed grown in Ireland. *Mar. Drugs* **2023**, *21*, 315. [CrossRef]
53. Hans, N.; Pattnaik, F.; Malik, A.; Naik, S. Comparison of different green extraction techniques and their influence on chemical characteristics of sulfated polysaccharide (fucoidan) from *Padina tetrastromatica* and *Turbinaria conoides*. *Algal Res.* **2023**, *74*, 103199. [CrossRef]
54. Marinho, G.S.; Sørensen, A.D.M.; Safafar, H.; Pedersen, A.H.; Holdt, S.L. Antioxidant content and activity of the seaweed *Saccharina latissima*: A seasonal perspective. *J. Appl. Phycol.* **2019**, *31*, 1343–1354. [CrossRef]
55. Atashrazm, F.; Lowenthal, R.M.; Woods, G.M.; Holloway, A.F.; Dickinson, J.L. Fucoidan and cancer: A multifunctional molecule with anti-tumor potential. *Mar. Drugs* **2015**, *13*, 2327–2346. [CrossRef] [PubMed]
56. Zhurishkina, E.V.; Stepanov, S.I.; Ayrapetyan, O.N.; Skorik, Y.A.; Vlasova, E.N.; Kruchina-Bogdanov, I.V.; Lebedev, D.V.; Kulminskaya, A.A.; Lapina, I.M. The effect of polydisperse fucoidans from *Fucus vesiculosus* on Hep G2 and Chang liver cells. *Bioact. Carbohydr. Diet. Fibre* **2020**, *21*, 100209. [CrossRef]
57. Cabral, E.M.; Mondala, J.R.; Oliveira, M.; Przyborska, J.; Fitzpatrick, S.; Rai, D.K.; Sivagnanam, S.P.; Garcia-Vaquero, M.; O'Shea, D.; Devereux, M.; et al. Influence of molecular weight fractionation on the antimicrobial and anticancer properties of a fucoidan rich-extract from the macroalgae *Fucus vesiculosus*. *Int. J. Biol. Macromol.* **2021**, *186*, 994–1002. [CrossRef]
58. Mathew, L.; Burney, M.; Gaikwad, A.; Nyshadham, P.; Nugent, E.K.; Gonzalez, A.; Smith, J.A. Preclinical evaluation of safety of fucoidan extracts from *Undaria pinnatifida* and *Fucus vesiculosus* for use in cancer treatment. *Integr. Cancer Ther.* **2017**, *16*, 572–584. [CrossRef]
59. Xia, X.; Wang, Y.; Shao, Y.; Xu, J.; Liang, B.; Liu, W.; Zheng, J.; Li, C.; Guan, H.; Wang, S.; et al. Marine sulfated polysaccharide PMGS synergizes with paclitaxel in inhibiting cervical cancer in vitro. *Mar. Drugs* **2023**, *21*, 259. [CrossRef]
60. Alboofetileh, M.; Rezaei, M.; Tabarsa, M.; You, S. Bioactivities of *Nizamuddinia zanardinii* sulfated polysaccharides extracted by enzyme, ultrasound and enzyme-ultrasound methods. *J. Food Sci. Technol.* **2019**, *56*, 1212–1220. [CrossRef]
61. Zhao, Y.M.; Wang, J.; Wu, Z.G.; Yang, J.M.; Li, W.; Shen, L.X. Extraction, purification and anti-proliferative activities of polysaccharides from *Lentinus edodes*. *Int. J. Biol. Macromol.* **2016**, *93*, 136–144. [CrossRef]
62. Harnedy, P.A.; FitzGerald, R.J. Extraction of protein from the macroalga *Palmaria palmata*. *LWT-Food Sci. Technol.* **2013**, *51*, 375–382. [CrossRef]
63. Garcia-Vaquero, M.; Ravindran, R.; Walsh, O.; O'Doherty, J.; Jaiswal, A.K.; Tiwari, B.K.; Rajauria, G. Evaluation of ultrasound, microwave, ultrasound–microwave, hydrothermal and high pressure assisted extraction technologies for the recovery of phytochemicals and antioxidants from brown macroalgae. *Mar. Drugs* **2021**, *19*, 309. [CrossRef]
64. Athukorala, Y.; Ahn, G.N.; Jee, Y.H.; Kim, G.Y.; Kim, S.H.; Ha, J.H.; Kang, J.S.; Lee, K.W.; Jeon, Y.J. Antiproliferative activity of sulfated polysaccharide isolated from an enzymatic digest of *Ecklonia cava* on the U-937 cell line. *J. Appl. Phycol.* **2009**, *21*, 307–314. [CrossRef]
65. Shao, P.; Chen, X.; Sun, P. Chemical characterization, antioxidant and antitumor activity of sulfated polysaccharide from *Sargassum horneri*. *Carbohydr. Polym.* **2014**, *105*, 260–269. [CrossRef] [PubMed]
66. Jose, G.M.; Kurup, G.M. Sulfated polysaccharides from *Padina tetrastromatica* arrest cell cycle, prevent metastasis and downregulate angiogenic mediators in HeLa cells. *Bioact. Carbohydr. Diet. Fibre* **2017**, *12*, 7–13. [CrossRef]
67. Zhao, S.; Tang, Y.; Wang, R.; Najafi, M. Mechanisms of cancer cell death induction by paclitaxel: An updated review. *Apoptosis* **2022**, *27*, 647–667. [CrossRef]
68. Asnaashari, S.; Amjad, E.; Sokouti, B. Synergistic effects of flavonoids and paclitaxel in cancer treatment: A systematic review. *Cancer Cell Int.* **2023**, *23*, 211. [CrossRef]

69. Panji, M.; Behmard, V.; Zare, Z.; Malekpour, M.; Nejadbiglari, H.; Yavari, S.; Nayerpour Dizaj, T.; Safaeian, A.; Bakhshi, A.; Abazari, O.; et al. Synergistic effects of green tea extract and paclitaxel in the induction of mitochondrial apoptosis in ovarian cancer cell lines. *Gene* **2021**, *787*, 145638. [CrossRef]
70. Zhang, Z.; Teruya, K.; Yoshida, T.; Eto, H.; Shirahata, S. Fucoidan extract enhances the anti-cancer activity of chemotherapeutic agents in MDA-MB-231 and MCF-7 breast cancer cells. *Mar. Drugs* **2013**, *11*, 81–98. [CrossRef]
71. Abudabbus, A.; Badmus, J.A.; Shalaweh, S.; Bauer, R.; Hiss, D. Effects of fucoidan and chemotherapeutic agent combinations on malignant and non-malignant breast cell lines. *Curr. Pharm. Biotechnol.* **2017**, *18*, 748–757. [CrossRef]
72. Thakur, V.; Lu, J.; Roscilli, G.; Aurisicchio, L.; Cappelletti, M.; Pavoni, E.; White, W.L.; Bedogni, B. The natural compound fucoidan from New Zealand *Undaria pinnatifida* synergizes with the ERBB inhibitor lapatinib enhancing melanoma growth inhibition. *Oncotarget* **2017**, *8*, 17887. [CrossRef]
73. Blaszczak, W.; Lach, M.S.; Barczak, W.; Suchorska, W.M. Fucoidan exerts anticancer effects against head and neck squamous cell carcinoma in vitro. *Molecules* **2018**, *23*, 3302. [CrossRef]
74. Kohen, R.; Nyska, A. Invited review: Oxidation of biological systems: Oxidative stress phenomena, antioxidants, redox reactions, and methods for their quantification. *Toxicol. Pathol.* **2002**, *30*, 620–650. [CrossRef] [PubMed]
75. Usov, A.I.; Smirnova, G.P.; Klochkova, N.G. Polysaccharides of algae: 55. Polysaccharide composition of several brown algae from Kamchatka. *Russ. J. Bioorg. Chem.* **2001**, *27*, 395–399. [CrossRef] [PubMed]
76. Dische, Z.; Shettles, L.B.; Osnos, M. New specific color reactions of hexoses and spectrophotometric micro-metods for their determination. *Arch. Biochem.* **1949**, *22*, 169–184. [PubMed]
77. Silvestri, L.J.; Hurst, R.E.; Simpson, L.; Settine, J.M. Analysis of sulfate in complex carbohydrates. *Anal. Biochem.* **1982**, *123*, 303–309. [CrossRef] [PubMed]
78. Scott, R.W. Colorimetric determination of hexuronic acids in plant materials. *Anal. Chem.* **1979**, *51*, 936–941. [CrossRef]
79. Obluchinskaya, E.D.; Voskoboinikov, G.M.; Galynkin, V.A. Contents of alginic acid and fucoidan in Fucus algae of the Barents Sea. *Appl. Biochem. Microbiol.* **2002**, *38*, 186–188. [CrossRef]
80. Uribe, E.; Pardo-Orellana, C.M.; Vega-Gálvez, A.; Ah-Hen, K.S.; Pastén, A.; García, V.; Aubourg, S.P. Effect of drying methods on bioactive compounds, nutritional, antioxidant, and antidiabetic potential of brown alga *Durvillaea antarctica*. *Dry. Technol.* **2020**, *38*, 1915–1928. [CrossRef]
81. Gómez-Ordóñez, E.; Jiménez-Escrig, A.; Rupérez, P. Molecular weight distribution of polysaccharides from edible seaweeds by high-performance size-exclusion chromatography (HPSEC). *Talanta* **2012**, *93*, 153–159. [CrossRef]
82. Rodríguez-Jasso, R.M.; Mussatto, S.I.; Pastrana, L.; Aguilar, C.N.; Teixeira, J.A. Extraction of sulfated polysaccharides by autohydrolysis of brown seaweed *Fucus vesiculosus*. *J. Appl. Phycol.* **2013**, *25*, 31–39. [CrossRef]
83. Bolanos de la Torre, A.; Henderson, T.; Nigam, P.; Owusu-Apenten, R. A universally calibrated microplate ferric reducing antioxidant power (FRAP) assay for foods and applications to Manuka honey. *Food Chem.* **2015**, *174*, 119–123. [CrossRef]
84. Johnson, S.; Nguyen, V.; Coder, D. Assessment of cell viability. *Curr. Protoc. Cytom.* **2013**, *64*, 9.2.1–9.2.26. [CrossRef] [PubMed]
85. Giliano, N.Y.; Noskin, L.A.; Zhurishkina, E.V.; Stepanov, S.I.; Ibatullin, F.M.; Torshin, B.I.; Yakunina, E.B.; Alchinova, I.B. The combination of low doses of glucosamine D and 2-DG enhances the cytotoxic effect in human tumor cells in culture. *Pathol. Physiol. Exp. Ther.* **2019**, *63*, 41–49. [CrossRef]
86. van Meerloo, J.; Kaspers, G.J.L.; Cloos, J. Cell Sensitivity Assays: The MTT Assay. In *Cancer Cell Culture*; Methods in Molecular Biology; Cree, I., Ed.; Humana Press: Totowa, NJ, USA, 2011; Volume 731, pp. 237–245. [CrossRef]
87. Sridhar, K.; Charles, A.L. In vitro antioxidant activity of Kyoho grape extracts in DPPH• and ABTS• assays: Estimation methods for EC50 using advanced statistical programs. *Food Chem.* **2018**, *275*, 41–49. [CrossRef] [PubMed]
88. Schrader, C.; Boehm, A.; Reiche, A.; Diet, A.; Mozet, C.; Wichmann, G. Combined effects of lapatinib and cisplatin on colony formation of head and neck squamous cell carcinoma. *Anticancer Res.* **2012**, *32*, 3191–3199.

marine drugs

MDPI

Article

Optimization of Nanoencapsulation of *Codium tomentosum* Extract and Its Potential Application in Yogurt Fortification

Micaela Costa [1], Cristina Soares [1,*], Aurora Silva [1,2], Maria Fátima Barroso [1], Pedro Simões [3], Mariana Ferreira [4], Paula Gameiro [4], Clara Grosso [1,*] and Cristina Delerue-Matos [1]

[1] REQUIMTE/LAQV, Instituto Superior de Engenharia do Porto, Instituto Politécnico do Porto, Rua Dr. António Bernardino de Almeida 431, 4249-015 Porto, Portugal; 1200125@isep.ipp.pt (M.C.); mass@isep.ipp.pt (A.S.); mfb@isep.ipp.pt (M.F.B.); cmm@isep.ipp.pt (C.D.-M.)
[2] Department of Analytical Chemistry and Food Science, Nutrition and Food Group (NuFoG), Instituto de Agroecoloxía e Alimentación (IAA)—CITEXVI, Universidade de Vigo, 36310 Vigo, Spain
[3] LAQV, REQUIMTE, Departamento de Química, Faculdade de Ciências e Tecnologia, Universidade NOVA de Lisboa, Quinta da Torre, 2829-516 Caparica, Portugal; pcs@fct.unl.pt
[4] LAQV, REQUIMTE, Departamento de Química e Bioquímica, Faculdade de Ciências da Universidade do Porto, Rua do Campo Alegre, 4169-007 Porto, Portugal; mariana.ferreira@fc.up.pt (M.F.); agsantos@fc.up.pt (P.G.)
* Correspondence: cds@isep.ipp.pt (C.S.); claragrosso@graq.isep.ipp.pt (C.G.)

Abstract: Marine macroalgae are excellent sources of bioactive compounds recognized by their pharmaceutical and biomedical potential. A subcritical water extraction (SWE) was applied to the macroalga *Codium tomentosum*, and the extract was used to prepare phytosomes. A Box–Behnken design was applied to optimize the entrapment efficiency. These phytosomes were further modified with DSPE-PEG (2000)-maleimide and apolipoprotein E and characterized by dynamic light scattering, UV spectrophotometry, octanol/water partition coefficient, differential scanning calorimetry, and Fourier transform infrared spectroscopy. As proof of concept, prototypes of functional food tailored to the elderly were produced. Yogurts were fortified with seaweed extract or phytosomes, and physicochemical properties and proximal composition (pH, acidity, syneresis, moisture, peroxides, proteins, total lipids, sugar content, ash, and mineral composition) were analyzed. The antioxidant and the inhibition capacity of two brain enzymes, cholinesterases (AChE and BuChE), involved in the pathogenesis of Alzheimer's disease, were also evaluated in the final prototypes. Despite their unappealing sensory characteristics, the results are promising for integrating marine extracts with potential neuroprotective effects into functional foods.

Keywords: Box–Behnken design; subcritical water extraction; phytosomes; seaweeds; food fortification

1. Introduction

Due to the increase in life expectancy, promoting active aging is crucial in the 21st century [1]. Therefore, searching for new neuroprotective drugs is urgent. Alzheimer's disease (AD) is the most prevalent neurodegenerative disorder, followed by Parkinson's disease (PD) [2]. Most people diagnosed are 60 years old or older. For people aged between 65 and 69, around 2 in every 100 people have dementia, with AD being the most common form. A person's risk then increases as they age, roughly doubling every five years [3]. Regarding PD, only 5 to 10 percent of people with this disease are diagnosed before the age of 50 [4].

Biris-Dorhoi [5] has reported a considerable variety of bioactive compounds identified in seaweed that may help prevent and treat many diseases. Seaweed consumption has been associated with a lower incidence of different chronic diseases, such as cancer, diabetes, neurodegenerative diseases, obesity-related disorders, and metabolic syndrome. Regarding specifically the neuroprotective activity of seaweeds, a broad class of compounds, such as polysaccharides, proteins, lipids, pigments, and polyphenols, isolated from macroalgae, have shown neuroprotective effects through mechanisms such as enzyme modulation or protection against amyloid-β (Aβ) or Tau-induced toxicity [6,7]. In AD patients, the degeneration of central cholinergic neurons reduces choline acetyltransferase (ChAT) activity, decreasing acetylcholine (Ach) synthesis. At the same time, increased cholinesterase activity accelerates Ach breakdown, worsening this neurotransmitter deficiency. In AD, AChE activity drops by up to 45%, but BuChE activity can double, making this cholinesterase a more significant target in the later stages of the disease. Thus, enhancing ChAT activity and reducing AChE and BuChE functions has become a critical strategy in AD treatment. Likewise, disrupting the balance between α-secretase and non-α-secretase pathways leads to increased BACE1 activity, resulting in Aβ oligomers and plaque accumulation, making BACE1 activity a critical therapeutic target in the AD treatment. Although tau protein hyperphosphorylation is an important therapeutic target for AD, only a few compounds have been identified that can effectively target tau protein [8].

The most promising result from seaweeds to date was achieved with sodium oligomannate, a mixture of oligosaccharides isolated from the marine algae *Ecklonia kurome* Okamura. Clinical trials have shown that it is safe and effective in treating mild-to-moderate AD, leading to its approval by the National Medical Products Administration (NMPA) of China in 2019 [9,10]. Recent studies suggest its neuroprotective effects are mediated through the microbiota–microglia–amyloid axis. It modulates gut microbiota while directly inhibiting Aβ fibril formation and neuroinflammation. Despite its therapeutic potential, the absorption, distribution, metabolism, and excretion (ADME) profile of sodium oligomannate remains poorly understood due to its complex high-molecular-weight and highly polar carbohydrate structure. Further research is necessary to elucidate its systemic bioavailability, brain penetration, and precise mechanisms of action in neurodegenerative diseases [9,11].

In addition, Peñalver et al. [12] described several studies reporting that incorporating seaweed and/or seaweed extracts into food products improves properties such as the shelf life, nutritional content, and textural and sensory aspects of the final products. However, some of these effects differ according to the seaweed species and the amount used in the formulation.

Codium tomentosum is a green macroalga with neuroprotective potential, as reported by Silva et al. [13], who have shown that several fractions obtained from the methanolic and dichloromethane extracts of *C. tomentosum* displayed neuroprotective activity in thrice-subcloned SH-SY5Y cells line exposed to the neurotoxin 6-hydroxydopamine (6-OHDA). The authors also investigated which mechanisms were triggered by these fractions, concluding that they mitigated reactive oxygen species (ROS) generation, counteracted mitochondrial dysfunctions and DNA damage, and reduced caspase-3 activity. Recently, a fraction obtained by subcritical water extraction (SWE) in the range of 190–250 °C was tested against several brain enzymes involved in the etiology of neurodegenerative and neuropsychiatric disorders, namely, cholinesterases, monoamine oxidase A and B and tyrosinase, revealing moderate inhibition (IC_{50} [AChE] = 239.8 μg/mL, IC_{50} [BuChE] = 430.1 μg/mL, IC_{50} [MAO-A] = 181.2 μg/mL, IC_{50} [MAO-B] = 422.5 μg/mL, and IC_{50} [tyrosinase] = 15.3 μg/mL). The same fraction was also demonstrated to be a strong superoxide radical anion ($O_2^{\bullet-}$) and nitric oxide radical ($^{\bullet}NO$) scavenger (IC_{50} = 85.7 μg/mL and 254.2 μg/mL, respectively) [14].

To counteract the low absorption of bioactive phytocompounds, nanosized drug delivery systems like phytosomes can enhance their penetration across biological barriers, such as the blood–brain barrier (BBB), thereby promoting their delivery to the desired target [15]. Phytosomes are innovative lipid-based nanocarriers with liposome-related structures but with some additional advantages. While hydrophilic biomolecules are just entrapped in the aqueous core of liposomes without chemical bonds being formed, in phytosomes, H-bonds are established between the extracts and the phosphate group of phospholipids, increasing their stability [15]. This approach has been successfully applied to encapsulate several plant-derived bioactive compounds [16].

While using natural extracts in functional food development is growing, incorporating seaweed or seaweed extracts remains problematic—mainly due to their strong sensory characteristics and limited consumer knowledge of their potential health benefits. Furthermore, regulatory requirements for substantiating health claims often necessitate preclinical or clinical evidence, adding complexity to commercialization efforts [17]. Luckily, new milk products have been produced by adding seaweed extracts and the impact on the product's final appearance has been evaluated. Roohinejad et al. [18] reported that the greenness and yellowing of fortified milk samples increased by adding ethanolic extracts prepared from seaweed also provided antioxidant functionality. Moreover, the type or concentration of seaweed extract did not influence quality parameters, e.g., microbiology. The sensory evaluation showed that the extract was accepted as a functional ingredient in milk. Seaweed extracts were found to be stable in milk, showing that their addition can improve certain milk qualities and shelf life characteristics.

This work aimed to extend the study developed by Soares et al. on the assessment of the bioactivities displayed by different subcritical water extraction (SWE) fractions of *C. tomentosum* [14], by designing and characterizing phytosomes containing the most active fraction, herein called *C. tomentosum* extract (CtE), to incorporate it into a neuroprotective functional food product—yogurt—targeted at senior citizens, who are at increased risk for neurodegenerative and neuropsychiatric disorders. The CtE (obtained through SWE at 190–250 °C, 100 bar) is abundant in phenolic compounds and Maillard reaction products (MRPs) [14]. Both classes of compounds are known for their antioxidant and neuroprotective properties [19–21], However, due to the high diversity of MRPs, some MRPs, such as acrylamide, toxic advanced glycation end products (TAGEs), and heterocyclic amines, have been implicated in the development of several diseases [22–24].

The phytosomes that were generated underwent characterization to identify key characteristics like size and composition. Furthermore, the nutritional profile of the food prototype, along with its antioxidant (DPPH$^{\bullet}$ and ABTS$^{\bullet+}$ scavenging activities and oxygen radical absorbance capacity (ORAC) assay) and neuroprotective (AChE and BuChE inhibition) properties, was assessed as well.

2. Results and Discussion

2.1. Box–Behnken Design

The entrapment efficiency of CtE varied according to the set of conditions tested, ranging from 25.19% (*A*—1 h, *B*—42.5 °C and *C*—1:4) and 45.70% (*A*—2.5 h, *B*—25 °C and *C*—1:4; and *A*—1 h, *B*—60 °C and *C*—1:2.5) (Table S1).

A reduced cubic model was fitted to the experimental results, and the most significant parameters ($p < 0.05$) were A, C, AB, AC, BC, B^2, A^2B, and A^2C (Table S2, Figure 1). The resulting model equation (Equation (1)) was:

$$\begin{aligned} \textit{Entrapment efficiency}(\%) \\ &= 29.12782 + 4.76425A + 0.428789B - 9.71050C - 0.873397AB + 13.17704AC - 0.167143BC \\ &-0.406866A^2 + 0.014842B^2 + 0.148889A^2B - 2.31630A^2C \end{aligned} \quad (1)$$

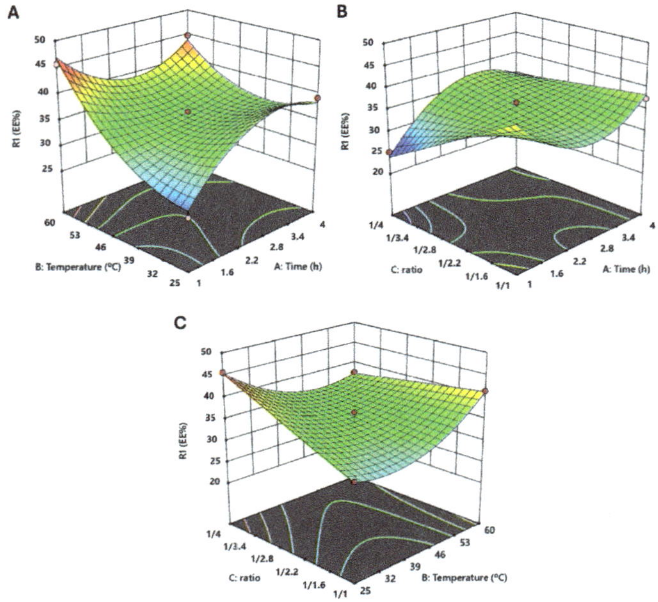

Figure 1. Three-dimensional surface graphics. (**A**)—Temperature vs. Time; (**B**)—Ratio vs. Time; (**C**)—Ratio vs. Temperature.

With the reduced cubic model, the calculated coefficients of determination (R^2), adjusted R^2, predicted R^2, and adeq precision were, respectively, 0.9666, 0.8832, 0.4041, and 12.1256. The model was significant (p = 0.0153), and the lack of fit was not significant (p = 0.4916) (Table S1). The diagnostic graphics (Figure S1) show a good fit of the model to the experimental results.

Two optimal conditions (Derringer's desirability function = 1.000) were retrieved from the model to obtain the highest % of complexation: condition 1 (A—1 h, B—59 °C, and C—1:1) and condition 2 (A—4 h, B—25 °C, and C—1:4), achieving a predicted value of 58.92% and 54.65%, respectively. At these optimal conditions, experimental values obtained were 61.76 ± 10.11% (n = 7) and 57.63 ± 10.65% (n = 7), respectively, showing that the model predictions were quite close to the actual values.

The optimal conditions for preparing phytosomes, as determined from the model, were consistent with those reported in previous studies [25–27]. Telange et al. [25] tested different conditions to prepare phytossomal complexes with apigenin, namely, different molar ratios of apigenin and phospholipid (1:1, 1:2, and 1:3) and temperatures (40, 50, and 60 °C). The reaction occurred during 2 h in a mixture of 1, 4–dioxane:methanol (14:6). A full-factorial design (3^2) was applied, revealing that a ratio = 1:2, and T = 60 °C were the optimal conditions to achieve the highest complex formation (93.7%). In another study, ginger or ginger plus rosehip and phosphatidylcholine (PC) were weighed in different ratios, dissolved in ethanol, and refluxed at 60 °C for 2 h. To determine the encapsulation efficiency of the phytosomal formulation, the non-entrapped free 6-gingerol and β-carotene were separated from the phytosomal complex by ultracentrifugation. The encapsulation efficiency of 6-gingerol and β-carotene in all preparations was between 83.3% and 94.3%. Although phytosomes containing 0.9 of ginger extract:0.1 of rosehip extract: 1 of PC displayed lower particle sizes (193.72 nm), phytosomes prepared with a ratio of 0.5:0.5:1 were chosen for further assays due to their strongest anti-inflammatory and antioxidant effects [26]. On the other hand, using room temperature was favorable for producing phytosomes with *Diospyros kaki* L. acetonic extract (acetone:water (80:20, v/v)) [27]. The authors mixed the extract with PC in a molar ratio of 1:1 or 1:2, in ethanol, for 2 h at 25 °C, obtaining entrapment efficiencies above 90%.

2.2. Characterization of Phytosomes

The phytosomes were functionalized before characterization. The DSPE-PEG (2000) peptide was employed to enhance the targeting specificity of the formulated nanoparticles, helping them evade digestive processes and immune responses [28], while ApoE was used to guide the nanoparticles to the BBB [15].

Concerning their size and polydispersity index (PDI), phytosomes produced through condition 1 (*A*—1 h, *B*—59 °C, and *C*—1:1) showed to be lower and less dispersed than those produced through condition 2 (*A*—4 h, *B*—25 °C, and *C*—1:4)—245.76 ± 49.00 nm and PDI = 0.26 ± 0.06 vs. 261.02 ± 70.46 nm and PDI = 0.32 ± 0.02, respectively. Therefore, condition 1 was selected for further characterization. This behavior is in line with the results reported by Direito et al. [27] who observed that phytosomes prepared with a ratio of 1:2 (extract:PC) tended to agglomerate more than those prepared using a ratio of 1:1 (193.3 nm and PDI = 0.347 vs. 177.1 nm and PDI = 0.184, respectively).

The study of the solubility in water and in n-octanol of the CtE and of the phytosomes produced showed that the isolated extract had high aqueous solubility (95%) and low solubility in n-octanol (5%), which would be expected due to the highly aqueous character of the extract. On the other hand, the complexation of the extract with PC conferred an amorphous character to the system and moderated its lipophilic character. This resulted in improved solubility in n-octanol and dissolution profile. This way, an increase in lipophilicity to 28% was observed for the phytosomes, resulting in a Kow = 0.382. These results align with previous studies reporting that phyto-phospholipid complexes have better lipophilicity and hydrophilicity than their active constituents [29,30]. Typically, these complexes demonstrate enhanced lipophilicity, which offers a significant advantage for the food and pharmaceutical industries in delivering polar compounds [29,30].

The UV spectra of the CtE and phytosomes were analyzed in the 200–700 nm range. As shown in Figure 2, the characteristic absorption peak of the CtE (280 nm) remained present in the phytosome, suggesting that weak physical interactions between the extract and PC occurred during the formation of the complex.

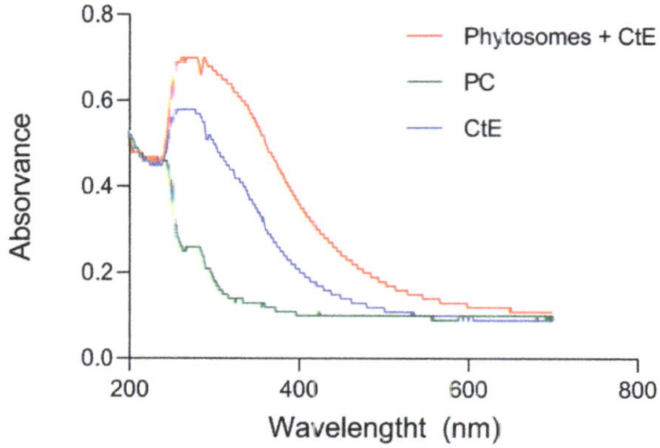

Figure 2. Spectra of samples in the UV and the visible spectrum [Blue] CtE; [Green] PC; [Red] Phytosomes containing CtE.

The thermograms of CtE, PC, and phytosome are represented in Figure 3. The extract exhibited a sharp endothermic peak at 377.5 °C corresponding to the sample melting. PC presented three low-intensity peaks (249.5, 355.8, and 391.4 °C) related to the fusion of the polar region and the melting of the hydrophobic tails of the phospholipids [30,31]. The phytosomal complex presents a new peak, completely different from those observed in the individual constituents of very low intensity at 462.5 °C, which could be related to the appearance of new hydrogen bonds between the -OH groups of the phenolic rings of the CtE with the phospholipid [30,31].

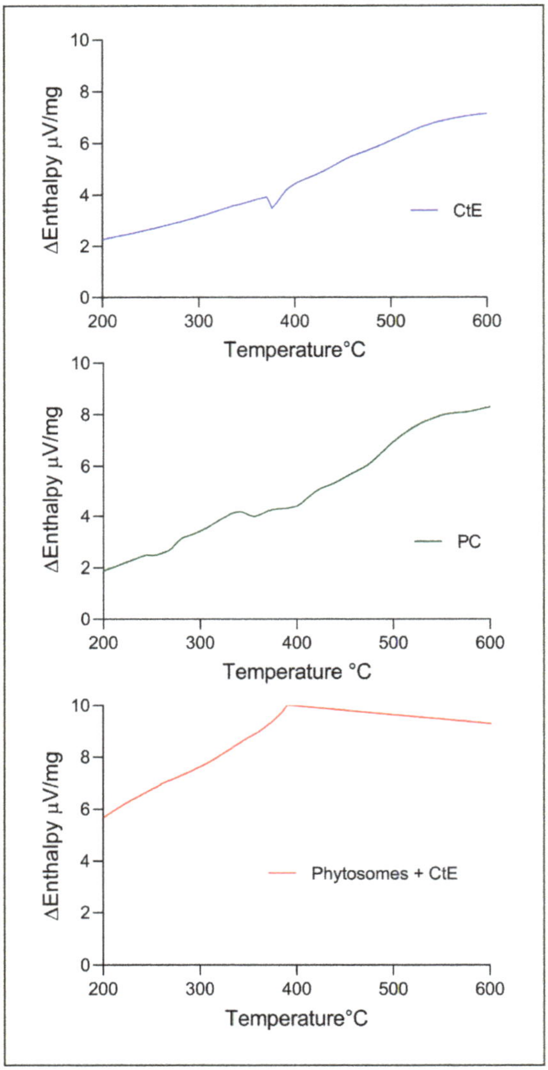

Figure 3. Differential scanning calorimetry spectra of samples: [Blue] CtE; [Green] PC; [Red] phytosomes with CtE.

The possible interaction between the CtE and PC in the phytosome was studied by FTIR (Figure 4). The peaks at 3416.62, 3369.38, and 3289.81 cm^{-1} represent hydroxyl (OH) stretching in the IR region of CtE, L-α-phosphatidylcholine, and the phytosome complex, respectively (Figure 4). The absorption signals at 2922.01 cm^{-1} of the CtE and 2854.92 cm^{-1} of the complex represent the characteristic C-H stretching of the long chain of fatty acids, and the peaks at 1664.39 cm^{-1} of the CtE and 1667.26 cm^{-1} of the complex represent the

C=O stretching, also alluding to the existence of aromaticity [32]. In the case of the CtE, a peak appears at 1079.99 cm^{-1} for the ether group (C-O-C) [32].

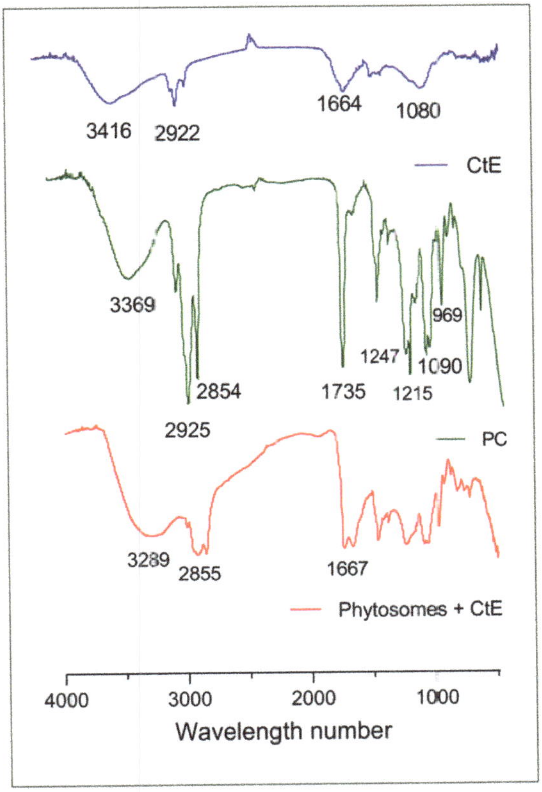

Figure 4. Fourier transform infrared spectroscopy of samples: [Blue] CtE; [Green] PC; [Red] phytosomes with CtE.

The FTIR spectrum of PC (Figure 4) marked the presence of multiple characteristic absorption signals: at 2925.81 and 2854.71 cm^{-1}, representing the characteristic C-H elongation band of the long fatty acid chain; at 1735.17 cm^{-1}, a characteristic of the carbonyl stretching of the fatty acid ester; at 1247.26 and 1215.94 cm^{-1}, corresponding to P=O stretching band (a characteristic of the phosphate functional group); at 1090.92 cm^{-1}, representing P-O-C elongation; and at 969.12 cm^{-1}, due to N-+$(CH_3)_3$ stretching [31–33].

No new significant peaks were observed in the complex (Figure 4). However, the C=O peak of the CtE was shifted in the complex to higher wavelengths, and there was also a clear absorption band at the 1234.51 cm^{-1} characteristic, in the case of complexes, of strong C–O bonds, proving the formation of new bonds. There was also a broadening of the characteristic phenolic band (OH) caused by the formation of hydrogen bonds, indicating that the phytosome formulation was successful [30].

2.3. Characterization of Fortified Yogurt

An initial sensory screening was conducted to eliminate yogurt formulations with undesirable organoleptic attributes. This step allowed us to focus on subsequent analyses (physicochemical, antioxidant, and bioavailability) of the most acceptable formulations in terms of taste, texture, and appearance.

2.3.1. Sensorial Analysis and Selection of Optimal Formulations for Further Analysis

Visual evaluation of yogurt samples (Figure 5) revealed that both the concentration and form of CtE significantly influenced surface texture, color, and sedimentation patterns. At low CtE concentrations (0.005–0.01%), yogurts maintained a smooth, uniform surface and minimal sedimentation, comparable to the control. However, at ≥0.05% CtE, surface cracking, gel destabilization, and visible sedimentation became evident, particularly at 0.2%, likely due to the interference of the extract's high polysaccharide and mineral content with the yogurt matrix [34]. Additionally, sedimentation was increasingly visible at higher concentrations, with dark deposits accumulating at the bottom of the containers. Yogurts containing more than 0.05% CtE fraction exhibited a yellowish, unappealing hue, similar to findings from previous studies on seaweed extract incorporation in yogurt [35].

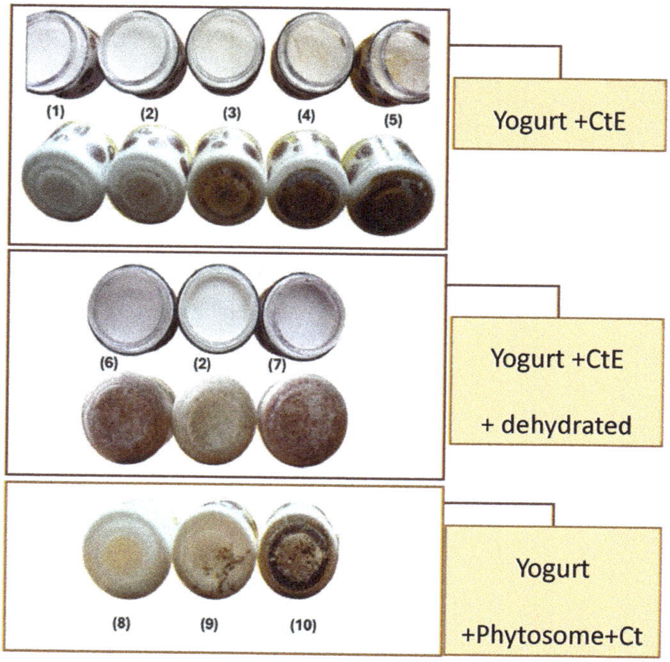

Figure 5. Visual appearance and sedimentation patterns of yogurts formulated with varying concentrations of CtE and phytosome-encapsulated CtE. Top section: Yogurts with 0.005% (1), 0.01% (2), 0.05% (3), 0.10% (4), and 0.2% (5) CtE, showing increasing surface cracking and instability at higher concentrations. Middle section: Yogurts with 0.01% CtE with (6) and without (2) dehydrated fruit and 0.15% CtE with dehydrated fruit (7), highlighting the masking effect of fruit on sedimentation. Bottom section: Yogurts with 0.01% (8) and 0.15% (9) CtE in phytosomes, as well as 0.15% unencapsulated CtE (10), demonstrating the effectiveness of phytosome encapsulation in reducing sedimentation at lower concentrations.

To counter these effects, two strategies were tested: phytosome encapsulation and dehydrated fruit addition. Phytosome encapsulation improved CtE dispersion and phase stability, particularly at 0.01%, where yogurts exhibited a homogeneous structure with minimal sedimentation. Even at 0.15% CtE, encapsulated samples showed reduced aggregation compared to their unencapsulated counterparts, confirming the technique's effectiveness [35–37]. Nevertheless, formulations with 0.15% CtE showed structural instability, indicating the potential need for hydrocolloids or stabilizers in future developments.

Dehydrated blackberry or raspberry enhanced visual appeal by masking sedimentation, likely due to particle coverage, which may also increase consumer acceptability [38]. Sensory analysis showed that CtE concentrations $\geq$ 0.10% increased acidity, partially balanced by fruit addition, while aroma remained consistent with standard yogurt.

Other studies using higher seaweed concentrations reported strong seaweed flavor and low flavor quality (e.g., 0.5% *Undaria pinnatifida* or *Saccharina latissima*) [39]. In contrast, our formulations using $\leq$0.15% CtE demonstrated moderate sensory impact and improved integration when paired with phytosomes or fruit. However, 0.15% CtE, samples still showed structural instability, suggesting the potential need for hydrocolloids or stabilizers.

Based on appearance, flavor, and texture, the following formulations were selected for further analysis: control yogurt (0% CtE); 0.01% CtE (unencapsulated); 0.01% CtE in phytosomes; 0.01% CtE + dehydrated fruit; 0.15% CtE; and 0.15% CtE + dehydrated fruit.

2.3.2. Inhibition Capacity of Brain Enzymes Cholinesterases (AChE and BuChE)

The control sample (yogurt without CtE) showed no or weak inhibition of cholinesterases. This result is in accordance with the study performed by Ramadan et al. [40]. These authors investigated the influence of three different treatments to reverse the neurotoxicity induced by $AlCl_3$ in rats: plain yogurt, microcapsules of triple omega 3-6-9, and fortified yogurt with those microcapsules. They concluded that treatments with fortified yogurt and microcapsules were more effective than plain yogurt in reverting the increase in AChE and BuChE activity promoted by $AlCl_3$.

Low AChE and BuChE inhibition percentages were obtained due to the low concentration of Cte or phytosomes incorporated in the yogurts (Figure 6). The best results (30% AChE inhibition) were shown in the yogurt containing 0.15% of CtE (4 mg/mL of sample) (Figure 6).

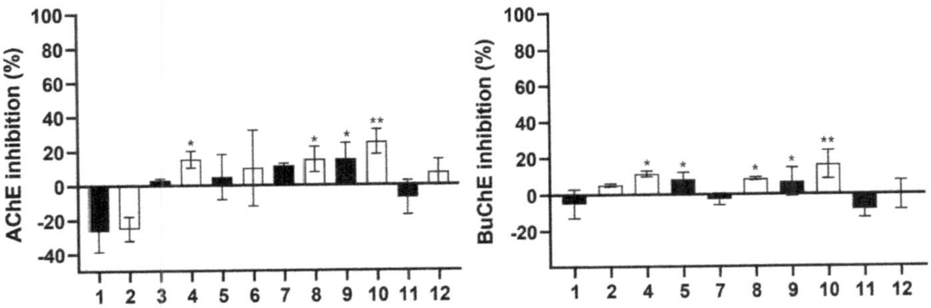

Figure 6. AChE and BuChE inhibition. 1—Control yogurt (2 mg/mL); 2—Control yogurt (4 mg/mL); 3—Yogurt with phytosomes 0.01% (2 mg/mL); 4—Yogurt with phytosomes 0.01% (4 mg/mL); 5—Yogurt with CtE 0.01% (2 mg/mL); 6—Yogurt with CtE 0.01% (4 mg/mL); 7—Yogurt with CtE 0.01%+ dehydrated fruit (2 mg/mL); 8—Yogurt with CtE 0.01%+ dehydrated fruit (4 mg/mL); 9—Yogurt with CtE 0.15% (2 mg/mL); 10—Yogurt with CtE 0.15% (4 mg/mL); 11—Yogurt with CtE 0.15%+ dehydrated fruit (2 mg/mL); 12—Yogurt with CtE 0.15%+ dehydrated fruit (4 mg/mL). Bars represent mean values, with significance indicated by * and ** for $p < 0.05$, representing samples that differ significantly from others

The percentages of inhibition obtained are relatively low due to the yogurt manufacturing integrating rather low percentages of the CtE and phytosomes. However, we have reported that the CtE shows a high percentage of inhibition of cholinesterases [14]. Therefore, by the cumulative effect, our results support that the possibility of achieving improved inhibition should not be discarded.

2.3.3. Antioxidant Activity

The prepared yogurts' radical scavenging ability was measured using the $ABTS^{\bullet+}$ and ORAC assays. The results are presented in Table 1.

Table 1. Antioxidant activity (ABTS and ORAC) of yogurt formulations containing CtE and phytosomes.

Samples	ABTS (mg TE/100 g)	ORAC (μmol TE/100 g)
Control (0%)	13.5 ± 0.3 [a]	62.1 ± 0.3 [a]
0.01% CtE	11.1 ± 0.1 [a]	118 ± 1 [b]
0.01% CtE + DF	24.2 ± 1.0 [c]	245 ± 1 [e]
0.15% CtE	18.4 ± 1.6 [b]	162 ± 3 [c]
0.15% CtE + DF	27.0 ± 0.7 [d]	167 ± 1 [d]
0.01% Phytosomes	12.9 ± 1.2 [a]	60.0 ± 0.1 [a]

Within columns, different letters correspond to significantly different values ($p < 0.05$).

Table 1 shows that the control yogurt had the lowest antioxidant activity (ABTS: 13.5 mg TE/100 g; ORAC: 62.1 μmol TE/100 g), providing a baseline. Yogurt containing 0.01% CtE in the phytosome form showed no significant improvement, suggesting a limited release of bioactives due to encapsulation. This may reflect strong interactions with yogurt components, stabilizing the formulation but limiting an immediate antioxidant action.

In contrast, adding 0.01% unencapsulated CtE markedly increased ORAC values (118 μmol TE/100 g), while ABTS remained like the control—implying assay sensitivity differences. When dehydrated fruit (DF) was added to this formulation, both ABTS (24.2 mg TE/100 g) and ORAC (245 μmol TE/100 g) increased significantly, suggesting a synergistic effect between fruit and seaweed-derived polyphenols. A higher CtE concentration (0.15%) further increased antioxidant values, especially ABTS (27.0 mg TE/100 g), though ORAC peaked at 0.01% CtE + DF.

Previous research has demonstrated the potential of seaweed extracts, such as those from *Ascophyllum nodosum* and *Fucus vesiculosus*, to enhance yogurt's antioxidant properties and shelf life. In a study where yogurts were formulated with 0.25% and 0.5% seaweed extracts, improvements in radical scavenging activity measured using the DPPH assay, lipid oxidation stability, and microbiological quality were observed over a 28-day storage period. The yogurt containing 0.5% *F. vesiculosus* extract exhibited a significantly higher radical scavenging activity ($p < 0.05$) compared to the control, reinforcing the role of seaweed bioactives in improving yogurt functionality [35].

2.3.4. pH, Titratable Acidity, and Peroxide Value

The pH, titratable acidity, and peroxide values of yogurt samples were evaluated during 7 days of storage at 4 °C to assess the impact of the CtE, phytosome encapsulation, and dehydrated fruit addition on yogurt stability over time. The results are presented in Table 2.

Initial pH (pH_0) values ranged from 4.26 to 4.40 ($p < 0.05$). The highest (4.40 ± 0.01) was observed in phytosome-encapsulated 0.01% CtE, suggesting delayed acidification. The lowest pH (4.26 ± 0.01) occurred in 0.01% CtE + DF, likely due to fruit-derived organic acids. These values are comparable to those in seaweed-fortified yogurts from previous studies [41].

By day 7 (pH_7), all samples showed a slight pH decline, with values ranging from 4.23 to 4.37 ($p < 0.05$). The control yogurt dropped from 4.36 to 4.31, showing a 1.2% reduction, while CtE- and phytosome-fortified samples exhibited smaller pH decreases (~0.7%), suggesting that phenolic compounds may inhibit bacterial metabolism and slow acidification [42,43]. The highest final pH (4.37 ± 0.01) remained in the phytosome sample, reinforcing its stabilizing effect on microbial activity. The lowest (4.23 ± 0.01) persisted in 0.01% CtE + DF, confirming accelerated acidification probably due to fruit sugars.

Table 2. Effect of seaweed extracts, dehydrated fruits, and phytosome encapsulation on pH, titratable acidity, and peroxide value in yogurt over 7 days at 4 °C.

Samples	pH_0	pH_7	TA_0 (g LA/100 g Yogurt)	TA_7 (g LA/100 g Yogurt)	PV_7 ($meqO_2$/100 g Yogurt)
Control (0%)	4.36 ± 0.01 ^{B,d}	4.31 ± 0.01 ^{A,d}	0.708 ± 0.003 ^{A,b}	0.850 ± 0.029 ^{B,b}	n.d.
0.01% CtE	4.37 ± 0.01 ^{A,d}	4.33 ± 0.01 ^{A,e}	0.683 ± 0.028 ^{A,b}	0.773 ± 0.089 ^{A,a,b}	0.0267 ± 0.0012 ^{b}
0.01% CtE + DF	4.26 ± 0.01 ^{B,a}	4.23 ± 0.01 ^{A,a}	0.820 ± 0.004 ^{B,c}	0.757 ± 0.022 ^{A,a,b}	0.0254 ± 0.0015 ^{b}
0.15% CtE	4.31 ± 0.01 ^{B,c}	4.29 ± 0.01 ^{A,c}	0.816 ± 0.001 ^{B,c}	0.801 ± 0.001 ^{A,b}	0.0418 ± 0.0033 ^{c}
0.15% CtE + DF	4.28 ± 0.01 ^{A,b}	4.24 ± 0.01 ^{B,b}	0.828 ± 0.001 ^{B,c}	0.800 ± 0.001 ^{A,b}	0.0483 ± 0.0044 ^{c}
0.01% Phytosomes	4.40 ± 0.01 ^{B,e}	4.37 ± 0.01 ^{A,f}	0.541 ± 0.002 ^{A,a}	0.679 ± 0.001 ^{B,a}	0.00635 ± 0.00032 ^{a}

0: initial time; 7: day 7; TA: titratable acidity; LA: lactic acid equivalents. Values are presented as mean ± standard deviation. Different lowercase letters in the same column indicate significant differences between samples ($p < 0.05$). Different uppercase letters in the same row indicate significant differences over time for pH and titratable acidity ($p < 0.05$).

Titratable acidity (TA_0) on day 0 ranged from 0.541 to 0.828 g lactic acid (LA)/100 g, with the lowest TA in the phytosome sample (0.541 ± 0.002 g LA/100 g) and the highest in 0.15% CtE + DF (0.828 ± 0.001 g LA/100 g, $p < 0.05$). After 7 days (TA_7), the control yogurt exhibited the highest acidity increase (0.850 ± 0.029 g LA/100 g, $p < 0.05$). CtE and DF-fortified samples ranged from 0.757 to 0.801 g LA/100 g, while the phytosome sample remained the lowest (0.679 ± 0.001 g LA/100 g, $p < 0.05$), confirming phytosome encapsulation mitigates acidification over time [37]. These values align with those observed in *Caulerpa racemosa*-fortified yogurts (0.64–0.85%) [41].

The decrease in pH and the increase in acidity over time resulted from the metabolism of lactic acid bacteria, including lactose hydrolysis and organic acid production [44]. Acidity values (0.541–0.850% lactic acid) remained within the Codex Alimentarius standard range (0.60–1.5%) [45].

Ghorbanzade et al. [37] evaluated pH and acidity changes in yogurt samples prepared with nano-encapsulated fish oil over 21 days at 4 °C and similarly observed that control yogurts exhibited the sharpest pH decline, while fortified samples showed slower acidification, consistent with our findings. Their study also confirmed that phytosome encapsulation helped regulate pH reduction and acidity increase, likely by moderating bacterial metabolism and acid production. Additionally, they reported that higher fat content contributed to increased acidity, possibly due to interactions with fermentation dynamics [37].

Lipid oxidation was assessed to evaluate the oxidative stability of the different yogurt formulations. Oxidation in dairy products can lead to off-flavors and reduced shelf life, making it a fundamental parameter for assessing yogurt quality [46].

Lipid oxidation was undetectable (n.d.) in the control yogurt on day 7, while fortified samples exhibited significant peroxide value (PV) increases ($p < 0.05$). The highest PV (0.0483 ± 0.0044 meq O_2/100 g) was found in 0.15% CtE + DF, indicating higher oxidative susceptibility at elevated extract concentrations. The lowest PV (0.00635 ± 0.00032 meq O_2/100 g, $p < 0.05$) in phytosome-fortified yogurt suggests that encapsulation significantly reduces lipid oxidation. Lipid peroxidation inhibition probably results from bioactive antioxidant activity (e.g., polyphenols in seaweed extracts) and membrane-stabilizing effects, which restrict oxygen penetration into lipid bilayers, slowing oxidation [47]. However, higher CtE concentrations increased oxidative susceptibility, likely due to the lipid content of algae (2.2 ± 0.1 g/100 g) [14], while nanoencapsulation effectively protected unsaturated fatty acids despite raising total lipid content [48].

Our findings align with previous studies on nanoencapsulation's role in preserving lipid stability. Ghorbanzade et al. [37] observed that peroxide values increased significantly in yogurts with unencapsulated fish oil. At the same time, nanoencapsulated samples maintained stable PV (~0.6 meq/kg) over 21 days, confirming encapsulation's protective barrier against oxidation.

These results confirm that phytosome encapsulation enhances oxidative stability, preserving unsaturated fatty acids and extending the shelf life of fortified dairy products.

2.3.5. Syneresis, Moisture, Total Solids, Organic, and Ash Contents in Yogurts

The physicochemical properties of the yogurt samples, including syneresis, moisture content, total solids, organic content, and ash percentage, are summarized in Table 3. Significant differences ($p < 0.05$) were observed among formulations, particularly in syneresis and total solids, which were influenced by the addition of CtE, dehydrated fruit (DF), and phytosome encapsulation.

Table 3. Physicochemical properties and proximate composition of yogurt samples with different formulations.

Samples	Syneresis (%)	Moisture (%)	Total Solids (%)	Organic Content (%)	Ash (%)
Control (0%)	19.8 ± 1.4 [a]	90.1 ± 0.1 [c]	9.92 ± 0.08 [a]	94.8 ± 0.2 [c]	5.20 ± 0.25 [a]
0.01% CtE	30.1 ± 2.4 [b]	90.4 ± 0.3 [c]	9.63 ± 0.30 [a]	94.1 ± 0.2 [b]	5.87 ± 0.24 [b]
0.01% CtE + DF	18.2 ± 0.7 [a]	87.9 ± 0.1 [a]	12.1 ± 0.1 [c]	92.6 ± 0.4 [a]	7.43 ± 0.38 [c]
0.15% CtE	52.5 ± 3.2 [d]	88.9 ± 0.1 [b]	11.1 ± 0.1 [b]	92.6 ± 0.2 [a]	7.38 ± 0.15 [c]
0.15% CtE + DF	39.6 ± 3.6 [c]	87.9 ± 0.1 [a]	12.1 ± 0.1 [c]	92.3 ± 0.3 [a]	7.73 ± 0.27 [c]
0.01% Phytosomes	17.2 ± 1.0 [a]	88.2 ± 0.1 [a]	11.8 ± 0.1 [c]	92.2 ± 0.1 [a]	7.82 ± 0.01 [c]

Values are presented as mean ± standard deviation. Different lowercase letters in the same column indicate significant differences between samples ($p < 0.05$).

Syneresis, a key indicator of whey separation and structural stability, varied significantly among samples ($p < 0.05$). The lowest values were observed in the control (19.8%), 0.01% CtE + DF (18.2%), and 0.01% Phytosome (17.2%), indicating better water retention and gel stability. In contrast, the highest syneresis occurred in 0.15% CtE (52.5%) and 0.15% CtE + DF (39.6%), suggesting that higher CtE concentrations disrupt the protein network, reducing water-holding capacity (WHC) and increasing whey separation [36].

These findings align with studies reporting that plant extracts can stabilize or weaken casein gels depending on concentration and protein interactions [49]. Additionally, phytosome encapsulation and increased total solids (via DF) enhanced WHC and reduced syneresis, likely due to emulsifier-stabilized water absorption and a reinforced protein matrix [36].

Moisture content significantly differed among formulations (87.9–90.4%, $p < 0.05$), with the lowest levels in dehydrated fruit-containing samples, likely due to the fruit's ability to absorb moisture from the yogurt, reducing overall water retention [50].

Total solids, which reflect the sum of organic and inorganic components, influence yogurt's nutritional density and texture. The lowest values were found in control (9.92%) and 0.01% CtE (9.63%). In comparison, the highest (11.8–12.1%, $p < 0.05$) were observed in CtE + DF and phytosome-containing samples, likely due to dehydrated fruit's fiber and sugar content, which also contributes to lower moisture content. These findings align with studies showing that fruit fortification increases dry matter, improving texture and reducing syneresis [51,52].

Organic content was the highest in control (94.8%) and slightly but significantly lower (92.2–94.1%) in fortified samples ($p < 0.05$), likely due to added mineral components from CtE and phytosomes.

Ash content, representing inorganic minerals, ranged from 5.20% to 7.82%, with the highest values in phytosome-containing samples. This reflects the mineral richness of seaweed extracts, especially in calcium, potassium, and magnesium [53].

2.3.6. Mineral Composition (Ca, K, Mg and Na)

The mineral composition of the yogurt samples, including calcium (Ca), potassium (K), magnesium (Mg), sodium (Na), and salt (NaCl) content, is presented in Table 4. Significant differences ($p < 0.05$) were observed for potassium, sodium, and salt content, while calcium and magnesium remained relatively stable across formulations.

Table 4. Mineral Composition of Yogurt Samples with Different Formulations.

Samples	Ca (mg/100 g Yogurt)	K (mg/100 g Yogurt)	Mg (mg/100 g Yogurt)	Na (mg/100 g Yogurt)	Salt (mg/100 g Yogurt)
Control (0%)	96.8 ± 3.9 ^{a}	104 ± 19 ^{a,b}	21.6 ± 1.1 ^{a}	87.5 ± 16.9 ^{a}	219
0.01% CtE	96.2 ± 3.0 ^{a}	93.4 ± 4.3 ^{a}	22.6 ± 2.3 ^{a}	85.3 ± 1.9 ^{a}	213
0.01% CtE + DF	96.4 ± 3.7 ^{a}	144 ± 3 ^{c}	22.9 ± 0.2 ^{a}	76.7 ± 1.8 ^{a}	192
0.15% CtE	106 ± 1 ^{a,b}	121 ± 4 ^{b,c}	22.1 ± 0.3 ^{a}	84.7 ± 4.5 ^{a}	212
0.15% CtE + DF	103 ± 4 ^{a,b}	137 ± 2 ^{c}	22.7 ± 0.4 ^{a}	75.7 ± 0.8 ^{a}	189
0.01% Phytosomes	113 ± 10 ^{b}	99.4 ± 7.4 ^{a,b}	19.3 ± 2.0 ^{a}	75.9 ± 6.4 ^{a}	190

Values are presented as mean ± standard deviation. Different lowercase letters in the same column indicate significant differences between samples ($p < 0.05$). Recommended daily intakes of minerals: Ca: 750 mg/day; K: 3500 mg/day; Mg: 300 mg/day; Na; 2000 mg/day (https://www.efsa.europa.eu/en/topics/topic/dietary-reference-values, accessed on 20 January 2023). Recommended maximum daily salt (NaCl) intake: <5000 mg/day, calculated from 2000 mg Na × 2.5 (https://www.who.int/data/gho/indicator-metadata-registry/imr-details/3082, accessed on 3 March 2025).

Calcium levels ranged from 96.2 to 113 mg/100 g, with the 0.01% phytosome sample exhibiting the highest concentration (113 ± 10 mg/100 g, $p < 0.05$). This suggests a potential contribution of phytosome encapsulation to calcium retention. Magnesium content remained relatively unchanged across formulations (19.3–22.9 mg/100 g, $p > 0.05$), indicating that CtE, DF, and phytosomes did not significantly impact Mg presence in yogurt.

Significant increases in potassium ($p < 0.05$) were observed in DF-containing formulations, with 0.01% CtE + DF (144 ± 3 mg/100 g) and 0.15% CtE + DF (137 ± 2 mg/100 g) showing the highest levels. These values were significantly higher than those in the control (104 ± 19 mg/100 g) and 0.01% CtE (93.4 ± 4.3 mg/100 g), suggesting that dehydrated fruit contributed to potassium enrichment, consistent with previous findings in fruit-fortified dairy products [54].

Sodium levels remained similar across formulations (75.7–87.5 mg/100 g, $p > 0.05$), indicating that CtE and phytosome encapsulation did not significantly alter Na content. However, salt content was significantly lower in DF-fortified samples (189–192 mg/100 g) compared to the control (219 mg/100 g), likely due to interactions between fruit-derived bioactives and ionic components affecting mineral solubility [55].

The mineral composition of these yogurts aligns with reported values for natural yogurts: Ca (129–155 mg/100 g), K (98.0–165 mg/100 g), Mg (10.6–15.0 mg/100 g), and Na (81.0–141 mg/100 g) [56]. While seaweed is generally rich in sodium [57], CtE in these formulations did not significantly increase the Na content.

The produced yogurts contribute modestly to the recommended daily intakes (RDAs) of sodium (3.78–4.38%), potassium (2.67–4.12%), and magnesium (6.43–7.62%). In contrast, calcium levels contribute more significantly (12.8–15.0%) than commercial natural yogurts (120 mg/100 g). The Na/K ratio remained below 1.0 in all samples (0.53–0.91), an important dietary metric associated with reduced cardiovascular disease risk [58].

These findings highlight the potential of DF and phytosome encapsulation to influence mineral retention and enhance the nutritional value of yogurt formulations.

2.3.7. Total Lipids, Proteins, Total Sugars, and Energetic Value

The nutritional composition of the yogurt formulations is summarized in Table 5, showing significant differences ($p < 0.05$) across all measured parameters, particularly total lipid content, which was notably influenced by CtE, dehydrated fruit (DF), and phytosome encapsulation.

Table 5. Nutritional composition of yogurt samples with different formulations.

Samples	Total Lipids (%)	Total Sugars (%)	Total Protein (%)	Caloric Content (kcal)
Control (0%)	1.05 ± 0.09 [a,b]	2.10 ± 0.19 [b]	3.17 ± 0.29 [a]	30.6
0.01% CtE	0.794 ± 0.056 [a]	1.51 ± 0.11 [a]	3.54 ± 0.25 [a,b]	27.3
0.01% CtE + DF	0.921 ± 0.037 [a,b]	1.27 ± 0.05 [a]	3.75 ± 0.15 [a,b,c]	28.4
0.15% CtE	1.49 ± 0.10 [b,c]	1.37 ± 0.10 [a]	4.28 ± 0.30 [b,c]	36.0
0.15% CtE + DF	1.89 ± 0.09 [c]	2.14 ± 0.11 [b]	4.40 ± 0.22 [c]	43.2
0.01% Phytosomes	5.35 ± 0.48 [d]	3.00 ± 0.27 [c]	4.45 ± 0.40 [c]	78.0

Values are presented as mean ± standard deviation. Different lowercase letters in the same column indicate significant differences between samples ($p < 0.05$). Caloric content was calculated using the Atwater general factor system where the energy values are 4.0 kcal/g for protein, 9.0 kcal/g for fat, and 4.0 kcal/g for sugars (https://www.fao.org/4/y5022e/y5022e04.htm#fn9, accessed on 21 January 2025). A daily caloric intake of 2000 kcal was adopted as a reference value, in line with general dietary guidelines provided by EFSA (https://www.efsa.europa.eu/en/topics/topic/dietary-reference-values, accessed on 4 March 2025).

Total lipids ranged from 0.794% to 5.35%, with the lowest values in 0.01% CtE yogurt (0.79%) and the highest in phytosome-encapsulated samples (5.35%, $p < 0.05$). This increase is attributed to the phospholipid-based encapsulation matrix, consistent with studies reporting elevated fat content in nanoencapsulated bioactives with enhanced oxidative stability [37]. Lower CtE concentrations slightly reduced fat content, possibly due to fat-binding interactions with bioactive compounds [59]. In contrast, higher CtE levels (0.15%) and DF addition increased lipid content (1.89%), likely due to fruit-derived lipids [60].

Protein content ranged from 3.17% in the control to 4.45% in phytosome-encapsulated yogurt, with significantly higher values observed in all fortified formulations ($p < 0.05$). Notably, 0.15% CtE + DF and phytosome samples reached 4.40% and 4.45%, respectively. This increase is likely due to interactions between seaweed bioactives and casein micelles, enhancing protein retention and structural stability [60,61]. Yogurts with 0.01% CtE and 0.01% CtE + DF showed moderate increases (3.54% and 3.75%, respectively), while 0.15% CtE reached 4.28%. The high protein values also reflect green algae's naturally high protein content (10–47% dry weight) [12] and the protective effect of nanoencapsulation during fermentation [36]. As all fortified samples exceeded typical commercial yogurt protein levels (~3.20 g/100 g), these formulations show strong potential as high-protein functional yogurts [62].

Total sugar content ranged from 1.27% to 3.00%, with significantly lower values in 0.01% CtE + DF (1.27%) and 0.15% CtE (1.37%) compared to the control (2.10%, $p < 0.05$). This reduction likely reflects increased carbohydrate metabolism by lactic acid bacteria in the presence of CtE and fruit polyphenols [63]. In contrast, the phytosome-encapsulated sample showed the highest sugar content (3.00%), possibly due to the encapsulation matrix contributing additional carbohydrates or altering fermentation kinetics [36,42,43]. These findings suggest that CtE and DF can reduce sugar content, supporting the development of low-sugar formulations, while phytosome-containing yogurts may require optimization to manage sugar levels. Compared to commercial yogurts (~4.6 g/100 g), the sugar content in all samples remained lower.

Caloric content varied significantly (27.3–78.0 kcal/100 g), with the lowest values in 0.01% CtE (27.3 kcal) and the highest in phytosome formulations (78.0 kcal, $p < 0.05$). The increased energy value in phytosome-encapsulated yogurts aligns with higher lipid content from the encapsulation system. Compared to commercial yogurts (~3% of daily energy intake), the phytosome formulation contributed 3.90% of the reference daily intake (RDI), whereas other formulations ranged from 1.37% to 2.16%.

Incorporating phytosomes significantly increased yogurt's caloric content, mainly due to the lipid-based composition of the encapsulation matrix. While low-calorie products are gaining popularity, consumer preferences are also shifting towards functional foods that provide improved bioavailability of bioactive compounds and health benefits. Studies indicate that consumers are willing to accept a moderate increase in caloric content if the product offers added functional properties, such as improved nutrient absorption, oxidative stability, and gut health benefits [64,65].

Furthermore, product formulation strategies can balance this caloric increase by adjusting portions, modifying sugar and fat content, or targeting health-conscious consumers seeking premium functional dairy products. Similar trends have been observed in fortified yogurts and nanoencapsulated bioactives where enhanced nutritional benefits offset higher caloric values [57,66].

These findings confirm that phytosome encapsulation significantly increases lipid and caloric content, while CtE and DF fortification enhance protein levels and reduce sugars. Together, these formulations show promise for functional dairy applications and can be positioned as high-value products for consumers seeking health benefits and innovative yogurt options.

3. Material and Methods

3.1. Reagents

L-α-phosphatidylcholine (egg yolk, Type XI-E, 100 mg/mL in chloroform, ≥99%, solution), human ApoE3 (recombinant, expressed in *E. coli*, ≥90% (SDS-PAGE), (HPLC), acetylthiocholine iodide ≥ 98% (TLC), butyrylthiocholine iodide ≥ 98%, butyrylcholinesterase from equine serum, acetylcholinesterase from electric eel, 5,5′-dithiobis(2-nitrobenzoic acid), Trizma® (St. Louis, MO, USA), ≥99.9% (titration), crystalline, bovine serum albumin, cold ethanol fraction, pH 5.2, ≥96%, 1-octanol ACS reagent, suitable for UV/vis spectroscopy, ≥99.5% (GC), 6-hydroxy-2,5,7,8-tetramethylchroman-2-carboxylic acid (Trolox), disodium fluorescein, potassium phosphate monobasic (KH_2PO_4), potassium phosphate dibasic trihydrate ($K_2HPO_4 \cdot 3H_2O$), and 2′,2′-azobis (2-amidinopropane) dihydrochloride (AAPH) were acquired from Sigma Chemicals Co. (). Anhydrous absolute ethanol and 96% sulfuric acid, RPE (for analysis—ISO) were acquired from Carlo Erba Reagents (Chau. du Vexin, Val-de-Reuil, France); ACS BASIC CL0217 chloroform, stabilised with ethanol from Scharlab (Barcelona, Spain), KBr—potassium bromide (IR) PAI and tablets for Kjeldahl (Catalyst with 0.3% $CuSO_4 \cdot 5H_2O$) from Panreac (Darmstadt, Germany); DSPE-PEG(2000) amine (chloroform 1,2-distearoyl-sn-glycero-3-phosphoethanolamine-N-[amino (polyethylene glycol)—2000]), from Avanti Polar Lipids (Alabaster, AL, USA); soluble starch GR ISO. CAS 9005-84-9, pH 6.0–7.5, sodium thiosulfate pentahydrate 99.5% for analysis, both from Merck (Darmstadt, Germany); potassium iodide RPE-ACS, sodium hydroxide AGR, and low metal micro-pearls, from Labbox (Barcelona, Spain); potassium hydrogenophthalate, ≥99.5%, from Honeywell (Charlotte, NC, USA). Potassium persulfate, and 2,2-azinobis (3-ethylbenzothiazoline-6-sulfonic acid) di-ammonium salt (ABTS) were purchased from Merck (Darmstadt, Germany).

3.2. Samples and Extraction

C. tomentosum extract was produced by subcritical water extraction as described by Soares, C. et al. [14]. In this study, only the E4 fraction was used, herein named CtE.

3.3. Box–Behnken Factorial Design

A Box–Behnken design with three independent variables [A—time (1–4 h), B—temperature (25–60 °C), and C—ratio CtE:phosphatidylcholine (1:1–1:4)] was applied to obtain the best conditions to maximize the phytosome complex formation. A total of 15 runs were performed, considering 3 central points. The software Design Expert (version 11, Stat-Ease Inc., Minneapolis, MN, USA) was used for experimental design, data analysis, and model building. After determining the model equation, Derringer's desirability function was used to maximize the modeled responses.

3.4. Phytosome Production and Characterization

The phytosomes were produced using the optimal conditions of temperature, time, and ratio CtE:phosphatidylcholine. Phytosome production started by mixing 3 mg of CtE and 30 µL of L-α-phosphatidylcholine (100 mg/mL in chloroform). After drying the chloroform under nitrogen flow, 3 mL of ethanol was added. To allow the reaction to occur, the mixture was placed in a water bath at 59 °C for 1 h. After this period, ethanol was evaporated under nitrogen, and 3 mL of chloroform was added to the dried complex. Then, the mixture was filtered twice through PTFE membranes (0.22 µm) to remove non-complexed extract. Phytosomes were stored dried, after chloroform evaporation, and used in a few days. The complex was further functionalized with 3% ApoE and 2.5% DSPE-PEG(2000) amine. Afterward, they were characterized by dynamic light scattering (DLS), UV spectrophotometry, octanol/water partition coefficient (Kow), differential scanning calorimetry (DSC), and Fourier transform infrared spectroscopy (FTIR), according to established procedures [30,33].

DLS analysis was performed in a Malvern Zetasizer ZS instrument (Worcestershire, UK), using disposable polystyrene cuvettes for each sample. Prior to each analysis, the samples were homogenized using an ultrasound bath. The intensity-distribution size was obtained with the Malvern Zetasizer v7.11 software.

CtE, L-α-phosphatidylcholine and phytosomes UV-vis spectra were traced in a UV-vis Shimadzu spectrophotometer (model UV-2101PC, Tokyo, Japan). For that, samples were diluted in chloroform and submitted to ultrasound to ensure correct solubilization. The UV-vis spectra were traced from 200 to 700 nm.

The solubility in water or in organic solvents was determined by adding 10 mL of water and 10 mL of n-octanol to the complex or to CtE, in a decantation funnel. The mixture was agitated for 24 h at room temperature. After phase separation, both phases were centrifuged for 20 min at 1000 rpm. The supernatant was filtered through PTFE membranes (0.22 µm). Sample concentration was determined at 280 nm (characteristic wavelength of CtE) in a microplate reader (BioTek Synergy HTX Multimode Reader, Winooski, VT, USA, EUA) using the calibration curves traced for CtE dissolved in water and CtE dissolved in n-octanol. The K_{ow} partition coefficient was calculated according to Equation (2):

$$K_{ow} = P = C_o/C_w \tag{2}$$

where C_o = concentration in the n-octanol phase and C_w = concentration in the aqueous phase.

To obtain L-phosphatidylcholine, CtE, and phytosomes thermograms, 3.0 ± 0.2 mg of each sample was placed into alumina crucibles. An empty alumina crucible was used as a reference. Thermograms and DSC results were obtained using a thermal analyzer STA 449 F3 Jupiter® (NETZSCH, Selb, Germany) with NETZSCH Proteus® 5.2 software.

The temperature program applied ranged from 25 °C to 1000 °C, with a rate of 20 °C per minute under a nitrogen flow of 50 mL/min.

For FTIR analysis, CtE was grounded with KBr (1:100) in a mortar. Transparent ultra-pure pellets were formed by applying a 10 Ton/nm^2 force. For L-α-phosphatidylcholine and phytosomes, producing KBr-sample pellets was not feasible, so the samples were directly placed between NaCl salt plates. The samples were analyzed using a Nicolet 6700 FT-IR (Thermo Fisher Scientific, Waltham, MA, USA) with OMNIC™ Spectra 8.3 software. The spectrum was obtained with a resolution of 4 cm^{-1} and analyzed within the wavenumber range of 400–4000 cm^{-1}.

3.5. Functional Yogurt Preparation and Characterization

The yogurt formulation followed a predefined recipe, was fermented for approximately 12 h in a yogurt maker, and then stored at 4 °C. A commercial ultra-pasteurized semi-skimmed milk containing 16 g of lipids, 49 g of sugars, 34 g of proteins, 1 g of salt, and 1.2 g of calcium per liter was used. Additionally, a commercial natural yogurt was employed as a source of lactic acid bacteria for fermentation, with 2.5 g of lipids, 4.6 g of sugars, 3.2 g of proteins, 0.14 g of salt, and 120 mg of calcium per 100 g. A total of ten yogurt samples were prepared, containing varying concentrations of the CtE: 0%, 0.005%, 0.01%, 0.05%, 0.1%, and 0.2%. Additional formulations included phytosome-encapsulated CtE at 0.01% and 0.15% and yogurts with 0.01% and 0.15% CtE combined with powdered dehydrated blackberry and raspberry. Physicochemical properties, such as pH, acidity, syneresis [37], moisture, total solids, organic and inorganic content [67], peroxides [68], proteins [69], total lipids [70], sugar content [71], and mineral composition [72], were analyzed according to established procedures. The in vitro inhibition capacity of the brain enzyme AChE and BuChE activities for each yogurt was measured according to a modified Ellman assay [14,73]. For antioxidant activity, the 2,2′-azino-bis(3-ethylbenzothiazoline-6-sulfonic acid radical (ABTS$^{•+}$) [74] and the oxygen radical absorbance capacity (ORAC) [14] assays were used. Trolox was used as standard in both assays. The results were expressed as mg Trolox equivalents (TE) per 100 g yogurt (mg TE/100 g) for ABTS and μmol Trolox equivalents per 100 g yogurt (μmol TE/100 g). For all the extracts, triplicate measurements were made.

For the sensorial analysis, a restricted group of informed, untrained, informal tasters was selected to verify possible alterations in fortified yogurts' aroma, taste, color, and texture using the affective method expressed by each taster's opinion.

3.6. Statistical Analysis

The data are presented as mean ± standard deviation and were evaluated using one-way ANOVA. Tukey's HSD post hoc test ($p < 0.05$) was employed to assess group differences. Analyses were conducted using SPSS (Version 29.0.2, IBM Corp., Armonk, NY, USA, 2023).

4. Conclusions

Phytosomes complexed with a neuroprotective seaweed fraction were successfully developed at the optimal conditions of temperature 59 °C, time 1 h, and ratio CtE:phosphatidylcholine of 1:1, offering a promising functional food ingredient designed for the elderly. FTIR and DSC analyses confirmed the formation of a phyto-phospholipid complex, while DLS analysis demonstrated a small particle size and low polydispersity, indicating favorable dispersion properties. Additionally, the octanol/water partition coefficient was higher for the phytosome complex than for the isolated CtE, suggesting improved bioavailability. Given the increasing need for neuroprotective dietary interventions in aging populations, these phytosomes hold the potential for being incorporated into functional yogurts and other food matrices aimed at supporting cognitive health in the elderly. Future research will focus on evaluating their stability, bioaccessibility, and long-term effects on cognitive function in aging individuals. Further studies, including in vitro digestion models and release profile assessments, are necessary to evaluate the liberation of the CtE under physiological conditions and optimize the formulation for enhanced functional benefits.

Supplementary Materials: The following supporting information can be downloaded at: https://www.mdpi.com/article/10.3390/md23040147/s1, Table S1: Entrapment efficiency (%) as a function of the three independent variables (t = time (h); T = temperature (°C); Ratio (CtE PC) = ratio (CtE:L-α-phosphatidylcholine)); Table S2: ANOVA analysis and statistical parameters of the reduced cubic model for the entrapment efficiency (%) using three parameters (A, B and C); Figure S1: Diagnostic graphs. A—Predicted vs Actual values; B—Normal Plot of Residuals; C—Residuals vs Predicted; D—Residuals vs Run; E—Residuals vs Time; F—Residuals vs Temperature; G—Residuals vs CtE:PC ratio.

Author Contributions: Conceptualization, C.S., C.G., P.S. and C.D.-M.; methodology, M.C., C.S., A.S., M.F. and C.G.; software, M.C. and C.G.; validation, C.S., C.G., M.F.B., P.S., M.F., P.G. and C.D.-M.; formal analysis, C.S., C.G., M.F.B., P.S. and C.D.-M.; investigation, M.C., C.S., A.S. and C.G.; resources, C.G. and C.D.-M.; writing—original draft preparation, M.C.; writing—review and editing, C.S., C.G., M.F.B., P.S., M.F., P.G. and C.D.-M.; supervision, C.S., C.G. and C.D.-M.; project administration, C.G. and C.D.-M.; funding acquisition, C.G. and C.D.-M. All authors have read and agreed to the published version of the manuscript.

Funding: This work was financed by FEDER—Fundo Europeu de Desenvolvimento Regional funds through the COMPETE 2020—Operacional Programme for Competitiveness and Internationalisation (POCI), and by Portuguese funds through FCT—Fundação para a Ciência e a Tecnologia in the framework of the project POCI-01-0145-FEDER-030240—PTDC/OCE-ETA/30240/2017—SilverBrain—From Sea to Brain: Green Neuroprotective Extracts for Nanoencapsulation and Functional Food Production.

Institutional Review Board Statement: Not applicable.

Informed consent Statement: Informed consent was obtained from all tasters involved in the study.

Data Availability Statement: The datasets analyzed in the current study are available from the corresponding author upon reasonable request.

Acknowledgments: This work was supported by project UID/50006—Laboratório Associado para a Química Verde—Tecnologias e Processos Limpos, financed by PT national funds (FCT/MECI, Fundação para a Ciência e Tecnologia and Ministério da Educação, Ciência e Inovação). Aurora Silva thanks the EU-FORA Fellowship Program (EUBA-EFSA-2023-ENREL-01) for the grant received. MF thanks FCT and LAQV-REQUIMTE for a post-doc fellowship (REQUIMTE 2019-34).

Conflicts of Interest: The authors declare no conflicts of interest.

References

1. Han, Y.; Kim, D.H.; Pack, S.P. Marine-Derived Bioactive Ingredients in Functional Foods for Aging: Nutritional and Therapeutic Perspectives. *Mar. Drugs* **2024**, *22*, 496. [CrossRef] [PubMed]
2. Jilani, M.G.; Hoque, M.; Tabrez, S.; Ali, S. The Genetic Basis of Neurodegenerative Disorders: Implications in Alzheimer's Disease. In *A New Era in Alzheimer' s Research*; Singh, S.K., Maccioni, R., Eds.; Elsevier: Amsterdam, The Netherlands, 2025; pp. 67–90.
3. Alzheimer's Society. *Factsheet Risk Factors for Dementia*; Alzheimer's Society: Belfast, UK, 2021.
4. NIH-NINDS. *Parkinson's Disease: Challenges, Progress, and Promise*; National Institute of Neurological Disorders and Stroke, National Institutes of Health: Bethesda, MD, USA, 2025.
5. Biris-Dorhoi, E.-S.; Michiu, D.; Pop, C.R.; Rotar, A.M.; Tofana, M.; Pop, O.L.; Socaci, S.A.; Farcas, A.C. Macroalgae—A Sustainable Source of Chemical Compounds with Biological Activities. *Nutrients* **2020**, *12*, 3085. [CrossRef] [PubMed]

6. Han, H.J.; Park, S.K.; Kang, J.Y.; Kim, J.M.; Yoo, S.K.; Kim, D.-O.; Kim, G.-H.; Heo, H.J. Mixture of Phlorotannin and Fucoidan from Ecklonia Cava Prevents the Aβ-Induced Cognitive Decline with Mitochondrial and Cholinergic Activation. *Mar. Drugs* **2021**, *19*, 434. [CrossRef] [PubMed]
7. Kannan, R.R.R.; Aderogba, M.A.; Ndhlala, A.R.; Stirk, W.A.; Van Staden, J. Acetylcholinesterase Inhibitory Activity of Phlorotannins Isolated from the Brown Alga, Ecklonia Maxima (Osbeck) Papenfuss. *Food Res. Int.* **2013**, *54*, 1250–1254. [CrossRef]
8. Jia, C.; Chai, J.; Zhang, S.; Sun, Y.; He, L.; Sang, Z.; Chen, D.; Zheng, X. The Advancements of Marine Natural Products in the Treatment of Alzheimer's Disease: A Study Based on Cell and Animal Experiments. *Mar. Drugs* **2025**, *23*, 91. [CrossRef]
9. Lu, J.; Pan, Q.; Zhou, J.; Weng, Y.; Chen, K.; Shi, L.; Zhu, G.; Chen, C.; Li, L.; Geng, M.; et al. Pharmacokinetics, Distribution, and Excretion of Sodium Oligomannate, a Recently Approved Anti-Alzheimer's Disease Drug in China. *J. Pharm. Anal.* **2022**, *12*, 145–155. [CrossRef]
10. Martins, B.; Vieira, M.; Delerue-Matos, C.; Grosso, C.; Soares, C. Biological Potential, Gastrointestinal Digestion, Absorption, and Bioavailability of Algae-Derived Compounds with Neuroprotective Activity: A Comprehensive Review. *Mar. Drugs* **2022**, *20*, 362. [CrossRef]
11. Bosch, M.E.; Dodiya, H.B.; Michalkiewicz, J.; Lee, C.; Shaik, S.M.; Weigle, I.Q.; Zhang, C.; Osborn, J.; Nambiar, A.; Patel, P.; et al. Sodium Oligomannate Alters Gut Microbiota, Reduces Cerebral Amyloidosis and Reactive Microglia in a Sex-Specific Manner. *Mol. Neurodegener.* **2024**, *19*, 18. [CrossRef]
12. Peñalver, R.; Lorenzo, J.M.; Ros, G.; Amarowicz, R.; Pateiro, M.; Nieto, G. Seaweeds as a Functional Ingredient for a Healthy Diet. *Mar. Drugs* **2020**, *18*, 301. [CrossRef]
13. Silva, J.; Martins, A.; Alves, C.; Pinteus, S.; Gaspar, H.; Alfonso, A.; Pedrosa, R. Natural Approaches for Neurological Disorders—The Neuroprotective Potential of Codium Tomentosum. *Molecules* **2020**, *25*, 5478. [CrossRef]
14. Soares, C.; Paíga, P.; Marques, M.; Neto, T.; Carvalho, A.P.; Paiva, A.; Simões, P.; Costa, L.; Bernardo, A.; Fernández, N.; et al. Multi-Step Subcritical Water Extracts of *Fucus vesiculosus* L. and *Codium tomentosum* Stackhouse: Composition, Health-Benefits and Safety. *Processes* **2021**, *9*, 893. [CrossRef]
15. Mancini, S.; Nardo, L.; Gregori, M.; Ribeiro, I.; Mantegazza, F.; Delerue-Matos, C.; Masserini, M.; Grosso, C. Functionalized Liposomes and Phytosomes Loading *Annona muricata* L. Aqueous Extract: Potential Nanoshuttles for Brain-Delivery of Phenolic Compounds. *Phytomedicine* **2018**, *42*, 233–244. [CrossRef] [PubMed]
16. Toma, L.; Deleanu, M.; Sanda, G.M.; Barbălată, T.; Niculescu, L.Ş.; Sima, A.V.; Stancu, C.S. Bioactive Compounds Formulated in Phytosomes Administered as Complementary Therapy for Metabolic Disorders. *Int. J. Mol. Sci.* **2024**, *25*, 4162. [CrossRef] [PubMed]
17. Matos, J.; Cardoso, C.; Serralheiro, M.L.; Bandarra, N.M.; Afonso, C. Seaweed Bioactives Potential as Nutraceuticals and Functional Ingredients: A Review. *J. Food Compos. Anal.* **2024**, *133*, 106453. [CrossRef]
18. Roohinejad, S.; Koubaa, M.; Barba, F.J.; Saljoughian, S.; Amid, M.; Greiner, R. Application of Seaweeds to Develop New Food Products with Enhanced Shelf-Life, Quality and Health-Related Beneficial Properties. *Food Res. Int.* **2017**, *99*, 1066–1083. [CrossRef]
19. Plaza, M.; Amigo-Benavent, M.; del Castillo, M.D.; Ibáñez, E.; Herrero, M. Facts about the Formation of New Antioxidants in Natural Samples after Subcritical Water Extraction. *Food Res. Int.* **2010**, *43*, 2341–2348. [CrossRef]
20. Xu, H.; Zhang, X.; Karangwa, E. Inhibition Effects of Maillard Reaction Products Derived from L-Cysteine and Glucose on Enzymatic Browning Catalyzed by Mushroom Tyrosinase and Characterization of Active Compounds by Partial Least Squares Regression Analysis. *RSC Adv.* **2016**, *6*, 65825–65836. [CrossRef]
21. Bagoudou, A.F.; Matsumoto, K.; Chawalitpong, S.; Park, H.Y.; Vattem, D.A.; Nakamura, S.; Katayama, S. Maillard Reaction Products Derived from Heat-Dried Green Tomato Increase Longevity and Neuroprotection in Caenorhabditis Elegans. *Food Sci. Technol. Res.* **2021**, *27*, 747–757. [CrossRef]
22. Zhao, M.; Zhang, B.; Deng, L. The Mechanism of Acrylamide-Induced Neurotoxicity: Current Status and Future Perspectives. *Front. Nutr.* **2022**, *9*, 859189. [CrossRef]
23. Ye, X.; Zhang, M.; Gong, Z.; Jiao, W.; Li, L.; Dong, M.; Xiang, T.; Feng, N.; Wu, Q. Inhibition of Polyphenols on Maillard Reaction Products and Their Induction of Related Diseases: A Comprehensive Review. *Phytomedicine* **2024**, *128*, 155589. [CrossRef]
24. Takeuchi, M. Toxic AGEs (TAGE) Theory: A New Concept for Preventing the Development of Diseases Related to Lifestyle. *Diabetol. Metab. Syndr.* **2020**, *12*, 105. [CrossRef] [PubMed]
25. Telange, D.R.; Patil, A.T.; Pethe, A.M.; Fegade, H.; Anand, S.; Dave, V.S. Formulation and Characterization of an Apigenin-Phospholipid Phytosome (APLC) for Improved Solubility, in Vivo Bioavailability, and Antioxidant Potential. *Eur. J. Pharm. Sci.* **2017**, *108*, 36–49. [CrossRef] [PubMed]
26. Deleanu, M.; Toma, L.; Sanda, G.M.; Barbălată, T.; Niculescu, L.Ş.; Sima, A.V.; Deleanu, C.; Săcărescu, L.; Suciu, A.; Alexandru, G.; et al. Formulation of Phytosomes with Extracts of Ginger Rhizomes and Rosehips with Improved Bioavailability, Antioxidant and Anti-Inflammatory Effects In Vivo. *Pharmaceutics* **2023**, *15*, 1066. [CrossRef] [PubMed]

27. Direito, R.; Reis, C.; Roque, L.; Gonçalves, M.; Sanches-Silva, A.; Gaspar, M.M.; Pinto, R.; Rocha, J.; Sepodes, B.; Rosário Bronze, M.; et al. Phytosomes with Persimmon (*Diospyros kaki* L.) Extract: Preparation and Preliminary Demonstration of In Vivo Tolerability. *Pharmaceutics* **2019**, *11*, 296. [CrossRef]
28. Tenchov, R.; Bird, R.; Curtze, A.E.; Zhou, Q. Lipid Nanoparticles–From Liposomes to MRNA Vaccine Delivery, a Landscape of Research Diversity and Advancement. *ACS Nano* **2021**, *15*, 16982–17015. [CrossRef]
29. Ghanbarzadeh, B.; Babazadeh, A.; Hamishehkar, H. Nano-Phytosome as a Potential Food-Grade Delivery System. *Food Biosci.* **2016**, *15*, 126–135. [CrossRef]
30. Kumar, S.; Baldi, A.; Sharma, D.K. Characterization and In Vitro Investigation of Antiscabietic Effect of Phytosomes Assimilating Quercetin and Naringenin Rich Fraction of Pistacia Integerrima Galls Extract against Sarcoptes Scabiei. *J. Drug Deliv. Sci. Technol.* **2022**, *67*, 102851. [CrossRef]
31. Telange, D.R.; Sohail, N.K.; Hemke, A.T.; Kharkar, P.S.; Pethe, A.M. Phospholipid Complex-Loaded Self-Assembled Phytosomal Soft Nanoparticles: Evidence of Enhanced Solubility, Dissolution Rate, Ex Vivo Permeability, Oral Bioavailability, and Antioxidant Potential of Mangiferin. *Drug Deliv. Transl. Res.* **2021**, *11*, 1056–1083. [CrossRef]
32. Semalty, A.; Tanwar, Y.S.; Singh, D.; Rawat, M.S.M. Phosphatidylcholine Complex in Improving Oral Drug Delivery of Epicatechin: Preparation and Characterization. *J. Drug Discov. Dev. Deliv.* **2014**, *1*, 46–55.
33. Singh, D.; Rawat, M.S.M.; Semalty, A.; Semalty, M. Chrysophanol–Phospholipid Complex. *J. Therm. Anal. Calorim.* **2013**, *111*, 2069–2077. [CrossRef]
34. Goh, K.K.T.; Sarkar, A.; Singh, H. Milk Protein–Polysaccharide Interactions. In *Milk Proteins*; Elsevier: Amsterdam, The Netherlands, 2014; pp. 387–419.
35. O'Sullivan, A.M.; O'Grady, M.N.; O'Callaghan, Y.C.; Smyth, T.J.; O'Brien, N.M.; Kerry, J.P. Seaweed Extracts as Potential Functional Ingredients in Yogurt. *Innov. Food Sci. Emerg. Technol.* **2016**, *37*, 293–299. [CrossRef]
36. Abdulqahar, F.W.; El-Messery, T.M.; Zaky, A.A.; El-Said, M.M. In Vitro Digestibility of Aucklandia Costus-Loaded Nanophytosomes and Their Use in Yoghurt as a Food Model. *Food Biosci.* **2022**, *50*, 102106. [CrossRef]
37. Ghorbanzade, T.; Jafari, S.M.; Akhavan, S.; Hadavi, R. Nano-Encapsulation of Fish Oil in Nano-Liposomes and Its Application in Fortification of Yogurt. *Food Chem.* **2017**, *216*, 146–152. [CrossRef] [PubMed]
38. Zahid, H.F.; Ranadheera, C.S.; Fang, Z.; Ajlouni, S. Functional and Healthy Yogurts Fortified with Probiotics and Fruit Peel Powders. *Fermentation* **2022**, *8*, 469. [CrossRef]
39. Nuñez, M.; Picon, A. Seaweeds in Yogurt and Quark Supplementation: Influence of Five Dehydrated Edible Seaweeds on Sensory Characteristics. *Int. J. Food Sci. Technol.* **2017**, *52*, 431–438. [CrossRef]
40. Ramadan, M.M.; El-Said, M.M.; El-Messery, T.M.; Mohamed, R.S. Development of Flavored Yoghurt Fortified with Microcapsules of Triple Omega 3-6-9 for Preventing Neurotoxicity Induced by Aluminum Chloride in Rats. *J. Food Process. Preserv.* **2021**, *45*, e15759. [CrossRef]
41. Dewi, E.N.; Purnamayati, L. Characterization of Caulerpa Racemosa Yogurt Processed Using Lactobacillus Bulgaricus and Streptococcus Thermophilus. *Food Res.* **2021**, *5*, 54–61. [CrossRef]
42. Yuan, X.; Wang, T.; Sun, L.; Qiao, Z.; Pan, H.; Zhong, Y.; Zhuang, Y. Recent Advances of Fermented Fruits: A Review on Strains, Fermentation Strategies, and Functional Activities. *Food Chem. X* **2024**, *22*, 101482. [CrossRef]
43. Savaghebi, D.; Ghaderi-Ghahfarokhi, M.; Barzegar, M. Encapsulation of Sargassum Boveanum Algae Extract in Nano-Liposomes: Application in Functional Mayonnaise Production. *Food Bioprocess Technol.* **2021**, *14*, 1311–1325. [CrossRef]
44. Gaspar, P.; Carvalho, A.L.; Vinga, S.; Santos, H.; Neves, A.R. From Physiology to Systems Metabolic Engineering for the Production of Biochemicals by Lactic Acid Bacteria. *Biotechnol. Adv.* **2013**, *31*, 764–788. [CrossRef]
45. FAO; WHO. *Codex Standard for Fermented Milks (CODEX STAN 243-2003) Milk and Milk Products*; FAO: Rome, Italy, 2015.
46. Clarke, H.J.; McCarthy, W.P.; O'Sullivan, M.G.; Kerry, J.P.; Kilcawley, K.N. Oxidative Quality of Dairy Powders: Influencing Factors and Analysis. *Foods* **2021**, *10*, 2315. [CrossRef] [PubMed]
47. Marín, D.; Alemán, A.; Montero, P.; Gómez-Guillén, M.C. Encapsulation of Food Waste Compounds in Soy Phosphatidylcholine Liposomes: Effect of Freeze-Drying, Storage Stability and Functional Aptitude. *J. Food Eng.* **2018**, *223*, 132–143. [CrossRef]
48. Ye, A.; Cui, J.; Taneja, A.; Zhu, X.; Singh, H. Evaluation of Processed Cheese Fortified with Fish Oil Emulsion. *Food Res. Int.* **2009**, *42*, 1093–1098. [CrossRef]
49. Öztürk, H.İ.; Aydın, S.; Sözeri, D.; Demirci, T.; Sert, D.; Akın, N. Fortification of Set-Type Yoghurts with *Elaeagnus angustifolia* L. Flours: Effects on Physicochemical, Textural, and Microstructural Characteristics. *LWT* **2018**, *90*, 620–626. [CrossRef]
50. Górnicki, K.; Choińska, A.; Kaleta, A. Effect of Variety on Rehydration Characteristics of Dried Apples. *Processes* **2020**, *8*, 1454. [CrossRef]
51. Greis, M.; Sainio, T.; Katina, K.; Nolden, A.A.; Kinchla, A.J.; Seppä, L.; Partanen, R. Physicochemical Properties and Mouthfeel in Commercial Plant-Based Yogurts. *Foods* **2022**, *11*, 941. [CrossRef]
52. Amal, A.; Eman, A.; Nahla, S.Z. Fruit Flavored Yogurt: Chemical, Functional and Rheological Properties. *Int. J. Environ. Agric. Res.* **2016**, *2*, 57–66.

53. Pereira, L. A Review of the Nutrient Composition of Selected Edible Seaweeds. In *Seaweed: Ecology, Nutrient Composition and Medicinal Uses*; Pomin, V.H., Ed.; Nova Science Publishers, Inc.: Hauppauge, NY, USA, 2011; pp. 15–47.
54. Salehi, F. Quality, Physicochemical, and Textural Properties of Dairy Products Containing Fruits and Vegetables: A Review. *Food Sci. Nutr.* **2021**, *9*, 4666–4686. [CrossRef]
55. Sánchez-Segarra, P. Influence of the Addition of Fruit on the Mineral Content of Yoghurts: Nutritional Assessment. *Food Chem.* **2000**, *71*, 85–89. [CrossRef]
56. Souza, S.O.; Santos, V.S.; Santos, E.S.; Ávila, D.V.L.; Nascimento, C.C.; Costa, S.S.L.; Garcia, C.A.B.; Araujo, R.G.O. Evaluation of the Mineral Content in Milk and Yogurt Types Using Chemometric Tools. *Microchem. J.* **2018**, *143*, 1–8. [CrossRef]
57. Gupta, S.; Abu-Ghannam, N. Recent Developments in the Application of Seaweeds or Seaweed Extracts as a Means for Enhancing the Safety and Quality Attributes of Foods. *Innov. Food Sci. Emerg. Technol.* **2011**, *12*, 600–609. [CrossRef]
58. Correia, H.; Soares, C.; Morais, S.; Pinto, E.; Marques, A.; Nunes, M.L.; Almeida, A.; Delerue-Matos, C. Seaweeds Rehydration and Boiling: Impact on Iodine, Sodium, Potassium, Selenium, and Total Arsenic Contents and Health Benefits for Consumption. *Food Chem. Toxicol.* **2021**, *155*, 112385. [CrossRef] [PubMed]
59. Silva, H.D.; Cerqueira, M.Â.; Vicente, A.A. Nanoemulsions for Food Applications: Development and Characterization. *Food Bioprocess Technol.* **2012**, *5*, 854–867. [CrossRef]
60. Jakobek, L. Interactions of Polyphenols with Carbohydrates, Lipids and Proteins. *Food Chem.* **2015**, *175*, 556–567. [CrossRef]
61. Thiviya, P.; Gamage, A.; Gama-Arachchige, N.S.; Merah, O.; Madhujith, T. Seaweeds as a Source of Functional Proteins. *Phycology* **2022**, *2*, 216–243. [CrossRef]
62. Pannerchelvan, S.; Rios-Solis, L.; Wasoh, H.; Sobri, M.Z.M.; Faizal Wong, F.W.; Mohamed, M.S.; Mohamad, R.; Halim, M. Functional Yogurt: A Comprehensive Review of Its Nutritional Composition and Health Benefits. *Food Funct.* **2024**, *15*, 10927–10955. [CrossRef]
63. Wang, Y.; Wu, J.; Lv, M.; Shao, Z.; Hungwe, M.; Wang, J.; Bai, X.; Xie, J.; Wang, Y.; Geng, W. Metabolism Characteristics of Lactic Acid Bacteria and the Expanding Applications in Food Industry. *Front. Bioeng. Biotechnol.* **2021**, *9*, 612285. [CrossRef]
64. Sloan, A.E. Top 10 Functional Food Trends: Reinventing Wellness. *Food Technol.* **2004**, *58*, 28–51.
65. Baker, M.T.; Lu, P.; Parrella, J.A.; Leggette, H.R. Consumer Acceptance toward Functional Foods: A Scoping Review. *Int. J. Environ. Res. Public Health* **2022**, *19*, 1217. [CrossRef]
66. Research, G.V. Functional Foods Market Size & Trends Analysis Report, 2030. 2022. Available online: https://www.grandviewresearch.com/industry-analysis/functional-food-market (accessed on 3 March 2025).
67. Saeed, M.; Ali, S.W.; Ramzan, S. Physicochemical Analysis of Mango Flavored Yogurt Supplemented with Moringa Oleifera Leaf Powder. *J. Food Sci. Technol.* **2021**, *58*, 4805–4814. [CrossRef]
68. Rabbani, M.; Pezeshki, A.; Ahmadi, R.; Mohammadi, M.; Tabibiazar, M.; Ahmadzadeh Nobari Azar, F.; Ghorbani, M. Phytosomal Nanocarriers for Encapsulation and Delivery of Resveratrol- Preparation, Characterization, and Application in Mayonnaise. *LWT* **2021**, *151*, 112093. [CrossRef]
69. European Parliament and Council of the European Union. Regulation (EU) No 1169/2011 of the European Parliament and of the Council of 25 October 2011 on the provision of food information to consumers. *Off. J. Eur. Union* **2011**, *L 304*, 18–63.
70. Ramalhosa, M.J.; Paíga, P.; Morais, S.; Rui Alves, M.; Delerue-Matos, C.; Oliveira, M.B.P.P. Lipid Content of Frozen Fish: Comparison of Different Extraction Methods and Variability during Freezing Storage. *Food Chem.* **2012**, *131*, 328–336. [CrossRef]
71. Masuko, T.; Minami, A.; Iwasaki, N.; Majima, T.; Nishimura, S.-I.; Lee, Y.C. Carbohydrate Analysis by a Phenol–Sulfuric Acid Method in Microplate Format. *Anal. Biochem.* **2005**, *339*, 69–72. [CrossRef] [PubMed]
72. Soares, C.; Tenreiro Machado, J.A.; Lopes, A.M.; Vieira, E.; Delerue-Matos, C. Electrochemical Impedance Spectroscopy Characterization of Beverages. *Food Chem.* **2020**, *302*, 125345. [CrossRef]
73. Ellman, G.L.; Courtney, K.D.; Andres, V.; Featherstone, R.M. A New and Rapid Colorimetric Determination of Acetylcholinesterase Activity. *Biochem. Pharmacol.* **1961**, *7*, 88–95. [CrossRef]
74. Mendes, M.; Carvalho, A.P.; Magalhães, J.M.C.S.; Moreira, M.; Guido, L.; Gomes, A.M.; Delerue-Matos, C. Response Surface Evaluation of Microwave-Assisted Extraction Conditions for Lycium Barbarum Bioactive Compounds. *Innov. Food Sci. Emerg. Technol.* **2016**, *33*, 319–326. [CrossRef]

marine drugs

Article

Wound Healing, Antioxidant, and Antiviral Properties of Bioactive Polysaccharides of Microalgae Strains Isolated from Greek Coastal Lagoons

Gabriel Vasilakis [1,†], Sofia Marka [2,3,†], Alexandros Ntzouvaras [2,4], Maria-Eleftheria Zografaki [2], Eirini Kyriakopoulou [5], Katerina I. Kalliampakou [2,5], Georgios Bekiaris [1], Evangelos Korakidis [5], Niki Papageorgiou [2], Stefania Christofi [1], Niki Vassilaki [5], Georgia Moschopoulou [3], Ioannis Tzovenis [4], Athena Economou-Amilli [4], Seraphim Papanikolaou [1] and Emmanouil Flemetakis [2,*]

1 Laboratory of Food Microbiology and Biotechnology, Department of Food Science and Human Nutrition, Agricultural University of Athens, 11855 Athens, Greece; vasilakis.gavriil@gmail.com (G.V.); giorgosbekiaris@yahoo.gr (G.B.); christofistefania@gmail.com (S.C.); spapanik@aua.gr (S.P.)
2 Laboratory of Molecular Biology, Department of Biotechnology, Agricultural University of Athens, 11855 Athens, Greece; smarka@aua.gr (S.M.); alexntzouv@gmail.com (A.N.); mzografaki@aua.gr (M.-E.Z.); kalliamp@yahoo.gr (K.I.K.); nikipapageorgiou99@gmail.com (N.P.)
3 Laboratory of Cell Technology, Department of Biotechnology, Agricultural University of Athens, 11855 Athens, Greece; geo_mos@aua.gr
4 Sector of Ecology & Systematics, Department of Biology, National and Kapodistrian University of Athens, 15784 Athens, Greece; itzoveni@biol.uoa.gr (I.T.); aamilli@biol.uoa.gr (A.E.-A.)
5 Laboratory of Molecular Virology, Hellenic Pasteur Institute, 11521 Athens, Greece; eirhnh63@gmail.com (E.K.); korakidis13@gmail.com (E.K.); nikiv@pasteur.gr (N.V.)
* Correspondence: mflem@aua.gr; Tel.: +30-21-0529-4343
† These authors contributed equally to this work.

Abstract: Microalgae have gained significant attention as sustainable sources of high value compounds, such as bioactive polysaccharides that are usually rich in sulfated groups and exhibit antioxidant properties. Here, 14 new microalgae strains of the genera *Tetraselmis*, *Dunaliella*, and *Nannochloropsis*, isolated from Greek coastal lagoons were analyzed to quantify and characterize their polysaccharide content. Heterogeneity was observed regarding the content of their total sugars (5.5–40.9 g/100 g dry biomass). The strains with a total sugar content above 20% were analyzed concerning the content of total, α- and β-glucans. *Tetraselmis verrucosa* f. *rubens* PLA1-2 and *T. suecica* T3-1 were rich in β-glucans (11%, and 8.1%, respectively). The polysaccharides of the two *Tetraselmis* strains were isolated and they were mainly composed of glucose and galactose. The isolated polysaccharides were fractionated using ion-exchange-chromatography. The anionic fraction from *T. verrucosa* f. *rubens* PLA1-2 was rich in sulfated polysaccharides, had antioxidant capacity, and exhibited healing properties. The anionic polysaccharides from the two *Tetraselmis* strains did not negatively influence the viability of human cells, while exhibiting antiviral properties against the replication of Hepatitis C Virus (HCV), with median efficient concentrations (EC50) at a range of 210–258 µg/mL.

Keywords: microalgae; bioactive polysaccharides; wound healing; antioxidants; antiviral properties; *Tetraselmis*

1. Introduction

Microalgae have gained significant scientific and industrial attention in recent years as alternative and sustainable sources of value-added metabolites, such as polysaccharides,

https://doi.org/10.3390/md23020077

lipids, proteins, vitamins and biopigments, due to their nutritional and pharmaceutical properties [1–12]. In parallel, the advantage of microalgae is the ease of cultivation, growth, and harvesting, independently of climatic or seasonal conditions [13].

Microalgal polysaccharides content varies between 15% and 75% across different species and are classified as intracellular polysaccharides, containing both the storage substances and the structural components of the cell walls, cell-bounded extracellular polysaccharides and released extracellular polysaccharides [14,15]. Both the production and composition of polysaccharides depend on the microalgal strain and are influenced by the nutritional and physicochemical conditions of the cultivation [16]. Polysaccharides present a diverse range of structures, determined by the composition of monosaccharides (40–50 hexoses, pentoses, and uronic acids), branches, and associated additives (such as sulfate groups, acyl groups, amino acids, or fatty acids) [17]. Bioactive polysaccharides, such as sulfated polysaccharides, beta-glucans (β-glucans), galactans, etc., are valuable in the food, feed, pharmaceutical, cosmetic, biomedical, and hydrocolloid industries, due to their hypolipidemic and hypoglycemic effects, as well as their antimicrobial, antiviral, antifungal, anti-inflammatory, antioxidant, and anticancer properties. These properties render them useful in various applications, owing to their biocompatibility, biodegradability, and non-toxicity [13,17–25].

Skin reconstruction and hydration products represent valuable assets in the field of cosmetology and pharmaceutical industries. Wound healing is a complex process involving tissue repair through several stages, including hemostasis, inflammation, proliferation, and remodeling. This process engages various cells and signaling molecules to regulate the cellular response and restore the structure of the injured tissue. Bioactive polysaccharides could contribute to the healing of wounds, especially in cases of extensive wounds or in patients with chronic wounds, that have difficult healing. Polysaccharides create an optimal environment for cell adhesion and proliferation by interacting with skin proteins, forming a barrier, which retains local moisture. Simultaneously, they exhibit antimicrobial and antiviral effects by stabilizing the skin's microflora, thus preventing infections and limiting reactive oxygen species (ROS) and inflammation in the wound. Otherwise, the unchecked inflammation could potentially lead to neoplastic differentiation [25,26].

In the present study, 14 newly isolated strains of microalgae from Greek coastal lagoons were initially evaluated for their polysaccharide content. Enzymatic determination of β-glucans content and subsequent polysaccharide extraction were performed on selected strains. After fractionation, the recovered eluates were characterized regarding their total sugars, sulfates concentration, and antioxidant capacity. Finally, cytotoxicity, antiviral activity, and wound healing properties of selected eluates were assessed.

2. Results

2.1. The Total Sugar and β-Glucan Contents Differ Significantly Among *Tetraselmis* Species

Polysaccharides are composed of sugar monomers; thus, we first determined the content of total sugars in the dry biomass (DB) of each microalgae strain. More information regarding the initial and final cell densities of the cultures, the maximum growth rates, and the final dry biomass concentration values after 10 days of growth is provided in the Supplemental Table S1. As shown in Table 1, the content of total sugars differed significantly among the different microalgae strains, with specific species of *Tetraselmis* exhibiting the highest and the lowest levels, respectively. Indeed, in the DB of *Tetraselmis verrucosa* f. *rubens* PLA1-2 the sugar content reached 40.9%, whereas the respective content in the DB of *Tetraselmis* spp. EST1-2 was only 5.5%.

Table 1. Quantitative determination of total sugars in the dry biomass (DB) of 14 microalgae strains, α- and β-glucans, and β-glucans to total sugars ratio in selected strains.

	Strain	Total Sugars (g/100 g DB)	Total Glucans (g/100 g DB)	α-Glucans (g/100 g DB)	β-Glucans (g/100 g DB)	β-Glucans (g) Per 100 g of Total Sugars
1	*Tetraselmis verrucosa* f. *rubens* PLA1-2	40.9 ± 2.6	28.7 ± 2.0	17.7 ± 0.8	11.0 ± 1.0	26.9 ± 0.9
2	*T. suecica* T3-1	32.6 ± 1.4	20.8 ± 1.1	12.7 ± 0.4	8.1 ± 0.7	24.8 ± 1.1
3	*T. verrucosa* f. *rubens* KSI1-3	27.8 ± 0.9	12.6 ± 0.7	8.6 ± 0.2	4.0 ± 0.5	14.4 ± 1.3
4	*T. suecica* ELO1-1	20.2 ± 1.8	15.5 ± 1.0	12.6 ± 0.6	2.9 ± 0.4	14.4 ± 0.6
5	*Tetraselmis* spp. Mes5	20.1 ± 1.1	13.6 ± 0.9	12.6 ± 0.7	1.0 ± 0.1	5.0 ± 0.2
6	*Dunaliela salina* 32	19.8 ± 1.3	-	-	-	-
7	*Tetraselmis* spp. Mes17	18.5 ± 1.3	-	-	-	-
8	*T. suecica* ELO1-2	17.8 ± 1.9	-	-	-	-
9	*T. verrucosa* f. *rubens* KLE1-3	14.9 ± 0.7	-	-	-	-
10	*Nannochloropsis gaditana* PLA1-1	12.6 ± 1.9	-	-	-	-
11	*D. salina* 30	12.5 ± 0.7	-	-	-	-
12	*T. verrucosa* f. *rubens* KLE1-4	11.8 ± 0.4	-	-	-	-
13	*D. salina* 31	6.5 ± 0.8	-	-	-	-
14	*Tetraselmis* spp. EST1-2	5.5 ± 0.2	-	-	-	-

-: not determined; Data represent mean ± SD of three independent samples.

The species exhibiting a total sugar amount in their DB above 20% (*w*/*w*) were further processed to determine the amounts of total glucans and alpha-glucans (α-glucans) and these were used to quantify the content of β-glucans, as molecules of increased interest. All microalgae exhibiting a total sugar content higher than 20% and thus further processed, belonged to *Tetraselmis* species. Of these strains, the *T. verrucosa* f. *rubens* PLA1-2 had the higher content of total glucans (28.7%, *w*/*w*), α-, and β-glucans (17.7% and 11 0%, *w*/*w*, respectively) in the DB, followed by *T. suecica* T3-1 (total glucans 20.8%, α-glucans 12.1%, and β-glucans 8.1%, *w*/*w*, in the DB). In general, we observed that the higher the total sugar content in the DB of microalgae, the higher the content of β-glucans. However, the ratio of β-glucans to total sugars was not constant ranging from 26.9% (*w*/*w*) in the case of *T. verrucosa* f. *rubens* PLA1-2 and 24.8% (*w*/*w*) in *T. suecica* T3-1 to 5.0% (*w*/*w*) in *Tetraselmis* spp. Mes5.

2.2. The Polysaccharides of the β-Glucan Rich Tetraselmis Strains Are Mainly Composed of Glucose and Galactose

To further characterize the polysaccharides of the two β-glucan-rich strains of *Tetraselmis* (*T. verrucosa* f. *rubens* PLA1-2 and *T. suecica* T3-1), these polysaccharides were isolated and hydrolysis was performed, followed by High Performance Liquid Chromatography (HPLC) analysis to detect and quantify their sugar monomers. To isolate the polysaccharides from the DB of microalgae, the lipophilic molecules were extracted using acetone. From the pellet of the defatted microalgal biomass, the water-soluble intracellular, structural, and bound molecules were extracted in pure water (ddH_2O), via the use of ultrasounds, thermal treatment, and vortexing. The proteins of this extract were denatured using a chloroform/n-butanol solution (Sigma-Aldrich, St. Luis, MO, USA) and from the deproteinated aqueous phase, the polysaccharides were precipitated using cold ethanol (Sigma-Aldrich, St. Luis, MO, USA). After their dissolution in ddH_2O (4 mg/mL), the isolated polysaccharides underwent thermal acidic hydrolysis, the resulting products were derivatized and subjected to HPLC analysis. Representative HPLC chromatograms from samples containing the hydrolyzed polysaccharides of the two microalgae strains are depicted in Figure 1A,B). The sugar monomers were identified and their relative percentage are shown in Table 2.

Our results showed that glucose was the most abundant sugar in the polysaccharides of both microalgal strains, followed by galactose (galactoglucans). The percentage of glucose in the polysaccharides of *T. verrucosa* f. *rubens* PLA1-2 and *T. suecica* T3-1 reached

71.9% and 66.4% (*w*/*w*), respectively, and the content of galactose was 19.8% and 20.9% (*w*/*w*) in these two cases, respectively. Thus, the glucose (glucans) content of the DB was approximately 29.4% and 21.6% (*w*/*w*), while the galactose (galactans) content was about 8.1% and 6.8% (*w*/*w*) for *T. verrucosa* f. *rubens* PLA1-2 and *T.* suecica T3-1, respectively. In addition to the above sugars, mannose, xylose, rhamnose, and ribose were detected in low quantities (<4%, *w*/*w*). The content of glucose in the above polysaccharides' extracts agreed with the high levels of glucans identified in the DB of these microalgae strains (see Table 1).

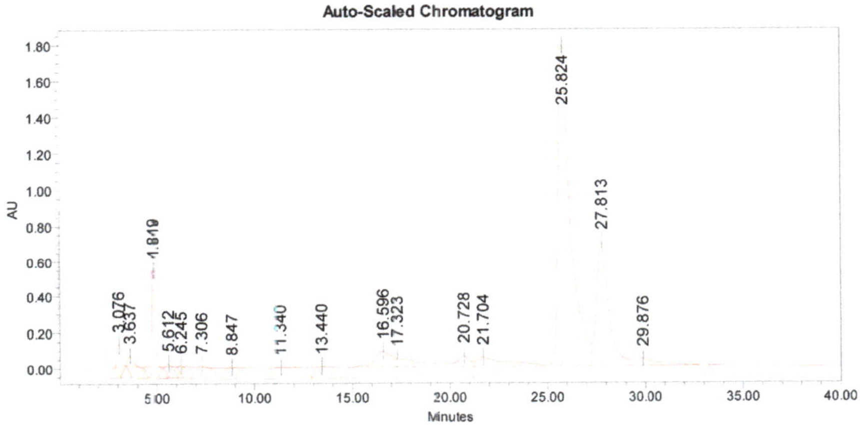

(A)

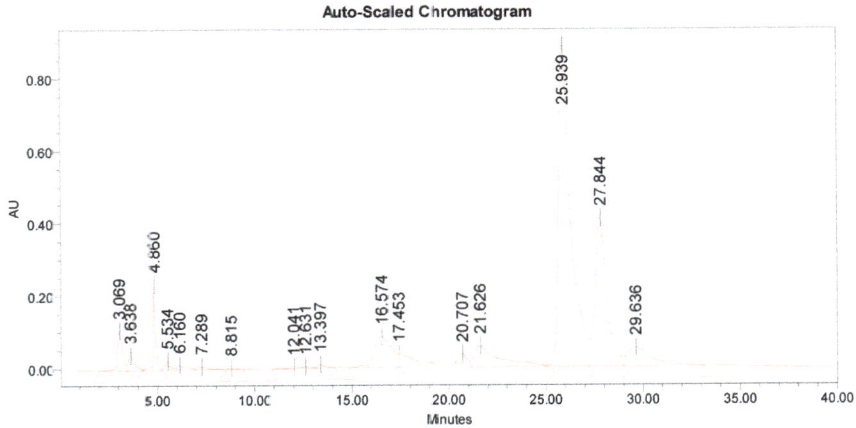

(B)

Figure 1. HPLC chromatogram of hydrolyzed polysaccharides. (**A**) HPLC chromatogram of hydrolyzed polysaccharides derived from *T. verrucosa* f. *rubens* PLA1-2. (**B**) HPLC chromatogram of hydrolyzed polysaccharides derived from *T. suecica* T3-1. Monosaccharides were identified based on the retention time of the respective standards as follows: mannose—16.5 min, ribose—17.4 min, rhamnose—20.7 min, glucuronic acid—21.6 min, galacturonic acid—23.3 min, glucose—25.8 min, galactose—27.8 min, xylose—29.6 min, arabinose—30.5 min, fucose—35.1 min. Based on the retention time of the sugar standards, the following sugars were identified in the above chromatograms of the hydrolyzed polysaccharides of the two microalgal strains: glucose, galactose, mannose, xylose, rhamnose, and ribose.

Table 2. Results from the HPLC analysis of polysaccharide hydrolysates derived from the selected microalgae strains: identified sugar monomers, their percentage content (% or mg/100 mg of total sugars), and molar ratio (mmol/100 mg of total sugars).

Monomers	Strains			
	***T. verrucosa* f. *rubens* PLA1-2**		***T. suecica* T3-1**	
	(%)	(mmol/100 mg)	(%)	(mmol/100 mg)
Glucose	71.9 ± 3.1	0.40 ± 0.02	66.4 ± 1.1	0.37 ± 0.01
Galactose	19.8 ± 1.6	0.11 ± 0.01	20.9 ± 1.3	0.12 ± 0.00
Glucuronic acid	2.7 ± 0.1	0.01 ± 0.00	3.7 ± 0.4	0.02 ± 0.00
Mannose	2.1 ± 0.3	0.01 ± 0.00	3.7 ± 0.6	0.02 ± 0.00
Xylose	1.3 ± 0.2	0.01 ± 0.00	2.9 ± 0.6	0.02 ± 0.00
Ramnose	1.3 ± 0.1	0.01 ± 0.00	1.0 ± 0.0	0.01 ± 0.00
Ribose	0.8 ± 0.2	0.01 ± 0.00	1.4 ± 0.2	0.01 ± 0.00
Arabinose	-	-	-	-
Fucose	-	-	-	-
Galacturonic acid	-	-	-	-

-: not detected; Data represent mean ± SD of three independent samples.

2.3. *The Anionic Fraction of Polysaccharides from T. verrucosa f. rubens PLA1-2 Contains a Significant Amount of Sulfated Polysaccharides and Exhibits Antioxidant Capacity*

To concentrate and separate the sulfated polysaccharides from the total polysaccharides content, the ddH_2O-dissolved polysaccharides (4 mg/mL) of the two *Tetraselmis* strains were fractionated via ion-exchange chromatography, to retain the negatively charged molecules. For each sample of ddH_2O-dissolved polysaccharides, four eluates were obtained. Eluate E_1 was recovered directly after loading the ddH_2O-dissolved polysaccharides onto the ion-exchange column. Next, the eluate E_2 was recovered from the column using pure water (ddH_2O) as eluent. Subsequently, the eluates E_3 and E_4 were obtained after loading the column with NaCl solutions (Sigma-Aldrich, St. Louis, MO, USA) using gradually increasing the NaCl concentration (0.2 and 1.0 M, respectively). The eluates were desalted and characterized concerning their total sugar content, their concentration of sulfates, and their antioxidant capacity expressed as Trolox equivalents. The results are displayed in Table 3.

Table 3. Total sugars, sulfates, sulfates to total sugars ratio (mmol SO_4^- per mg of total sugars), and antioxidant capacity (Trolox equivalents) of the fractions obtained by ion-exchange chromatography from the H_2O-dissolved polysaccharides of the two *Tetraselmis* strains.

Strain	Eluates	Total Sugars (mg/mL)	SO_4^- (mg/mL)	SO_4^-/ Total Sugars (mmol/mg)	Antioxidant Capacity (μM Trolox Eq.)
T. verrucosa f. *rubens* PLA1-2	E_1	0.68 ± 0.04	-	-	-
	E_2	2.06 ± 0.35	-	-	-
	E_3	0.66 ± 0.02	-	-	-
	E_4	0.66 ± 0.06	0.485 ± 0.010	7.65 ± 0.93	3.00 ± 0.71
T. suecica T3-1	E_1	0.59 ± 0.01	-	-	-
	E_2	2.06 ± 0.07	-	-	-
	E_3	1.09 ± 0.05	-	-	-
	E_4	0.59 ± 0.07	0.014 ± 0.004	0.25 ± 0.11	-

-: not detected; Data represent mean ± SD of three independent samples.

The highest concentration of total sugars (2.06 mg/mL) was observed in the case of E_2 eluates of the fractionated ddH_2O-dissolved polysaccharides for both *Tetraselmis* strains. In the E_1, the solvent was also pure water (ddH_2O), thus 0.68 mg/mL and 0.59 mg/mL of neutral polysaccharide molecules were from *T. verrucosa* f. *rubens* PLA1-2 and *T. suecica* T3-1, respectively. The weak and strong anionic polysaccharides of E_3 and E_4 eluates were determined as 0.66 mg/mL for both eluates, in the case of *T. verrucosa* f. *rubens* PLA1-2 and 1.09 mg/mL and 0.59 mg/mL, respectively, in the case of *T. suecica* T3-1. The recovered eluates were characterized concerning the presence of sulfates, while their putative antioxidant capacity was determined by using the Ferric Reducing Antioxidant Power (FRAP) assay. The eluates E_1, E_2, and E_3 did not contain sulfated polysaccharides, nor did they exhibit antioxidant capacity. Similarly, the E_4 eluate from *T. suecica* T3-1 had a low content of sulfated polysaccharides (0.014 mg/mL) and did not exhibit antioxidant capacity. On the contrary, the E_4 eluate of the fractionated ddH_2O-dissolved polysaccharides from *T. verrucosa* f. *rubens* PLA1-2 contained a remarkable concentration of sulfated polysaccharides (0.485 mg/mL) and exhibited antioxidant capacity (3.00 μM Trolox). The presence of sulfated and sugar groups was also confirmed by Fourier transform infrared (FTIR) spectroscopy (see Supplemental Figure S1). Specifically, the observation of the full range spectrum (Supplemental Figure S1a) allowed the identification of three strong peaks at 3390, 1644, and 667 cm^{-1}. These peaks could be assigned to a plethora of bond vibrations such as the -OH and $-NH_2$ group vibrations for the former peak or the C=O, C-N, N-H stretching for the peak at 1644 cm^{-1}. However, due to the aqueous nature of the polysaccharide extracts, these peaks possibly correspond to water bond vibrations and are more specific to the O-H symmetric and asymmetric stretching and the H-O-H bending for the observed peaks at 3390 and 1644 cm^{-1}, respectively [27]. The isolation of the region between 1400 and 900 cm^{-1} (Supplemental Figure S1b), which is less affected by water bond vibrations, allowed the identification of peaks at 1338, 1227, 1123, 1080, 1064, and 996 cm^{-1}. The weak peak at 1338 cm^{-1} could be assigned to the asymmetric stretching vibration of CCO- of carboxylic acid salts, in combination with the respective symmetric stretching vibration at 1644 cm^{-1}. This peak could also be assigned to some proteinic residues (Amide III region; C=N stretching, C=O stretching, N-H bending vibration) [28]. The peak at 1227 cm^{-1} could be associated with the S=O stretching of the sulfated groups in sulfated polysaccharides [29], while the peaks at 1200–900 cm^{-1} are mostly related to polysaccharides and especially the C-O stretching (1123 cm^{-1}), the pyranose ring stretching (1080 and 1064 cm^{-1}) and the alkene C-H stretching of the ring (996 cm^{-1}) [28].

2.4. Biological Properties of the Strongly Anionic Polysaccharides of the Two Tetraselmis Strains

The E_4 eluates (strongly anionic polysaccharides) of both *Tetraselmis* strains that were found to contain high and low levels of sulfated polysaccharides in the case of *T. verrucosa* f. *rubens* PLA1-2 and *T. suecica* T3-1, respectively, were subsequently assessed for effects on the viability of human cells, and for putative wound healing and antiviral properties.

2.4.1. The Strongly Anionic Polysaccharides from the Two Tetraselmis Strains Do Not Negatively Influence the Viability of Human Primary Cells

Normal human dermal fibroblasts (NHDF) cells (primary cells) were used to check for putative effects of E_4 eluates derived from *T. suecica* T3-1 and *T. verrucosa* f. *rubens* PLA1-2 strains, on cell viability. The viability of cells was evaluated using the 3-[4,5-dimethylthiazol-2-yl]-2,5 diphenyl tetrazolium bromide (MTT) colorimetric assay. The cells were incubated with a culture medium containing various concentrations of the E_4 eluates (i.e., 50, 100, 250, and 500 μg/mL) for 24 and 48 h. Control cells were incubated with a culture medium supplemented with the respective volume of ddH_2O. The MTT assay was performed at the end of the incubation period and the results are presented in Figure 2.

As shown in Figure 2, the viability of the normal human primary cells was not negatively affected by the 48-h incubation of cells with the E_4 eluates, even when a concentration of 500 μg anionic polysaccharides per mL of cell culture medium was used. Actually, in several cases, the presence of the anionic polysaccharides had a slight positive effect on the cell viability, compared to the control cells.

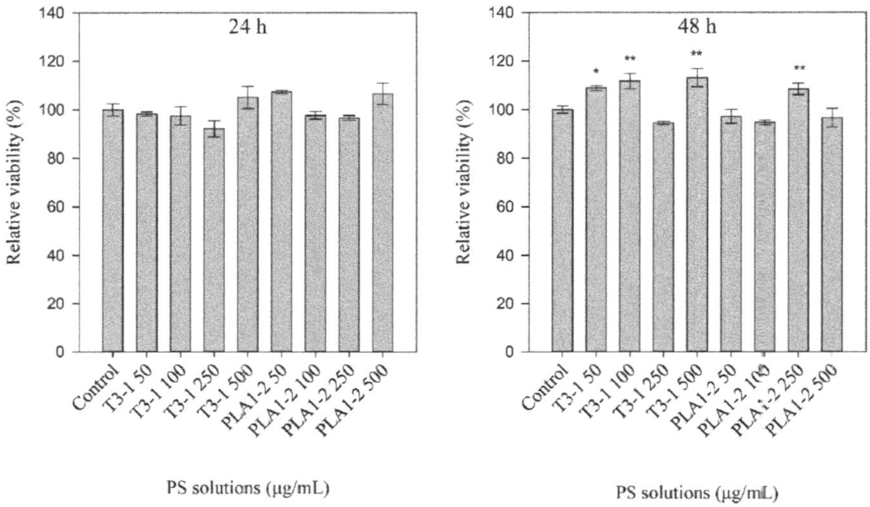

Figure 2. Effect of E4 eluates on cell viability. Relative viability of normal human dermal fibroblasts (NHDF) when incubated (for 24 h-left panel, for 48 h-right panel) in the presence of various concentrations of E_4 eluates derived from the microalgae strains *T. suecica* T3-1 (T3-1) and *T. verrucosa* f. *rubens* PLA1-2 (PLA1-2). The different concentrations of 50, 100, 250, and 500 μg of anionic polysaccharides/mL of cell culture medium, used are mentioned. Control cells were incubated with culture medium supplemented with the respective volume of ddH_2O (which was equal to the volume added in the case of the E_4 eluates). The viability of the cells at the control assay was set to 100%. Bars represent mean values from three independent experiments in triplicate. Error bars indicate standard deviations. * $p < 0.05$, ** $p < 0.01$, versus control assay's results.

2.4.2. The Strongly Anionic Polysaccharides from the *T. verrucosa* f. *rubens* PLA1-2 Strain Exhibit Wound Healing Properties

As cell migration governs the wound healing process to restore the integrity and function of the injured tissue, an in vitro assay using normal human dermal fibroblasts (NHDF) cells was performed to simulate the wound healing procedure [30], in order to test the E_4 eluates from *T. verrucosa* f. *rubens* PLA1-2 and *T. suecica* T3-1 for potential wound healing properties. In brief, NHDF cells seeded in wells were allowed to reach a confluency of almost 80%. Then, a scratch was made in the layer of cells and the migration of cells to close the produced gap, in the presence (or not, control cells) of different concentrations of the strongly anionic polysaccharides of the two *Tetraselmis* strains, was monitored. The closure of the gap due to the migration of cells simulated the wound healing procedure. Two concentrations, 300 μg and 500 μg of the strongly anionic polysaccharides per mL of cell culture medium were tested. The cells used as control were incubated with a culture medium supplemented with the respective volume of ddH_2O. The results are presented in Figure 3.

The E_4 eluate from *T. suecica* T3-1 did not affect the wound healing procedure negatively but also did not exhibit any wound healing properties, neither at 300 nor at 500 μg/mL, compared to the control (approximately 20% relative wound density) after 48 h of incubation. A significant positive effect on the simulated wound healing procedure was observed when the cells were treated with the E_4 eluate from *T. verrucosa* f. *rubens* PLA1-2, at both concentrations used. About 58% relative wound density was achieved when a concentration of 500 μg/mL was applied, while 44% relative wound density was observed in the case of 300 μg/mL. This positive effect was also dose-dependent, as the use of a higher concentration of the E_4 eluate from *T. verrucosa* f. *rubens* PLA1-2 resulted in greater wound density.

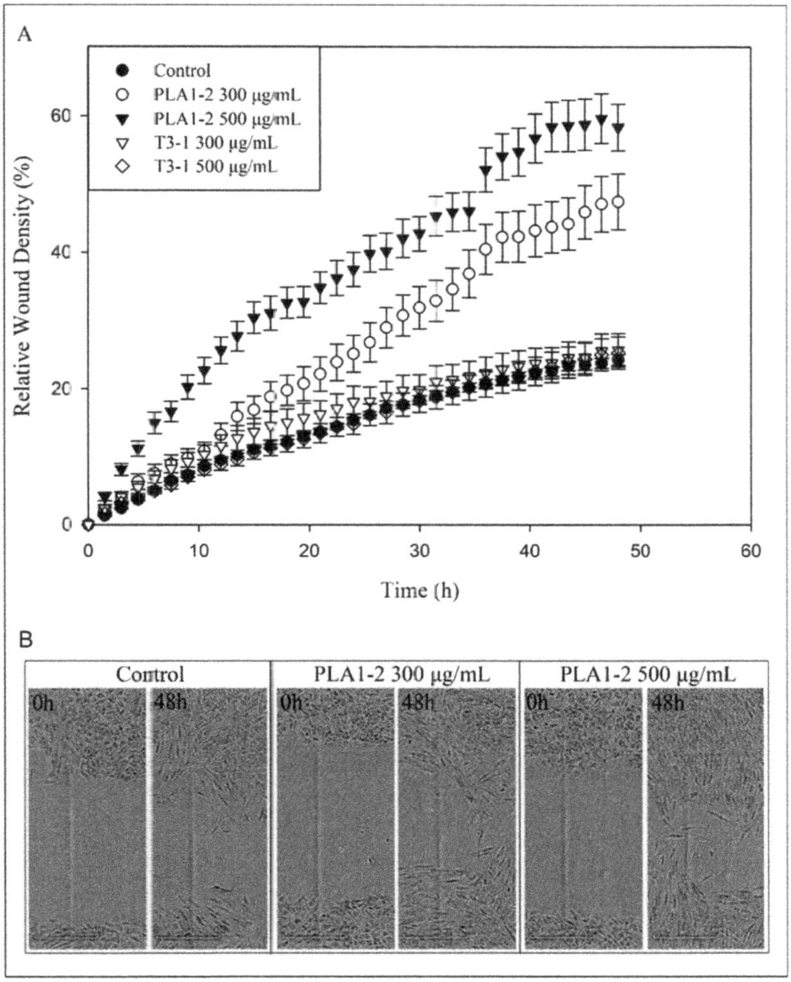

Figure 3. Effect of E4 eluates on wound healing. At t = 0 h a scratch was produced in the layer of NHDF cells, and the culture medium was changed with new one supplemented, or not (control cells), with 300 µg or 500 µg of the strongly anionic polysaccharides of a *Tetraselmis* strain per mL of cell culture medium, and the migration of cells, to close the scratch-produced gap in the cell layer, was monitored every 3 h for 48 h. (**A**) Quantification results of cell migration based on the images of the gap in the layer of cells, at 3 h-intervals post treatment and up to 48 h. Relative wound density achieved using E_4 extracts from *T. verrucosa* f. *rubens* PLA1-2 and *T. suecica* T3-1 as healing agents. The relative wound density is the ratio of the cell occupied area to the area of the initial gap (set at 100%) in the layer of cells. Bars represent mean values from three independent experiments in triplicate. Error bars indicate standard deviations. (**B**) Representative images of the gap in the layer of cells at 0 h and 48 h post treatment. Control cells and cells treated with300 µg, and 500 µg, of the strongly anionic polysaccharides from *T. verrucosa* f. *rubens* PLA1-2. Control cells were incubated with culture medium supplemented with the respective volume of ddH_2O (which was equal to the volume added in the case of the E_4 eluates).

2.4.3. The Strongly Anionic Polysaccharides from the Two Tetraselmis Strains Exhibit Antiviral Activity Against the Replication of Hepatitis C Virus (HCV)

In this study, we tested the E_4 eluates from *T. verrucosa* f. *rubens* PLA1-2 and *T. suecica* T3-1 for antiviral properties against the Hepatitis C Virus (HCV). To test the E_4 eluates for potential effects on HCV replication, we used the human hepatoma Huh5-2 cell line that stably harbors the subgenomic reporter replicon of the HCV genotype 1b (Con1 strain) [31]. The HCV genotype 1 and especially the subtype 1b is the most prevalent group worldwide. This HCV replicon expresses the reporter protein firefly luciferase (F-Luc) the activity of which is directly correlated with the replication level of the replicon, and it has been used extensively for the testing/development of new treatments for HCV [32].

To check for effects on HCV replication by the E_4 eluates from *T. verrucosa* f. *rubens* PLA1-2 and *T. suecica* T3-1, the Huh5-2 cells harboring the HCV reporter replicon, were treated for 72 h with the indicated concentrations (i.e., 50, 100, and 200 μg of the strongly anionic polysaccharides per mL of cell culture medium) of these E_4 eluates. The cells used as control were incubated with a culture medium supplemented with the respective volume of ddH_2O. Then, the cells were lysed, and the viral RNA replication-derived firefly luciferase activity was determined and normalized to the cell's total protein amount. The results are presented in Figure 4A,B.

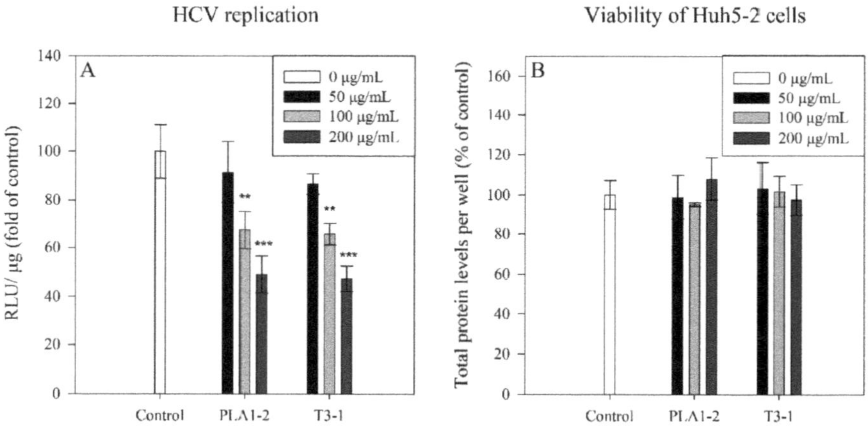

Figure 4. Effect of E4 eluates on HCV replication. Huh5-2 cells stably harboring the subgenomic reporter replicon of HCV that expresses the firefly luciferase (F-Luc), were treated for 72 h with different concentrations, 50 μg, 100 μg, or 200 μg of the strongly anionic polysaccharides of a *Tetraselmis* strain per mL of cell culture medium. Control cells were incubated with culture medium supplemented with the respective volume of ddH_2O (which was equal to the volume added in the case of the E_4 eluates). (**A**) Viral RNA replication-derived firefly luciferase activity in the presence of various concentrations of E_4 eluates derived from the microalgae strains *T. suecica* T3-1 (T3-1) and *T. verrucosa* f. *rubens* PLA1-2 (PLA1-2). The different concentrations of 50, 100, and 200 μg of anionic polysaccharides per mL of cell culture medium, used are mentioned. The mean value of the firefly luciferase activity of control cells (expressed as relative light units (RLU)/μg of protein) was set to 100%. (**B**) Viability of cells in the presence of the anionic polysaccharides from the two *Tetraselmis* strains expressed as total protein levels per well. Bars represent mean values from three independent experiments in triplicate. Error bars indicate standard deviations. ** $p < 0.01$, *** $p < 0.001$, versus control.

As shown, both microalgal E4 eluates exhibited dose-dependent antiviral activity against the HCV replicon without affecting the viability of Huh5-2 cells. Specifically, in the higher concentrations tested (i.e., 100 and 200 μg/mL), the strongly anionic polysaccharides from the *Tetraselmis* strains reduced the HCV replication with the highest inhibition (more than 40%) observed in the case of 200 μg/mL. The median effective concentration (EC_{50}) of the strongly anionic polysaccharides of E4 eluates, from *T. suecica* T3-1 and *T. verrucosa* f. *rubens* PLA1-2 strains, was calculated at 257.3 μg/mL and 210.8 μg/mL, respectively.

3. Discussion

Polysaccharides isolated from microalgae have been shown to exhibit many desirable properties and have applications in the food industry, medicine, and cosmetology. The synthesis and composition of polysaccharides depend upon the microalgae strain and the conditions of cultivation such as nutrient availability, light quality and intensity, salinity, and temperature. Usually, stress conditions induce the production of polysaccharides but at the same time compromise the growth of microalgae [33]. *Tetraselmis* species have been shown to produce large amounts of bioactive polysaccharides [24]. In the present study, many *Tetraselmis* species initially isolated from Greek coastal lagoons, were included to select the ones that produce high amounts of polysaccharides under standard conditions of cultivation. To do so, the different microalgae strains were grown under standard conditions and the microalgae dry biomass (DB) was characterized concerning the total sugar content and the presence of α- and β-glucans.

Interestingly, a high level of sugars in the DB of *Tetraselmis verrucosa* f. *rubens* PLA1-2 was achieved using a cultivation medium (Walne's solution of adjusted salinity 40‰) which was not supplemented with carbohydrates. Similar levels of sugars have been observed for *Arthrospira platensis* (41.1%), *Chlorella vulgaris* (47.9%), and *Dunaliella salina* (31.7%) species but only when their cultivation medium was supplemented with carbohydrates (0.05 g/L) [34]. This stain exhibited also the highest amount of α- and b-glucans in the DB. α-glucans, produced by microalgae as exopolysaccharides or found as wall components or as energy storage compounds, have been shown to act as prebiotics and to exhibit antiproliferative and immunostimulatory properties [35]. β-glucans, found in microalgae as storage compounds, cell-bounded, or as wall components, can positively affect human metabolism due to their antioxidant, hypoglycemic, and hypocholesterolemic properties, while can also modulate the immune responses acting as immunostimulants, anti-inflammatory and anti-cancer agents [36,37].

Previous studies comparing several microalgae species, with respect to β-glucan content in the DB, had revealed that *Scenedesmus ovalternus* 52.80, *Porphyridium purpureum* 1380-1d, *Cylindrotheca fusiformis* 1017/2, and *Tetraselmis suecica* 66/22c strains produced very high amounts of β-glucans (24.2%, 22.4%, 17.9%, and 16.1%, respectively) under standard conditions of cultivation, whereas most of the rest microalgae species studied showed a β-glucan content between 5 and 10% of DB [38]. In the same study, several of the above β-glucans-rich microalgae strains exhibited also very high levels of total carbohydrates in their DB, with *Porphyridium purpureum* 1380-1d reaching 59.2%, while the maximum content of α-glucans was up to 12% and was observed in the same strain. Based on the above, in our study, the maximum amounts of α-glucans (17.7%) and β-glucans (11.0%) in the DB, detected in the case *T. verrucosa* f. *rubens* PLA1-2, represented values close to the typical ones for most microalgae strains.

The composition of the polysaccharides derived from *T. suecica* T3-1 and *T. verrucosa* f. *rubens* PLA1-2 consisted of a significant proportion of galactose, in addition to glucans. Previous studies involving the microalgae species *Chlorella vulgaris, Phaeodactylum tricornutum, Porphyridium purpureum, Scenedesmus ovalternus, Nannochloropsis salina*, and *Dunaliella salina* have revealed that the sugars detected in our *Tetraselmis* strains are often found in polysaccharide extracts of microalgae, glucose and galactose are usually the most abundant sugars detected, and their percentage can vary considerably between microalgal species [13,39].

Galactan polymers and especially their sulfated forms have attracted scientific interest, due to their various properties, such as rheological, antimicrobial, antioxidant, anticoagulant, antithrombotic, and anticancer activities. These properties are directly linked to the structure of the compounds. Typically, galactans are sourced from plants and algae, particularly macroalgae and specifically Rhodophyta, they have a high molecular weight (>100 kDa), demonstrating significant biological activity as hydrocolloids and exhibit distinctive rheological behavior. They are commonly used as stabilizers in various food products, including dairy, bakery, confectionery, etc. [40,41]. Studies have also demonstrated that sulfated carrageenans possess immunomodulatory properties and antitumor activity against Ehrlich-Lettre ascitic carcinoma (EAC) and breast adenocarcinoma [40,42].

Moreover, in our study, the polysaccharides' extracts of *T. verrucosa* f. *rubens* PLA1-2 and *T. suecica* T3-1 were fractionated and checked for the presence of sulfates and for putative antioxidant properties. As in the E_1 and E_2 eluates, the eluent was pure water (ddH_2O), these fractions were rich in neutral polysaccharides that can not bind to the positively charged column. The weak and strong anionic polysaccharides were recovered at the E_3 and E_4 eluates, respectively. Based on the results, the amount of the anionic polysaccharides is lower than that of the neutral polysaccharides in both *Tetraselmis* strains. All polysaccharides' eluates were characterized concerning the presence of sulfates and their putative antioxidant capacity and only the E_4 eluate of *T. verrucosa* f. *rubens* PLA1-2 exhibited high content of sulfated polysaccharides and antioxidant activity. The water-soluble polysaccharides from *Tetraselmis* spp. strains have been shown to present significant antioxidant, antifungal, and tyrosinase inhibitory activities [24]. Moreover, sulfated polysaccharides from microalgae have attracted interest due to their medicinal properties. Sulfated polysaccharides are found mainly in marine organisms, specifically as a key component of cell walls and have significant physiological roles, such as helping to retain moisture protecting the microalgae against drying or acting as a protective barrier against pathogens [43]. Sulfated polysaccharides encompass a diverse group of anionic polymers of high pharmaceutical interest. Actually, the sulfated polysaccharides isolated from *T. suecica* have been shown to exhibit anti-inflammatory activity against NO and IL-6 [22], while those from *Isochrysis galbana*, which is a strain rich in glucans, inhibited the proliferation of human leukemia cells [23]. Moreover, the sulfated polysaccharides from the genus *Porphyridium* spp., have been shown to prevent the accumulation and action of free radicals (ROS), acting protectively against oxidative stress [20,21].

The recovered E4 eluates of *T. verrucosa* f. *rubens* PLA1-2 and *T. suecica* T3-1 were evaluated for putative biological properties such as effects on the viability of human cells, on wound-healing, and on viral replication. Based on our results, there were no negative effects on the viability of primary or of cancer human cells, by the use of the anionic polysaccharides-containing fractions of the two *Tetraselmis* strains, irrespectively of their content of sulfated polysaccharides. In several studies, high and dose-dependent cytotoxicity has been observed when cancerous cell lines were treated with polysaccharides' extracts obtained from microalgae (e.g., *Crypthecodinium cohnii, Galdieria sulphuraria, Isochrysis galbana, Nannochloropsis oculate, Porphyridium cruentum, Dixoniella grisea, Dunaliella salina*, etc.). Therefore, the microalgae-derived polysaccharides' extracts are considered natural compounds bearing anti-cancer properties based on their effects on many human cancer cell lines; indicatively, MCF-7 (breast adenocarcinoma), HeLa (cervical carcinoma), HCT 116 (colorectal carcinoma), U-937 and HL-60 (leukemia), NCI-H460 (lung carcinoma), and HepG2 (hepatocellular liver carcinoma) [44–48]. Interestingly, studies involving non-cancerous cell lines have reported a lack of cytotoxic effects in cells treated with microalgal-derived polysaccharides. For example, no effects on cell viability were observed when Vero cells were treated with *Cladophora* spp. derived sulfated polysaccharides up to a concentration of 625 μg per mL of cell culture medium [49]. Moreover, fractions of polysaccharides from the red microalgae *Porphyridium cruentum* were shown to exhibit cytotoxic effects against several cancerous cell lines (colon carcinoma HT-29 cells, breast adenocarcinoma MCF-7 cells and triple negative mammary adenocarcinoma MDA-MB-231 cells), but did not reduce the viability of a non-cancerous cell line (mammary epithelial MCF-10A cells), when the same concentrations of polysaccharides were used to supplement the cells' culture medium [50].

The absence of cytotoxic effects of E_4 eluates of both *Tetraselmis* strains on the normal human dermal fibroblast cells, gave us the opportunity to use an in vitro assay, that simulates the wound healing procedure by examining the effects on cell migration, to investigate the putative wound healing properties of these fractions. The results showed that the E_4 eluate from *T. suecica* T3-1 did not affect the migration of the normal human dermal fibroblast cells neither positively nor negatively, at any concentration applied. Interestingly, as shown in Table 3, the E_4 eluate from *T. suecica* T3-1 had a low content of sulfated polysaccharides and did not exhibit antioxidant capacity. In contrast, a significant positive effect was observed when the E_4 eluate from *T. verrucosa* f. *rubens* PLA1-2 was used, at both concentrations tested and this effect was also dose-dependent. The E_4 eluate from *T. verrucosa* f. *rubens* PLA1-2 was characterized by notable antioxidant capacity and concentration of sulfated polysaccharides, thus these characteristics seemed to increase the migration of cells towards the scratched area. In vivo, studies should undoubtedly prove the efficacy of the specific eluate on wound healing.

Antioxidant, anti-inflammatory, antimicrobial, antiviral, and hygroscopic effects of sulfated polysaccharides are considered mandatory in skin regeneration [51,52]. By comparing the cell-migration effects of E4 eluates from the two microalgae strains, we conclude that the presence of sulfated polysaccharides bearing antioxidant capacity is crucial for enhancing the migration of the dermal fibroblast cells to restore the gap in the cell layer. Thus, our results are in agreement with numerous studies [53] showing the significant role of sulfated polysaccharides in wound treatment approaches. Indeed, microalgal (especially species belonging to *Chlorophyceae*, *Eustigmatophyceae*, *Chlorodendrophyceae*, and *Porphyridium* spp.) and cyanobacterial biologically active compounds, such as pigments, peptides, fatty acids, and polysaccharides have been widely used in the production of wound dressings for skin regeneration applications. Indicatively, extracts from *Spirulina* spp., *Aphanothece* spp., *Chlorella* spp., *Chlamydomonas* spp., *Tetraselmis* spp., and *Porphyridium* spp. have been examined for various potential effects (including biocompatibility, proliferation and migration of fibroblast cells, antithrombogenicity, antitumor effects against UVB irradiation, anti-photoaging effect, wound angiogenesis, and collagen deposition increase, IgE, TNF-α, IL-4, IL-5, INF-γ reduction, antimicrobial effects, etc.) in aqueous, ethanolic, or methanolic solutions, in simple, synthetic, or hydrogel form [26].

Extracellular polysaccharides isolated from *Nostoc* spp. PCC7936 strain, when cultivated under acetate ions supplementation in the medium were used for hydrogel formation in the presence of 0.4% (*w*/*v*) $FeCl_3$. These biocompatible hydrogels promoted fibroblast migration and wound healing of scratches in NHDF [54]. Water-soluble extracts derived from *Chlorella vulgaris* and *Arthrospira platensis*, containing polysaccharides and proteins, and microencapsulated with sericin, presented cytocompatibility and significant human fibroblast cell migration and complete wound closure, especially when the extract from *A. platensis* was used [55]. In another study, Melo et al. [56] used extracts from *Chlorella vulgaris* cultivated auto- and mixotrophically. Hydrogels were prepared using Carbopol and tested for healing dermal wounds in Swiss albino mice. The hydrogel based on the extract from the mixotrophic cultivation resulted in an accelerated healing process.

In the current study, the E_4 eluates from *T. verrucosa* f. *rubens* PLA1-2 and *T. suecica* T3-1 presented also significant antiviral properties against the Hepatitis C Virus (HCV). HCV has a positive sense single stranded RNA (+ssRNA) as a genome, and it is a blood-borne virus that infects the human liver causing acute or chronic hepatitis, which may progress to liver cirrhosis and hepatocellular carcinoma. According to Word Health Organization (WHO), about 50 million people are infected by HCV worldwide [57]. The viral RNA-dependent RNA-polymerase is error prone, thus, the virus circulates in the blood of the patient in the form of quasispecies making it difficult to develop a vaccine and increasing the likelihood of failure of the direct-acting antivirals, currently used as antiviral therapy, due to the emergence of new mutations. Thus, new agents with multi-level modes of action against HCV are needed.

The putative antiviral activity is probably the most studied property of microalgae-derived sulfated polysaccharides and these compounds have been shown to act as antiviral agents against many enveloped and non-enveloped viruses [43,58]. The proposed mechanisms of action of sulfated polysaccharides include possible changes on the surface of the virion or of the cell, and/or changes on the cell gene expression and metabolism, that could inhibit the virion attachment/penetration and uncoating, and/or suppress the expression and replication of the virus genome, respectively. As the E_4 eluates from both *Tetraselmis* strains reduced the HCV replication, we conclude that this effect is irrespective of the content of sulfated polysaccharides or the presence of antioxidant capacity in these fractions. Extracts with a high degree of sulfation present anionic properties and usually act as protective agents against viruses [33]. Especially, extracellular polysaccharides derived from strains belonging to *Arthrospira* spp., *Porphyridium* spp., *Gyrodinium* spp., *Rhodella* spp., and *Cochlodinium* spp. have exhibited antiviral activity against viruses indicatively belonging in *Herpesviridae, Poxviridae, Paramyxoviridae, Orthomyxoviridae, Retroviridae, Hepadnaviridae*, etc. [13].

4. Materials and Methods

4.1. Microalgae Strains and Cultivation Conditions

Fourteen microalgae strains previously isolated from Greek coastal lagoons and deposited in the AthU-Al (Athens University Algae) strain bank (http://phycotheca.biol.uoa.gr) of the NKUA (National and Kapodistrian University of Athens, Greece), were used in this study. These strains included *Tetraselmis verrucosa* f. *rubens* PLA1-2, *T. verrucosa* f. *rubens* KSI1-3, *T. verrucosa* f. *rubens* KLE1-3, *T. verrucosa* f. *rubens* KLE1-4, *T. suecica* ELO1-1, *T. suecica* ELO1-2, *T. suecica* T3-1, *T.* spp. Mes5, *T.* spp. Mes17, *T.* spp. EST1-2, *Dunaliela salina* 30, *D. salina* 31, *D. salina* 32, and *Nannochloropsis gaditana* PLA1-1. The above microalgae were cultivated for 10 days in rigorously aerated 2-L flasks, using Walne's solution of adjusted salinity 40‰ as a growth medium. The cultivated microalgae were incubated at 21–23 °C, air supplied through a pump at a flow rate of 0.5–1 vvm, at ~35% relative humidity, using a light period of 12 h day/12 h night and a light intensity of 100–150 μmoles × photons × m^{-2} × s^{-1} [59]. To obtain the dry biomass (DB), the grown microalgae were centrifuged at 5000× *g* for 10 min and the microalgae containing pellet was freeze-dried at −45 °C (VirTis Freezemobile 12SL, The Virtis Company, New York, NY, USA) to constant weight. Three independent cultivations and harvests were performed for each microalgae strain.

4.2. Determination of Total Sugars and β-Glucan Content of Microalgae

The total sugar content of microalgae was determined as described by Ntzouvaras et al. [59]. Briefly, the microalgae DB was suspended in ultra-pure water (ddH_2O), 1 mL of the resulting suspension was mixed with 6 mL of phenol-sulfuric acid, incubated at 20 °C with continuous vortexing, and then, the absorbance was measured at 490 nm. A standard curve generated by the absorbance of known amounts of glucose was used to determine the total sugar content of microalgae as glucose equivalents. The results were expressed as g of sugars/100 g of microalgae DB (%, *w*/*w*).

The determination of β-glucans content (g/100 g DB) was conducted using the β-glucan enzyme assay kit (K-YBGL) of Megazyme® (Wicklow, Ireland), following the manufacturer's instructions. Only microalgae that exhibited a total sugar content above 20% *w*/*w* were checked with this assay. The β-glucan enzyme assay determines directly the total and α-glucans and indirectly the β-glucans, and it has been previously used to quantify the β-glucans of microalgae [38,60–62]. Briefly, the quantification of total glucans involved hydrolysis of the microalgae DB in the presence of concentrated sulfuric acid (H_2SO_4, acidic hydrolysis), followed by heating at 100 °C for 2 h to release the monosaccharides. After pH adjustment, the remaining glucan fragments were quantitatively hydrolyzed to glucose molecules using a mixture of highly purified exo-1,3-β-glucanase and β-glucosidase enzymes. Then, the released glucose molecules were incubated with glucose oxidase and peroxidase in the presence of 4-aminoantipyrine and p-hydroxybenzoic acid, and the absorbance of the resulting product was measured at 510 nm against the reagent blank, using a Hitachi U-2000 spectrophotometer (Hitachi Ltd., Tokyo, Japan). Known concentrations of glucose were treated as above (with glucose oxidase and peroxidase) and the measured values of absorbance at 510 nm were used to create a standard curve. The total glucan content (% *w*/*w*) of each microalgae sample was estimated based on the following type:

$$\text{Total glucan content } (\%\ w/w) = \Delta A \times F/W \times 90 \quad (1)$$

where: ΔA = sample reaction absorbance − reagent blank absorbance, F = absorbance value of the D-glucose 100 μg standard, W = weight of sample analyzed.

For the quantification of α-glucans, the microalgae DB was hydrolyzed in the presence of concentrated sodium hydroxide (NaOH, alkaline hydrolysis), followed by adjustment of pH and enzymatic treatment with amyloglucosidase and invertase. The released glucose molecules were treated and quantified as described above. The α-glucan content (% *w*/*w*) of each microalgae sample was estimated based on the following type: α-glucan (% *w*/*w*) = $\Delta A \times F/W \times 9.315$

The β-glucan content of each microalgae sample was calculated indirectly as the difference between total glucan content and α-glucan content. In each process, three independent DB samples were analyzed per microalgae strain.

4.3. Extraction and Isolation of Crude Polysaccharides from Microalgae

The isolation of crude polysaccharides of microalgae involves several steps: (1) the removal of lipophilic molecules from the microalgae DB, (2) the disruption of microalgae to release the water-soluble intracellular, structural, and bound molecules, (3) the deproteinization process, and finally, (4) the recovery of extracts containing the crude polysaccharides.

4.3.1. Extraction of Lipophilic Molecules from the Microalgae DB

Lipophilic molecules (lipids, chlorophyll, and other pigments) are extracted in organic solvents [63]. Thus, the microalgal DB was suspended in acetone under continuous vortexing and centrifuged at 5000× *g* for 10 min at 4 °C (Hettich Universal Centrifuge,

Model 320-R, Merck KGaA, Darmstadt, Germany). The resulting pellet was suspended in acetone and treated again as above. The procedure was repeated several times until the complete decolorization of the microalgal biomass. Residual acetone in the defatted microalgal biomass was removed by evaporation, after drying the biomass at 50 °C under vacuum, using a Flash Evaporator/Rotavapor R-114 system (BÜCHI Labortechnik AG, St. Gallen, Switzerland), for several rounds of 30 min (until biomass weight stabilization).

4.3.2. Microalgae Cells' Disruption Process

To facilitate microalgae cell disruption and molecule extraction, the defatted microalgal biomass was suspended in ddH_2O, and ultrasounds, thermal treatment (incubation in hot water—100 °C), and vortexing techniques were used, according to a slightly modified protocol based on Kurd and Samavati [64] and Huo et al. [65]. The high-frequency ultrasounds were produced by an Ultraschallprozessor Hielscher UP200S device (Hielscher Ultrasonics, Teltow, Germany) (power: 200 W), set at 80% of its power. Ultrasound treatment of each sample lasted 10–15 min with intermediate pauses, while the temperature remained between 80–100 °C, due to the ultrasounds. Then, each sample was centrifuged at 5000× *g* for 10 min. The supernatant containing the crude water-soluble fraction was kept for further treatment, whereas the pellet was treated once again as above to maximize the extraction of molecules. After centrifugation, the new supernatant was kept and mixed with the previous one and further processed.

4.3.3. Deproteinization Process of the Crude Water-Soluble Fraction of the Defatted Microalgal Biomass

The deproteinization procedure was carried out using a 5:1 chloroform/n-butanol solvent mixture (Sevag method) to insolubilize and remove the proteins from the extract through centrifugation. Briefly, the method involved the mixing of the crude water-soluble fraction of the defatted microalgal biomass and the solvent mixture at a 2:1 ratio, followed by vigorous vortexing and centrifugation at 15,000× *g* for 10 min at 4 °C. This resulted in the formation of two phases (an aqueous upper phase and an organic lower phase) and an interface containing the denatured protein precipitate. The interface and the organic phase were removed, while the aqueous phase was mixed with solvent mixture at a 2:1 ratio, vortexed, and centrifuged, and the procedure was repeated until the interface was no longer visible. At least six repetitions were required for the specific extracts, as recommended by Huo et al. [65].

The removal of proteins was confirmed by using the Bradford assay (with detection limits of 0.1–1.0 mg/mL) [66]. Specifically, for each deproteinated sample a small volume (100 μL) was mixed with 5 mL of Bradford reagent 1X (Sigma-Aldrich, St. Louis, MO, USA), vortexed, incubated for 5 min, and then its absorbance was measured at 595 nm. A standard curve generated by the absorbance at 595 nm of known amounts of bovine serum albumin (BSA) protein (Panreac, Barcelona, Spain) was produced and used to quantify the total protein content of the sample as albumin equivalents (g/L). All samples were analyzed in triplicates.

4.3.4. Isolation of Crude Polysaccharides Extract from the Deproteinated Samples

To isolate the polysaccharides, the deproteinated sample was mixed with cold absolute ethanol (96% *v*/*v* purity) in a 1:4 ratio. The mixture was vortexed for 1 h, incubated for 24 h at 4 °C, and then centrifuged at 15,000× *g* for 10 min at 4 °C, to precipitate the polysaccharides. The pellet of polysaccharides was dissolved in ddH_2O and frozen.

4.4. Detection and Quantification of Sugar Monomers of the Polysaccharide Extracts

The polysaccharide extracts were further analyzed to detect the quantity of their respective sugar monomers. For each sample (10.0 mg/mL concentration), 0.5 mL underwent acidic hydrolysis using 1 mL of trifluoroacetic acid (TFA) 4 M, combined with heat treatment (100 °C for 3 h), to release sugar monomers. The resulting hydrolysates were neutralized using an equal volume of NaOH 4 M. Identification and quantification of monosaccharides were carried out using a modified protocol based on 1-phenyl-3-methyl-5-pyrazolone (PMP)-derivatization process adapted from Dai et al. [67] and Ai et al. [68]. Briefly, 0.5 mL of the hydrolyzed sample was mixed with 0.8 mL of 0.5 M PMP and 1.2 mL of 0.3 M NaOH and heated in a water bath at 70 °C for 1 h, to facilitate PMP-derivatives. The sample then was cooled using a cold-water bath and 1.2 mL of 0.3 M HCl was added to neutralize the pH and terminate the reaction. To remove excess PMP, 1 mL of chloroform was added to the mixture, followed by vortexing and centrifugation at 17,000× *g* for 10 min, resulting in the formation of two phases. The lower phase (organic) that contained the PMP was removed. For the complete removal of PMP the above process was repeated 2–3 times and then, the aqueous phase was subjected to High Performance Liquid Chromatography (HPLC) using a Waters Alliance 2695 apparatus (Waters Corporation, Milford, MA, USA) equipped with a RP-HPLC Column SVEA C18 Plus (4.6 mm × 250.0 mm, 5.0 µm) (Thermo Fisher Scientific, Waltham, MA, USA) and a Waters 2696 PhotoDAD (Diode Array Detector) (Waters Corporation, Milford, MA, USA) for UV detection at 245 nm. The injection volume was 20 µL with an eluant flow rate of 0.8 mL/min. Two mobile phases were used, and gradient elution was performed. Mobile phase A was 100% acetonitrile and phase B was a mixture of ddH_2O and acetonitrile (9:1, *v*/*v*) with 0.045% KH_2PO_4 and 0.05% triethylamine buffer (pH 7.5), as described by Ai et al. [68]. The identification of the sugar monomers was based on the retention time of each substance, compared to the retention time of standards (i.e., arabinose, fucose, galactose, glucose, mannose, rhamnose, ribose, glucuronic acid, galacturonic acid, and xylose). The peak area ratio of the analyte relative to that of the respective standard and the concentration of the standard were used to calculate the content (%, *w*/*w*) of each sugar monomer in the polysaccharide extract. Three independent samples were analyzed per microalgae strain.

4.5. Fractionation of Polysaccharide Extracts and Eluates Characterization

For each polysaccharide extract, fractionation was performed via ion-exchange chromatography, using as an anion exchanger the diethylaminoethyl cellulose resin (DEAE Cellulose 52) (Sigma-Aldrich, St. Louis, MO, USA), to retain the negatively charged molecules. Chromatography was performed using a 15.0 mm × 100 mm Glass Fritted Chromatography Column (Bio-Rad, Hercules, CA, USA) with 5 mL of stationary phase. The resin layer was washed with 20 mL of ddH_2O, then 1 mL of the polysaccharide extract was added to the column, and the eluate was recovered (E1). Then, 1 mL pure water (ddH_2O) was loaded onto the column and the eluate (E2) was obtained. Next, the eluates E3 and E4 were obtained after loading the column with NaCl solutions using a gradually increasing NaCl concentration (0.2 and 1.0 M, respectively), to elute the negatively charged molecules bound to the column. The NaCl was removed from the eluates through filtration using Amicon Ultra-2 centrifugal filters (with cut-off 3 kDa) (Sigma-Aldrich, St. Louis, MO, USA), according to the manufacturer's instructions. The eluates were analyzed to determine the total sugars as described above (Materials and Methods Section 4.2), and further characterized concerning the concentration of sulfates and their antioxidant activity (see below).

4.5.1. Quantification of Eluates' Sulfates of the Polysaccharide Extracts

The determination of sulfates (SO_4^-, mg/mL) in the eluates derived from the fractionation of the polysaccharide extracts, was carried out based on the protocol developed by Torres et al. [69]. Briefly, 20 μL of appropriately diluted eluate (detection limits of sulfates: 0.01–1.22 mg/mL) was mixed with 140 μL of 0.5 M HCl and 40 μL of barium chloride-gelatin reagent, in a flat-bottom 96-well clear plate (SPL Lifescience, Pocheon, Republic of Korea). After 30 min of incubation, the absorbance was measured at 405 nm. Three independent samples were analyzed per microalgae strain. The quantification of sulfates (mg/mL) was based on a standard curve generated by the absorbance at 405 nm of known concentrations of SO_4^-, derived from Na_2SO_4 (0.676 mg SO_4^- per mg Na_2SO_4). To produce the barium chloride-gelatin reagent, 25 mg of gelatin (Sigma-Aldrich, St. Louis, MO, USA) was mixed with 25 mL of ddH_2O and incubated for 10 min under gentle agitation at 80 °C. Subsequently, 250 mg of $BaCl_2$ (Sigma-Aldrich, St. Louis, MO, USA) was added and stirred to homogenize.

4.5.2. Antioxidant Capacity of the Eluates of the Polysaccharide Extracts

The antioxidant capacity of the eluates of the polysaccharide extracts was evaluated using the Ferric Reducing Antioxidant Power (FRAP) assay, by monitoring the capacity of the extract to reduce ferric tripyridyl triazine to ferrous triazine, as previously described by Wang et al. [70], with minor modifications. Briefly, 10 μL of appropriately diluted eluate (detection limits: 20–200 μM Trolox equivalents, see below) was mixed with 190 μL of FRAP reagent, vortexed, and incubated at 37 °C for 30 min. Absorbance was measured at 593 nm using a microplate reader (Tecan, Männedorf, Switzerland). A standard curve of the FRAP assay was generated using known amounts of the 6-hydroxy-2,5,7,8-tetramethylchroman-2-carboxylic acid (Trolox) (Sigma-Aldrich, St. Louis, MO, USA) and used to quantify the total antioxidant capacity of the eluates as Trolox equivalents (μM). Three independent samples were analyzed per microalgae strain.

4.5.3. Attenuated Total Reflection—Fourier Transform Infrared (ATR-FTIR) Analysis

The ATR-FTIR spectra of the *T. verrucosa* f. *rubens* PLA1-2 polysaccharide extract (E4 eluate) were obtained by a Perkin Elmer Spectrum-Two spectrometer equipped with a Diamond ATR compartment (Perkin Elmer, Hopkinton, MA, USA) using the Spectrum 10 software (v.10.5.1.581) provided by the manufacturer. The recorded spectrum was an average of 64 scans in the mid-infrared region (4000 and 400 cm^{-1}) at a resolution of 4 cm^{-1}. The recorded spectrum was then ATR-corrected using a refractive index of 1.5 for diamond, to be comparable to the available spectral libraries for facilitating the interpretation of spectra, linear baseline was corrected and then normalized by the mean using The Unscrambler X v.10.5 software (CAMO software, Oslo, Norway).

4.6. Biological Properties of the Eluates of the Polysaccharide Extracts

Selected eluates (E1-4) of the polysaccharide extracts were subsequently assessed for effects on the viability of human cells and for putative antiviral and wound healing properties. To do so the polysaccharide extract eluates were freeze-dried and then a specific amount was dissolved in ddH_2O.

4.6.1. Effects on the Viability of Human Cells

Putative effects of the polysaccharide extract eluates on human cell viability were assessed in vitro using normal human dermal fibroblasts (NHDF-Ad—Human Dermal Fibroblasts, Adult) (Lonza Group, Brussels, Switzerland) cells (primary cells), whereas the cell viability was evaluated with the 3-[4,5-dimethylthiazol-2-yl]-2,5 diphenyl tetrazolium bromide (MTT) assay. This assay is based on the conversion of the yellow MTT into purple formazan crystals, by the mitochondrial activity of the living cells. Formazan crystals are dissolved in DMSO and the absorbance at 560 nm of the resulting solution is used to estimate the viability of cells.

Prior to the assay, NHDF cells were routinely cultivated in a Fibroblast Growth Medium-2 (FGM-2 Bulletkit, Lonza Group, Brussels, Switzerland) at 37 °C and 5% CO_2 and subcultured with ReagentPack™ Subculture kit (Lonza Group, Brussels, Switzerland), following the instructions of the manufacturer. To check for effects of a polysaccharide extract eluate on cell viability, NHDF cells were seeded in 96-wells sterile culture plates (Nunc™, Thermo Fisher Scientific, Rockford, IL, USA) (10,000 cells/well) and cultivated in fibroblast growth media-2 (FGM-2 medium; Lonza, Walkersville, MD, USA) for 24 h. Then, the culture medium was replaced with a new one containing different amounts of the polysaccharide extract eluate (concentrations used: 50–500 μg/mL) or the equal volume of ddH_2O (control), and the cells were further incubated for 24 and 48 h. Subsequently, 20 μL of MTT (Sigma-Aldrich, St. Louis, MO, USA) (5 mg/mL) was added to each well, the cells were incubated for 2 h, then 200 μL dimethylsulfoxide (DMSO; Panreac, Barcelona, Spain) was added, to dissolve the formed purple formazan crystals, and the absorbance was measured at 560 nm. Background control wells contained only the culture medium and MTT reagent, without cells, to account for any non-specific absorbance and ensure accurate measurement of cell viability. All samples were analyzed in quadruplicate and the cell viability was calculated according to the following equation:

$$\text{Cell Viability due to tested sample (\%)} = (\text{Absorbance of the test at 560 nm})/(\text{Absorbance of the control at 560 nm}) \times 100)$$

4.6.2. Wound Healing Effects

For the assessment of the putative wound healing properties of the polysaccharide extract eluates, approximately 20,000 NHDF cells per well were seeded in the Incucyte® Imagelock 96-Well Plate (Essen BioScience, Sartorius, Royston, UK) and incubated for 24 h. Then, standardized wounds were created using Wound Maker™ (Essen BioScience, Sartorius, Royston, UK). The culture medium was carefully removed, the cells were washed with PBS 1X and a new culture medium that contained a lower amount of fetal calf serum (FCS) (1%) to reduce cell proliferation, and was supplemented with a polysaccharide extract eluate, was added. Two different concentrations (300 and 500 μg/mL) of polysaccharide extract eluates were used, whereas the cells used as controls in the respective new culture medium were supplemented with an equal volume of ddH_2O. Then, the cells were incubated at 37 °C, 5% (v/v) CO_2 in a humidified incubator connected with IncuCyte S3 apparatus (Essen BioScience, Sartorius, Royston, UK) to monitor cell migration (magnification ×10, photo shooting every three hours for 48 h). After this period, the results of each time point were collected and analyzed, and the relative healing of the wound was determined using the Incucyte® ZOOM™ software (v2009B) (Essen BioScience, Sartorius, Royston, UK).

4.6.3. Antiviral Activity Properties

The putative antiviral activity of the polysaccharide extract eluates was examined in the human hepatoma Huh5-2 cell line stably harboring the subgenomic reporter replicon of the Hepatitis C virus (HCV) genotype 1b (Con1 strain) [31]. This HCV subgenomic reporter replicon autonomously replicates in the Huh5-2 cells and expresses a selectable marker (the neo gene), which encodes the enzyme aminoglycoside 3′-phosphotransferase conferring resistance to geneticin (G418), and the reporter protein firefly luciferase (F-Luc). The level of F-Luc activity directly correlates with the level of the replication of this HCV replicon [31]. The Huh5-2 cells harboring the HCV reporter replicon were routinely cultured using high glucose (25 mM) Dulbecco's modified minimal essential medium (Thermo Fisher Scientific, Waltham, MA, USA), supplemented with 0.1 mM non-essential amino acids, 2 mM L-glutamine, 100 U/mL penicillin, 100 μg/mL streptomycin, 10% (*v*/*v*) heat inactivated FCS, and 500 μg/mL geneticin (G418) [71] and incubated at 37 °C, 5% (*v*/*v*) CO_2 in a humidified incubator.

To check for the effects of a polysaccharide extract eluate on the replication of the HCV, the cells were seeded in 96-wells plates. At 24 h the culture medium was replaced with a new one which did not contain geneticin but contained different amounts of the polysaccharide extract eluate (concentrations used: 50, 100, or 200 μg/mL) or the equal volume of ddH_2O (control). The cells were further incubated for 72 h and then, the cells were washed twice with phosphate buffered saline (PBS) 1X and lysed in 40 μL of Luciferase Cell Culture Lysis Reagent 1X (Promega Corporation, Madison, WI, USA). F-Luc activity was determined in cell lysates, using the Luciferase Assay system (Promega Corporation, Madison, WI, USA) according to the manufacturer's instructions. Briefly, 4 μL of the cell lysate was mixed with 30 μL of Luciferase Assay Reagent, vortexed immediately and the produced bioluminescence was measured using a GloMax 20/20 single tube luminometer (Promega Corporation, Madison, WI, USA) for 10 s. Luciferase activity was normalized to the total protein amount quantified with the Bradford assay and expressed as relative light units per μg of protein (RLU/μg). The median effective concentration (EC_{50}) of the polysaccharide extract eluate, refers to the concentration that reduces the F-Luc signal by 50% compared to the control and it was determined by nonlinear regression analysis using the Prism 6.0 software (GraphPad Software Inc., La Jolla, CA, USA).

5. Conclusions

Microalgae have been demonstrated to be valuable sources of molecules, including bioactive polysaccharides. The microalgae strains studied here exhibited heterogeneity regarding the total sugar content. Among them, *T. suecica* T3-1 and *T. verrucosa* f. *rubens* PLA1-2 contained significant amounts of β-glucans, followed by galactans. The anionic eluates of both microalgae showed no cytotoxicity in normal (NHDF) and cancer (Huh5-2) cells even in high concentrations but displayed significant antiviral activity against the Hepatitis C virus replicon. The anionic eluate of *T. verrucosa* f. *rubens* PLA1-2 contained notable sulfates, presented antioxidant capacity, and was found to increase the migration of the NHDF cells in a wound healing simulating assay, thus it could be potentially utilized as a wound healing agent in skin regeneration.

Supplementary Materials: The following supporting information can be downloaded at: https://www.mdpi.com/article/10.3390/md23020077/s1, Table S1: Growth parameters of the various microalgae strains used in the present study. Starting cell density (CDs), final cell density (CDf), growth rate during exponential phase (μmax) and final dry biomass (X) concentration after 10 days of cultivation of microalgae on using Walne's culture medium under specific conditions.; Figure S1: ATR-FTIR spectrum of the *Tetraselmis verrucosa* f. *rubens* PLA1-2 extracts at (**a**) 4000–400 cm^{-1} and (**b**) 1400–900 cm^{-1}. The peaks of interest are marked.

Author Contributions: Conceptualization, G.V., S.M., I.T., A.E.-A. and E.F.; methodology, G.V., S.M., A.N., M.-E.Z., E.K. (Eirini Kyriakopoulou), K.I.K., G.B., S.C., N.V., G.M., I.T., A.E.-A., S.P. and E.F.; software, G.V., S.M., M.-E.Z., G.B., S.C., N.V., G.M. and E.F.; validation, S.M., M.-E.Z., K.I.K., S.C., N.V., G.M., I.T., A.E.-A., S.P. and E.F.; formal analysis, G.V., S.M., A.N., M.-E.Z., E.K. (Eirini Kyriakopoulou), K.I.K., G.B., E.K. (Evangelos Korakidis) and S.C.; investigation, G.V., S.M., A.N., M.-E.Z., E.K. (Eirini Kyriakopoulou), E.K. (Evangelos Korakidis) and N.P.; resources, N.V., G.M., I.T., A.E.-A., S.P. and E.F.; data curation, G.V., S.M., A.N., M.-E.Z., E.K. (Eirini Kyriakopoulou), K.I.K., G.B., E.K. (Evangelos Korakidis), N.P., S.C., N.V. and E.F.; writing—original draft preparation, G.V. and K.I.K.; writing—review and editing, S.M., A.N., M.-E.Z., E.K. (Eirini Kyriakopoulou), K.I.K., G.B., E.K. (Evangelos

Korakidis); N.P., S.C., N.V., G.M., I.T., A.E.-A., S.P. and E.F.; visualization, G.V., S.M., M.-E.Z., E.K. (Eirini Kyriakopoulou), K.I.K., G.B. and S.C.; supervision, N.V., G.M., I.T., A.E.-A., S.P. and E.F.; project administration, I.T., A.E.-A. and E.F.; funding acquisition, I.T., A.E.-A. and E.F. All authors have read and agreed to the published version of the manuscript.

Funding: This research was co-funded by the European Regional Development Fund of the European Union and Greek national funds through the Operational Program Competitiveness, Entrepreneurship and Innovation under the call "SPECIAL ACTIONS 'AQUACULTURE—INDUSTRIAL MATERIALS—OPEN INNOVATION IN CULTURE' (Project Code: T6YBΠ-00377, Project Acronym: PhyCosmetic-GR)".

Institutional Review Board Statement: Not applicable.

Data Availability Statement: The original data presented in the study are included in the article/Supplementary Material; further inquiries can be directed to the corresponding author.

Acknowledgments: We would like to express our gratitude to R. Bartenschlager (Heidelberg University, Germany) for kindly providing the Huh5-2 replicon cell line to the Molecular Virology laboratory of the Hellenic Pasteur Institute, where the antiviral activity experiments were conducted under the supervision of Niki Vassilaki. We would like, also, to express our gratitude to A. C. Kaliora for kindly providing access to the FTIR analysis equipment at the Laboratory of Food Chemistry, Biochemistry and Physical Chemistry, Harokopio University of Athens.

Conflicts of Interest: The authors declare no conflict of interest. The funders had no role in the design of the study; in the collection, analyses, or interpretation of data; in the writing of the manuscript; or in the decision to publish the results.

References

1. Markou, G.; Nerantzis, E. Microalgae for high-value compounds and biofuels production: A review with focus on cultivation under stress conditions. *Biotechnol. Adv.* **2013**, *31*, 1532–1542. [CrossRef] [PubMed]
2. Tsiplakou, E.; Abdullah, M.A.M.; Skliros, D.; Chatzikonstantinou, M.; Flemetakis, E.; Labrou, N.; Zervas, G. The effect of dietary *Chlorella vulgaris* supplementation on micro-organism community, enzyme activities and fatty acid profile in the rumen liquid of goats. *J. Anim. Physiol. Anim. Nutr.* **2016**, *101*, 275–283. [CrossRef] [PubMed]
3. Letsiou, S.; Kalliampakou, K.; Gardikis, K.; Mantecon, L.; Infante, C.; Chatzikonstantinou, M.; Labrou, N.E.; Flemetakis, E. Skin protective effects of *Nannochloropsis gaditana* extract on H_2O_2-stressed human dermal fibroblasts. *Front. Mar. Sci.* **2017**, *4*, 221. [CrossRef]
4. Chatzikonstantinou, M.; Kalliampakou, A.; Gatzogia, M.; Flemetakis, E.; Katharios, P.; Labrou, N. Comparative analyses and evaluation of the cosmeceutical potential of selected *Chlorella* strains. *J. Appl. Phycol.* **2017**, *29*, 179–188. [CrossRef]
5. Barkia, I.; Saari, N.; Manning, S.R. Microalgae for high-value products towards human health and nutrition. *Mar. Drugs* **2019**, *17*, 304. [CrossRef]
6. Ntzouvaras, A. Commercial cultivation of *Dunaliella salina* for the production of beta-carotene. In *Algae for Food Cultivation, Processing and Nutritional Benefits*; Raja, R., Hemaiswarya, S., Arunkumar, K., Carvalho, I., Eds.; CRC Press: Boca Raton, FL, USA, 2021; pp. 47–53.
7. Sijil, P.V.; Cherita, C.; Jethani, H.; Chauhan, V.S. Microalgae as a Renewable and Sustainable Source of High Value Metabolites. In *Microalgae for Sustainable Products: The Green Synthetic Biology Platform*; Shekh, A., Dasgupta, S., Eds.; The Royal Society of Chemistry: London, UK, 2022; pp. 1–26.
8. Zisis, F.; Kyriakaki, P.; Satolias, F.F.; Mavrommatis, A.; Simitzis, P.E.; Pappas, A.C.; Surai, P.F.; Tsiplakou, E. The Effect of dietary inclusion of microalgae *Schizochytrium* spp. on ewes' milk quality and oxidative status. *Foods* **2022**, *11*, 2950. [CrossRef]
9. Chantzistrountsiou, X.; Ntzouvaras, A.; Papadaki, S.; Tsirigoti, A.; Tzovenis, I.; Economou-Amilli, A. Carotenogenic activity of two hypersaline Greek *Dunaliella salina* strains under nitrogen deprivation and salinity stress. *Water* **2023**, *15*, 241. [CrossRef]
10. Kyriakaki, P.; Mavrommatis, A.; Tsiplakou, E. *Schizochytrium* spp. dietary supplementation modulates immune-oxidative transcriptional signatures in monocytes and neutrophils of dairy goats. *Antioxidants* **2023**, *12*, 497. [CrossRef]
11. Kyriakaki, P.; Mavrommatis, A.; Tsiplakou, E. The interaction of microalgae dietary inclusion and forage-to-concentrate ratio on the lipid metabolism-related gene expression in subcutaneous adipose tissue of dairy goats. *Animals* **2024**, *14*, 3291. [CrossRef]
12. Udayan, A.; Pandey, A.K.; Sirohi, R.; Sreekumar, N.; Sang, B.-I.; Sim, S.-J.; Kim, S.-H.; Pandey, A. Production of microalgae with high lipid content and their potential as sources of nutraceuticals. *Phytochem. Rev.* **2023**, *22*, 833–860. [CrossRef]

13. Raposo, M.D.J.; de Morais, R.; Bernardo de Morais, A. Bioactivity and applications of sulphated polysaccharides from marine microalgae. *Mar. Drugs* **2013**, *11*, 233–252. [CrossRef] [PubMed]
14. Gaignard, C.; Gargouch, N.; Dubessay, P.; Delattre, C.; Pierre, G.; Laroche, C.; Fendri, I.; Abdelkafi, S.; Michaud, P. New horizons in culture and valorization of red microalgae. *Biotechnol. Adv.* **2019**, *37*, 193–222. [CrossRef] [PubMed]
15. Tounsi, L.; Hentati, F.; Hlima, H.-B.; Barkallah, M.; Smaoui, S.; Fendri, I.; Michaud, P.; Abdelkafi, S. Microalgae as feedstock for bioactive polysaccharides. *Int. J. Biol. Macromol.* **2022**, *221*, 1238–1250. [CrossRef]
16. Prybylski, N.; Toucheteau, C.; El Alaoui, H.; Bridiau, N.; Maugard, T.; Abdelkafi, S.; Fendri, I.; Delattre, C.; Dubessay, P.; Pierre, G.; et al. Bioactive polysaccharides from microalgae. *Handb. Microalgae-Based Process. Prod.* **2020**, *20*, 533–571.
17. Delattre, C.; Pierre, G.; Laroche, C.; Michaud, P. Production, extraction and characterization of microalgal and cyanobacterial exopolysaccharides. *Biotechnol. Adv.* **2016**, *34*, 1159–1179. [CrossRef]
18. Dvir, I.; Chayoth, R.; Sod-Moriah, U.; Shany, S.; Nyska, A.; Stark, A.H.; Madar, Z.; Arad, S.M. Soluble polysaccharide of red microalga *Porphyridium* sp. alters intestinal morphology and reduces serum cholesterol in rats. *Br. J. Nutr.* **2000**, *84*, 469–476. [CrossRef]
19. Umemura, K.; Yanase, K.; Suzuki, M.; Okutani, K.; Yamori, T.; Andoh, T. Inhibition of DNA topoisomerases I and II, and growth inhibition of human cancer cell lines by a marine microalgal polysaccharide. *Biochem. Pharmacol.* **2003**, *66*, 481–487. [CrossRef]
20. Tannin-Spitz, T.; Bergman, M.; van Moppes, D.; Grossman, S.; Arad, S.M. Antioxidant activity of the polysaccharide of the red microalga *Porphyridium* sp. *J. Appl. Phycol.* **2005**, *17*, 215–222. [CrossRef]
21. Sun, L.; Wang, C.; Shi, Q.; Ma, C. Preparation of different molecular weight polysaccharides from *Porphyridium cruentum* and their antioxidant activities. *Int. J. Biol. Macromol.* **2009**, *45*, 42–47. [CrossRef]
22. Jo, W.S.; Choi, Y.J.; Kim, H.J.; Nam, B.H.; Hong, S.H.; Lee, G.A.; Lee, S.W.; Seo, S.Y.; Jeong, M.H. Anti-inflammatory effect of microalgal extracts from *Tetraselmis suecica*. *Food Sci. Biotechnol.* **2010**, *19*, 1519–1528. [CrossRef]
23. Sadovskaya, I.; Souissi, A.; Souissi, S.; Grard, T.; Lencel, P.; Greene, C.M.; Duin, S.; Dmitrenik, P.S.; Chizhov, A.O.; Shashkov, A.S.; et al. Chemical structure and biological activity of a highly branched (1→3,1→6)-β-d-glucan from *Isochrysis galbana*. *Carbohydr. Polym.* **2014**, *111*, 139–148. [CrossRef] [PubMed]
24. Kashif, A.S.; Hwang, Y.J.; Park, J.K. Potent biomedical applications of isolated polysaccharides from marine microalgae *Tetraselmis* species. *Bioprocess Biosyst. Eng.* **2018**, *41*, 1611–1620. [CrossRef] [PubMed]
25. Colusse, G.A.; Carneiro, J.; Duarte, M.E.R.; Carvalho, J.C.; Noseda, M.D. Advances in microalgal cell wall polysaccharides: A review focused on structure, production, and biological application. *Crit. Rev. Biotechnol.* **2022**, *42*, 562–577. [CrossRef]
26. Miguel, S.P.; Ribeiro, M.P.; Otero, A.; Coutinho, P. Application of microalgae and microalgal bioactive compounds in skin regeneration. *Algal Res.* **2021**, *58*, 102395. [CrossRef]
27. Mercantili, L.; Davis, F.; Higson, S.P.J. Ultrasonic initiation of the alkaline hydrolysis of triglycerides (saponification) without phase catalysis. *J. Surfactants Deterg.* **2014**, *17*, 133–141. [CrossRef]
28. Socrates, G. *Infrared and Raman Characteristic Group Frequencies: Tables and Charts*, 3rd ed.; John Wiley & Sons Ltd.: Chichester, UK, 2001.
29. Pereira, L.; Amado, A.M.; Critchley, A.T.; van de Velde, F.; Ribeiro-Claro, P.J.A. Identification of selected seaweed polysaccharides (phycocolloids) by vibrational spectroscopy (FTIR-ATR and FT-Raman). *Food Hydrocoll.* **2009**, *23*, 1903–1909. [CrossRef]
30. Cappiello, F.; Casciaro, B.; Mangoni, M.L. A novel in vitro wound healing assay to evaluate cell migration. *J. Vis. Exp.* **2018**, *133*, e56825. [CrossRef]
31. Vrolijk, J.M.; Kaul, A.; Hansen, B.E.; Lohmann, V.; Haagmans, B.L.; Schalm, S.W.; Bartenschlager, R. A replicon-based bioassay for the measurement of interferons in patients with chronic hepatitis C. *J. Virol. Methods* **2003**, *110*, 201–209. [CrossRef]
32. Khan, S.; Soni, S.; Veerapu, N.S. HCV replicon systems: Workhorses of drug discovery and resistance. *Front. Cell. Infect. Microbiol.* **2020**, *10*, 325. [CrossRef]
33. Costa, J.A.V.; Lucas, B.F.; Alvarenga, A.G.P.; Moreira, J.B.; de Morais, M.G. Microalgae polysaccharides: An overview of production, characterization, and potential applications. *Polysaccharides* **2021**, *2*, 759–772. [CrossRef]
34. Andreeva, A.; Budenkova, E.; Babich, O.; Sukhikh, S.; Dolganyuk, V.; Michaud, P.; Ivanova, S. Influence of carbohydrate additives on the growth rate of microalgae biomass with an increased carbohydrate content. *Mar. Drugs* **2021**, *19*, 381. [CrossRef]
35. Reddy Shetty, P.; Batchu, U.R.; Buddana, S.K.; Sambasiva Rao, K.; Penna, S. A comprehensive review on α-D-Glucans: Structural and functional diversity, derivatization and bioapplications. *Carbohydr. Res.* **2021**, *503*, 108297. [CrossRef] [PubMed]
36. Vetvicka, V.; Vannucci, L.; Sima, P.; Richter, J. Beta Glucan: Supplement or drug? From laboratory to clinical trials. *Molecules* **2019**, *24*, 1251. [CrossRef] [PubMed]
37. Varnosfaderani, S.M.N.; Ebrahimzadeh, F.; Oryani, M.A.; Khalili, S.; Almasi, F.; Heris, R.M.; Payandeh, Z.; Li, C.; Afjade, M.N.; Bahrami, A.A. Potential promising anticancer applications of β-glucans: A review. *Biosci. Rep.* **2024**, *44*, BSR20231686.
38. Schulze, C.; Wetzel, M.; Reinhardt, J.; Schmidt, M.; Felten, L.; Mundt, S. Screening of microalgae for primary metabolites including β-glucans and the influence of nitrate starvation and irradiance on β-glucan production. *J. Appl. Phycol.* **2016**, *28*, 2719–2725. [CrossRef]

39. Ortiz-Tena, J.G.; Rühmann, B.; Schieder, D.; Sieber, V. Revealing the diversity of algal monosaccharides: Fast carbohydrate fingerprinting of microalgae using crude biomass and showcasing sugar distribution in *Chlorella vulgaris* by biomass fractionation. *Algal Res.* **2016**, *17*, 227–235. [CrossRef]
40. Delattre, C.; Fenoradosoa, T.A.; Michaud, P. Galactans: An overview of their most important sourcing and applications as natural polysaccharides. *Braz. Arch. Biol. Technol.* **2011**, *54*, 1075–1092. [CrossRef]
41. Pierre, G.; Delattre, C.; Laroche, C.; Michaud, P. Galactans and its applications. In *Polysaccharides*; Ramawat, K., Mérillon, J.M., Eds.; Springer: Cham, Switzerland, 2014; pp. 1–37.
42. Yuan, H.; Song, J.; Li, X.; Li, N.; Dai, J. Immunomodulation and antitumor activity of kappa carrageenan oligosaccharides. *Cancer Lett.* **2006**, *243*, 228–234. [CrossRef]
43. Panggabean, J.A.; Adiguna, S.P.; Rahmawati, S.I.; Ahmadi, P.; Zainuddin, E.N.; Bayu, A.; Putra, M.Y. Antiviral activities of algal-based sulfated polysaccharides. *Molecules* **2022**, *27*, 1178. [CrossRef]
44. Gardeva, E.; Toshkova, R.; Yossifova, L.; Minkova, K.; Gigova, L. Cytotoxic and apoptogenic potential of red microalgal polysaccharides. *Biotechnol. Biotechnol. Equip.* **2012**, *26*, 3167–3172. [CrossRef]
45. Hafsa, M.B.; Ismail, M.B.; Garrab, M.; Aly, R.; Gagnon, J.; Naghmouchi, K. Antimicrobial, antioxidant, cytotoxic and anti-cholinesterase activities of water-soluble polysaccharides extracted from microalgae *Isochrysis galbana* and *Nannochloropsis oculate*. *J. Serb. Chem. Soc.* **2017**, *82*, 509–522.
46. Singab, A.N.; Ibrahim, N.; Elsayed, A.E.; El-Senousy, W.; Aly, H.; Abd Elsamiae, A.; Matloub, A. Antiviral, cytotoxic, antioxidant and anti-cholinesterase activities of polysaccharides isolated from microalgae *Spirulina platensis*, *Scenedesmus obliquus* and *Dunaliella salina*. *Arch. Pharm. Sci. Ain Shams Univ.* **2018**, *2*, 121–137. [CrossRef]
47. Gürlek, C.; Yarkent, Ç.; Köse, A.; Tuğcu, B.; Gebeloğlu, I.K.; Öncel, S.; Elibol, M. Screening of antioxidant and cytotoxic activities of several microalgal extracts with pharmaceutical potential. *Health Technol.* **2020**, *10*, 111–117. [CrossRef]
48. Casas-Arrojo, V.; Decara, J.; de los Ángeles Arrojo-Agudo, M.; Pérez-Manríquez, C.; Abdala-Díaz, R.T. Immunomodulatory, antioxidant activity and cytotoxic effect of sulfated polysaccharides from *Porphyridium cruentum*. (S.F.Gray) Nägeli. *Biomolecules* **2021**, *11*, 488. [CrossRef]
49. Srisai, P.; Suriyaprom, S.; Panya, A.; Pekkoh, J.; Tragoolpua, Y. Inhibitory effects of algal polysaccharide extract from *Cladophora* spp. against herpes simplex virus infection. *Sci. Rep.* **2024**, *14*, 11914. [CrossRef]
50. Ivanova, J.; Konstantinidou, A.; Kabaivanova, L.; Georgieva, A.; Vladov, I.; Petkova, S. Examination of exopolysaccharides from *Porphyridium cruentum* for estimation of their potential antitumour activity in vitro. *Proc. Bulg. Acad. Sci.* **2022**, *75*, 1146–1155. [CrossRef]
51. Ma, X.-T.; Sun, X.-Y.; Yu, K.; Gui, B.-S.; Gui, Q.; Ouyang, J.-M. Effect of content of sulfate groups in seaweed polysaccharides on antioxidant activity and repair effect of subcellular organelles in injured HK-2 cells. *Oxidative Med. Cell. Longev.* **2017**, *2017*, 2542950. [CrossRef]
52. Lakhrem, M.; Eleroui, M.; Boujhoud, Z.; Feki, A.; Dghim, A.; Essayagh, S.; Hilali, S.; Bouhamed, M.; Kallel, C.; Deschamps, N.; et al. Anti-vasculogenic, antioxidant, and anti-inflammatory activities of sulfated polysaccharide derived from *Codium tomentosum*: Pharmacokinetic assay. *Pharmaceuticals* **2024**, *17*, 672. [CrossRef]
53. Andryukov, B.G.; Besednova, N.N.; Kuznetsova, T.A.; Zaporozhets, T.S.; Ermakova, S.P.; Zvyagintseva, T.N.; Chingizova, E.A.; Gazha, A.K.; Smolina, T.P. Sulfated polysaccharides from marine algae as a basis of modern biotechnologies for creating wound dressings: Current achievements and future prospects. *Biomedicines* **2020**, *8*, 301. [CrossRef]
54. Montero, X.A.; Alves, A.; Ribeiro, M.; Lazari, M.; Coutinho, P.; Otero, A. Biochemical characterization of *Nostoc* sp. exopolysaccharides and evaluation of potential use in wound healing. *Carbohydr. Polym.* **2020**, *254*, 117303.
55. Bari, E.; Arciola, C.R.; Vigani, B.; Crivelli, B.; Moro, P.; Marrubini, G.; Sorrenti, M.; Catenacci, L.; Bruni, G.; Chlapanidas, T.; et al. In vitro effectiveness of microspheres based on silk sericin and *Chlorella vulgaris* or *Arthrospira platensis* for wound healing applications. *Materials* **2017**, *10*, 983. [CrossRef] [PubMed]
56. Melo, D.R.G.; de Andrade, A.F.; Bezerra, R.P.; Marques, D.A.V.; Silva, V.A.D., Jr.; Paz, S.T.; Filho, J.L.D.L.; Porto, A.L.F. Hydrogel-based *Chlorella vulgaris* extracts: A new topical formulation for wound healing treatment. *J. Appl. Phycol.* **2019**, *31*, 3653–3663. [CrossRef]
57. WHO. Hepatitis C. 2024. Available online: https://www.who.int/news-room/fact-sheets/detail/hepatitis-c (accessed on 13 December 2024).
58. Hans, N.; Malik, A.; Naik, S. Antiviral activity of sulfated polysaccharides from marine algae and its application in combating COVID-19: Mini review. *Bioresour. Technol. Rep.* **2021**, *13*, 100623. [CrossRef] [PubMed]
59. Ntzouvaras, A.; Chantzistrountsiou, X.; Papageorgiou, N.; Koletti, A.; Adamakis, I.-D.; Zografaki, M.-E.; Marka, S.; Vasilakis, G.; Tsirigoti, A.; Tzovenis, I.; et al. New records of *Tetraselmis* sp. strains with biotechnological potential isolated from Greek coastal lagoons. *Water* **2023**, *15*, 1698. [CrossRef]
60. Rojo-Cebreros, A.H.; Ibarra-Castro, L.; Martinez-Brown, J.M.; Velasco-Blanco, G.; Martinez-Tellez, M.A.; Medina-Jasso, M.A.; Nieves-Soto, M.; Quintanna-Zavala, D. Potential of *Nannochloropsis* in beta glucan production. In *Nannochloropsis: Biology, Biotechnological Potential and Challenges*; Jan, M., Kazik, P., Eds.; Nova Science Publishers, Inc.: New York, NY, USA, 2017; pp. 181–225.

61. Markou, G.; Eliopoulos, C.; Argyri, A.; Arapoglou, D. Production of *Arthrospira* (*Spirulina*) *platensis* enriched in β-glucans through phosphorus limitation. *Appl. Sci.* **2021**, *11*, 8121. [CrossRef]
62. Ocaranza, D.; Balic, I.; Bruna, T.; Moreno, I.; Díaz, O.; Moreno, A.A.; Caro, N. A modeled high-density fed-batch culture improves biomass growth and β-glucans accumulation in *Microchloropsis salina*. *Plants* **2022**, *11*, 3229. [CrossRef]
63. Sati, H.; Mitra, M.; Mishra, S.; Baredar, P. Microalgal lipid extraction strategies for biodiesel production: A review. *Algal Res.* **2019**, *38*, 101413. [CrossRef]
64. Kurd, F.; Samavati, V. Water soluble polysaccharides from *Spirulina platensis*: Extraction and in vitro anti-cancer activity. *Int. J. Biol. Macromol.* **2015**, *74*, 498–506. [CrossRef]
65. Huo, S.; Wang, H.; Chen, J.; Hu, X.; Zhang, C.; Qian, J.; Zhu, F.; Ma, H.; Elshobary, M. A preliminary study on polysaccharide extraction, purification, and antioxidant properties of sugar-rich filamentous microalgae *Tribonema minus*. *J. Appl. Phycol.* **2022**, *34*, 2755–2767. [CrossRef]
66. Bradford, M.M. A rapid and sensitive method for the quantitation of microgram quantities of protein utilizing the principle of protein-dye binding. *Anal. Biochem.* **1976**, *72*, 248–254. [CrossRef]
67. Dai, J.; Wu, Y.; Chen, S.; Zhu, S.; Yin, H.; Wang, M.; Tang, J. Sugar compositional determination of polysaccharides from *Dunaliella salina* by modified RP-HPLC method of precolumn derivatization with 1-phenyl-3-methyl-5-pyrazolone. *Carbohydr. Polym.* **2010**, *82*, 629–635. [CrossRef]
68. Ai, Y.; Yu, Z.; Chen, Y.; Zhu, X.; Ai, Z.; Liu, S.; Ni, D. Rapid determination of the monosaccharide composition and contents in tea polysaccharides from Yingshuang green tea by pre-column derivatization HPLC. *J. Chem.* **2016**, *2016*, 6065813. [CrossRef]
69. Torres, P.B.; Nagai, A.; Palacios Jara, C.E.; Santos, J.P.; Chow, F.; dos Santos, D.Y.A.C. Determination of sulfate in algal polysaccharide samples: A step-by-step protocol using microplate reader. *Ocean Coast. Res.* **2021**, *69*, e21021. [CrossRef]
70. Wang, N.; Pei, H.; Xiang, W.; Li, T.; Lin, S.; Wu, J.; Chen, Z.; Wu, H.; Li, C.; Wu, H. Rapid screening of microalgae as potential sources of natural antioxidants. *Foods* **2023**, *12*, 2652. [CrossRef] [PubMed]
71. Mpekoulis, G.; Tsopela, V.; Panos, G.; Siozos, V.; Kalliampakou, K.I.; Frakolaki, E.; Sideris, C.D.; Vassiliou, A.G.; Sideris, D.C.; Vassilacopoulou, D.; et al. Association of Hepatitis C virus replication with the catecholamine biosynthetic pathway. *Viruses* **2021**, *13*, 2139. [CrossRef]

marine drugs

Article

New Green Biorefinery Strategies to Valorize Bioactive Fractions from *Palmaria palmata*

Melis Cokdinleyen [1,2], Gloria Domínguez-Rodríguez [1,3,*], Huseyin Kara [2], Elena Ibáñez [1] and Alejandro Cifuentes [1]

1 Laboratory of Foodomics, Institute of Food Science Research (CIAL, CSIC), Nicolás Cabrera 9, 28049 Madrid, Spain; melis.cokdinleyen@cial.uam-csic.es (M.C.); elena.ibanez@csic.es (E.I.); a.cifuentes@csic.es (A.C.)

2 Faculty of Sciences, Department of Chemistry, Selçuk University, Arciçh, Ismetpasa Cad, Selçuklu, Konya 42250, Turkey; hkara@selcuk.edu.tr

3 Departamento de Química Analítica, Química Física e Ingeniería Química, Facultad de Ciencias, Universidad de Alcalá, Ctra. Madrid-Barcelona Km. 33.600, Alcalá de Henares, 28871 Madrid, Spain

* Correspondence: gloria.dominguezr@uah.es

Abstract: A biorefinery process was developed to isolate phycobiliproteins, sulfated polysaccharides, and phenolic compounds from *Palmaria palmata*. The extraction process was carried out in three stages using ultrasound-assisted extraction (UAE) and pressurized liquid extraction (PLE) integrated with different natural deep eutectic solvents (NaDESs). In general, PLE provided higher phycobiliprotein contents than UAE in the first step of the process. In fact, the hydrolysis product of the PLE-NaDES extracts achieved a higher antioxidant capacity than that of the UAE-NaDES extracts. Particularly, glycerol:glucose (2:1) with 50% water in combination with PLE was the most suitable NaDES to recover the highest phycobiliprotein, protein, and sulfated polysaccharide contents from *Palmaria palmata* in the first and second steps of the biorefinery process. Finally, a PLE-NaDES using choline chloride:glycerol (1:2) with 60% water as the NaDES was employed for the recovery of antioxidant and neuroprotective phenolic compounds from the residue of the second step, obtaining a higher total phenolic content than employing PLE with ethanol/water (70:30, *v*/*v*) as the extraction solvent. Moreover, a forced stability study revealed that the NaDESs provided a protective effect compared to the water extracts against the degradation of phycobiliproteins, preserving their color over time. This study contributes to the recovery of high-value components from an undervalued biomarine source through a sustainable biorefinery process.

Keywords: biorefinery; phycobiliproteins; sulfated polysaccharides; proteins; phenolic compounds; *Palmaria palmata*; natural deep eutectic solvents; ultrasound-assisted extraction; pressurized liquid extraction

1. Introduction

Currently, the Food and Drug Administration (FDA) as well as the European Food Safety Authority (EFSA) are introducing regulations to limit the use of synthetic colors in foods due to health concerns, such as quinoline yellow colorant, which induces toxicity by protein aggregation [1]. Red macroalgae have recently attracted significant attention in the exploration of natural colorants with bioactive properties for their inclusion as innovative additives for pharmaceutical and food products [2,3].

P. palmata is a red macroalga that grows from the middle of the intertidal zone (the region between high and low tide), in both sheltered and exposed coastal areas [4]. The current availability of *P. palmata* depends on harvesting wild populations, but it is difficult to meet growing demand [5]. Currently, *P. palmata* aquaculture is largely small-scale, lacks significant mechanization, and is primarily carried out during spring and summer, when the plants are more easily harvested by hand [6]. Thus, different researchers have focused their efforts on the development of the vegetative propagation and cultivation processes of *P. palmata* to enhance its use in commercial-scale operations [6,7]. However, the current cultivation of this alga has been scarcely exploited as a source of natural pigments and phenolic compounds despite its interesting content [2,8]. Particularly, the major constituents of *P. palmata* are pigment proteins called phycobiliproteins.

Phycobiliproteins are light-harvesting pigment proteins with high levels of solubility that are found intracellularly in red algae [9]. These proteins consist of apoproteins and chromophores linked by thioether bonds, which exhibit different color properties due to the presence of four different chromophores in their structure. According to their structure and absorption spectra, phycobiliproteins are divided into phycoerythrin (490–570 nm), phycocyanin (610–625 nm), phycoerythrocyanin (560–600 nm), and allophycocyanin (650–660 nm) [10,11]. Frequently, they are obtained from red algae such as *P. palmata* to be included in food as colorants and functional ingredients [9,11]. In fact, phycobiliprotein hydrolysates from *P. palmata* have shown interesting anti-inflammatory and antihypertensive capacities [12–14]. However, the bioactivity of these compounds obtained from *P. palmata* has scarcely been studied.

These compounds are usually recovered from algae employing conventional extraction, such as maceration, with water as the solvent; however, this approach has several limitations [10]. Phycobiliproteins are found intracellularly, and their extraction implies the rupture of the rigid cell wall of red macroalgae to break the polysaccharide barrier, releasing phycobiliproteins as well as valuable proteins and sulfated polysaccharides to the extraction solvents [15–17]. In this sense, conventional extractions with water are often inefficient, and more aggressive extraction treatments are necessary to break down the cell wall. For that, freeze grinding or maceration with liquid nitrogen, freezing, and thawing processes are employed to break down the algae cell wall, improving the recovery of phycobiliproteins [10,17,18]. Nevertheless, these treatments require the use of costly specific instruments as well as large extraction times, implying that phycobiliproteins are exposed to light and oxygen for long times, increasing their susceptibility to degradation [10,19]. For this reason, advanced extraction techniques such as enzymatic-assisted extraction (EAE), ultrasound-assisted extraction (UAE), or pressurized liquid extraction (PLE) have been proposed by several authors as more intense, selective extraction techniques that require lower extraction times and temperatures compared with conventional extractions [18,20–22]. Particularly, considering the composition of the cell wall of the algae, specific enzymes can be selected to break it down and release target compounds by EAE; however, this type of extraction technique requires the precise control of pH, temperature, and substrate concentration. Moreover, the use of specific enzymes makes the process more expensive [2]. On the other hand, the use of ultrasonic waves in UAE and the high pressure employed in PLE have demonstrated the breakdown of the biomass of different algae, favoring the release of phycobiliproteins [17,23,24]. In fact, Gallego et al. [24] developed a biorefinery process to obtain phycobiliproteins, proteins, and sulfated polysaccharides from *Porphyridium cruentum* biomass by PLE using water as an extraction solvent. In addition, the biorefinery process developed by Gallego et al. [24] revealed the importance of the use of a biorefinery process to extract and fractionate valuable compounds from algae for their integration into sustainable biomass production procedures.

Advanced extraction techniques such as UAE and PLE have been employed with water as the extraction solvent for the recovery of phycobiliproteins, proteins, and sulfated polysaccharides [23,24]. Phycobiliproteins are hydrosoluble molecules, and this makes water an ideal solvent for releasing these proteins from the algae cells. Nevertheless, solvent selection is not only a crucial parameter for achieving a high extraction efficiency but it also impacts the stability of target compounds after extraction. In this sense, water has not demonstrated a protective effect on the degradation of bioactive compounds from different matrices [25], and considering that the phycobiliproteins' color is unstable to heat and light, the selection of solvents with preservative effects could be an interesting approach [19]. In particular, sustainable, biodegradable, non-toxic, and economic solvents with preservative effects on the degradation of bioactive compounds have emerged in the past few years: natural deep eutectic solvents (NaDESs) [25,26].

NaDESs are mixtures of natural components, such as sugars, amino acids, or organic acids, among others, which have demonstrated a significant potential for the extraction process due to the strong hydrogen bonds formed between the solvent components and the extracted compounds [26]. These interactions provide higher extraction yields of bioactive compounds compared to the use of conventional solvents such as water as well as a protective effect against their degradation [27]. Moreover, NaDESs possess a higher viscosity than water; this reduces the mobility of target compounds within the solution, limiting their exposure to oxygen and consequently the oxidative reactions [28]. Even though these solvents have been widely employed for the recovery of bioactive compounds (such as phenolics) from several food matrices using maceration or combined with advanced extraction techniques, such as UAE and PLE [29], studies about the recovery of bioactive compounds from algae are very limited [30,31]. In fact, there are no studies about the recovery of phycobiliproteins, proteins, sulfated polysaccharides, and phenolic compounds from *P. palmata* by NaDESs combined with advanced extraction techniques.

Thus, this study proposes, for the first time, the development of a biorefinery process for the recovery of phycobiliproteins, proteins, sulfated polysaccharides, and phenolic compounds from *P. palmata* based on the combination of UAE and PLE with NaDESs. In the first and second steps of the biorefinery process, different NaDESs were tested to maximize the extraction of phycobiliproteins, proteins, and sulfated polysaccharides with antioxidant capacity in combination with UAE and PLE. Finally, in the third step, phenolic compounds were obtained employing PLE-NaDESs with choline chloride:glycerol (1:2) as the NaDES. The extraction efficiency of the NaDES was evaluated by comparison with water extracts, together with its preservative effect on the degradation of phycobiliproteins during a forced stability study.

2. Results

To develop a biorefinery approach for extracting valuable compounds from *P. palmata* biomass, a sequential downstream process was established according to Figure 1. For that, the characteristics of the target compounds, the use of environmentally friendly solvents, and the need for a rapid and efficient extraction method were investigated. Based on these considerations, experiments were conducted to identify the optimal advanced extraction technique for maximizing thermolabile phycobiliproteins' recovery (step 1) followed by maximizing the recovery of residual non-thermolabile phycobiliproteins along with proteins and sulfated polysaccharides (step 2), and finally, phenolic compounds (step 3).

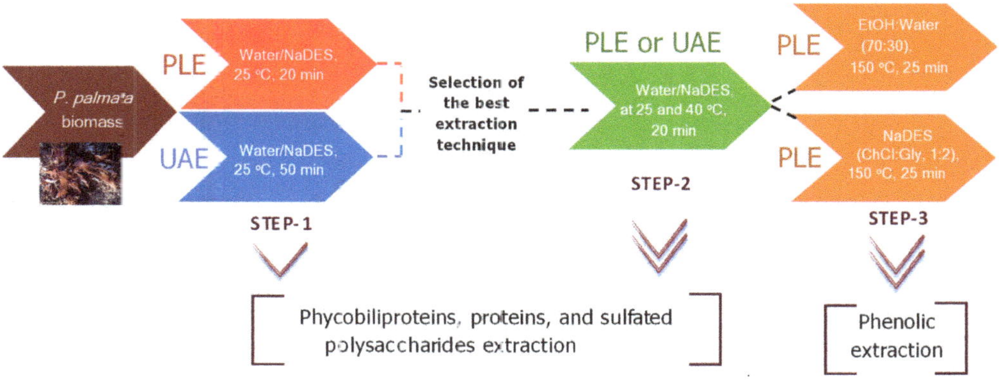

Figure 1. Workflow followed for the valorization of *Palmaria palmata* biomass through a biorefinery process using UAE and PLE combined with NaDES.

2.1. Optimization of Biorefinery Process

2.1.1. UAE-NaDES and PLE-NaDES Extraction of Bioactive Phycobiliproteins, Proteins, and Sulfated Polysaccharides from *P. palmata* (Step 1)

One of the most important physicochemical parameters that determine the extraction efficiency is the solvent viscosity, which is widely modified by the addition of water. For this reason, different NaDESs were synthesized with two different water percentages (25% and 50%), considering that hydrogen bonds of NaDESs are able to stay stable up to this percentage [32].

NaDES viscosity was measured at 25 °C and 40 °C (see Table S1), observing that when the temperature and the percentage of water in the NaDES increased, the NaDES viscosity decreased. However, different authors have reported that the optimal extraction conditions for the recovery of thermolabile phycobiliproteins such as phycoerythrin are 25 °C using water for the extraction [24,33]. For this reason, step 1 of the biorefinery process was focused on the extraction of phycobiliproteins at low temperatures, avoiding their degradation.

UAE-NaDES and PLE-NaDES extractions were compared in terms of phycobiliprotein contents; however, due to the chemical composition of *P. palmata* [5,34], other compounds such as proteins and sulfated polysaccharides can be co-extracted. Thus, these compounds were also analyzed.

In particular, Gly:Glu:Bet and Gly:Glu:Pro NaDESs with 25% water could not be implemented in step 1 of the biorefinery process using PLE by obstruction problems.

As can be observed in Table 1, the use of higher percentages of water in NaDESs increased the recovery of phycobiliproteins for both extraction techniques, except for the recovery of APC by UAE, in which 25% water in the NaDES allowed us to obtain higher APC contents than using 50% water. Particularly, the PLE-NaDES using Gly:Glu with 50% water as the NaDES was the best extraction technique for the recovery of phycobiliproteins from *P. palmata* compared to the UAE-NaDESs. Moreover, the efficiency of the NaDES as a solvent extraction to obtain phycobiliproteins was confirmed by comparisons with UAE-water and PLE-water extractions. As can be seen in Table 1, the use of water as an extraction solvent provided lower phycobiliprotein values than using the Gly:Glu NaDES. Nevertheless, the UAE-NaDES achieved the highest protein and sulfated polysaccharide contents compared to the PLE extractions, except for the PLE-water extraction.

Table 1. Total phycobiliprotein contents (μg/mg sample, R-phycocyanin, allophycocyanin, and B-phycoerythrin), total protein content (μg/mg sample), and total sulfated polysaccharide contents (μg/mg sample) from extracts obtained by UAE-NaDES and PLE-NaDES at 25 °C during step 1.

STEP 1	R-Phycocyanin (R-PC) (μg/mg Sample)		Allophycocyanin (APC) (μg/mg Sample)		B-Phycoerythrin (B-PE) (μg/mg Sample)		Total Protein Content (μg/mg Sample)		Total Sulfated Polysaccharide Content (μg/mg Sample)	
Solvents	UAE	PLE	UAE	PLE	UAE	PLE	UAE	PLE	UAE	PLE
Gly:Glu, 50% H_2O	11 ± 2^{Aa}	12.4 ± 0.7^{Ab}	14 ± 2^{ABb}	18 ± 2^{Aa}	17 ± 2^{Aa}	18 ± 1^{Aa}	173 ± 15^{Aa}	126 ± 5^{Cb}	54.3 ± 0.8^{Aa}	50 ± 2^{Bb}
Gly:Glu:Bet, 50% H_2O	10.7 ± 0.6^{Aa}	10.5 ± 0.1^{Ba}	13 ± 2^{Bb}	15.4 ± 0.9^{ABa}	15.6 ± 0.9^{ABa}	15.3 ± 0.5^{ABa}	158 ± 9^{Aa}	85 ± 9^{Db}	53.4 ± 0.3^{Aa}	44 ± 2^{Cb}
Gly:Glu:Pro, 50% H_2O	10.5 ± 0.4^{ABa}	10.7 ± 0.5^{Ba}	16 ± 2^{ABa}	13 ± 1^{Bb}	15.8 ± 0.4^{ABa}	15.6 ± 0.6^{ABa}	164 ± 6^{Aa}	145 ± 14^{Bb}	44 ± 2^{Bb}	50 ± 2^{Ba}
Gly:Glu, 25% H_2O	8 ± 1^{BCa}	8.9 ± 0.6^{Ca}	17 ± 2^{Ba}	9 ± 2^{Cb}	13 ± 2^{CDa}	12.8 ± 1.0^{Ba}	94 ± 13^{Bb}	131 ± 15^{Ca}	37 ± 5^{Ca}	30 ± 2^{Db}
Gly:Glu:Bet, 25% H_2O	6.8 ± 0.4^{C}	-	14 ± 2^{AB}	-	10.5 ± 0.9^{D}	-	18 ± 1^{D}	-	32 ± 4^{C}	-
Gly:Glu:Pro, 25% H_2O	8.6 ± 0.2^{ABC}	-	17 ± 1^{A}	-	14.1 ± 0.1^{BC}	-	59 ± 8^{C}	-	37 ± 4^{C}	-
H_2O	9.7 ± 0.4^{ABa}	10.7 ± 0.5^{Bb}	13.8 ± 0.6^{ABa}	13 ± 1^{Ba}	16.5 ± 0.2^{ABa}	15.6 ± 0.6^{ABa}	152 ± 7^{Ab}	189 ± 7^{Aa}	38.4 ± 0.2^{BCa}	61.7 ± 0.7^{Ab}

A,B,C,D Letters indicate statistically significant differences in the same column ($p \leq 0.05$). a,b Letters indicate statistically significant differences between extraction techniques ($p \leq 0.05$).

In agreement with the phycobiliprotein extraction, the NaDES composed of Gly:Glu with 50% water allowed us to obtain the highest total protein and sulfated polysaccharide contents by UAE, but without statistically significant differences with the UAE-water extraction in terms of protein content. Lower protein and sulfated polysaccharide contents were achieved by PLE than by UAE, with the PLE-water extracts having higher contents than the PLE-NaDES extracts. Probably, an increase in the extraction temperature could improve the recovery of proteins and sulfated polysaccharides by PLE.

On the other hand, considering that the NaDES with 50% water provided extracts containing high phycobiliprotein, protein, and sulfated polysaccharide contents, these extracts were hydrolyzed with trypsin in order to investigate their antioxidant capacity. To determine the optimum hydrolysis time with trypsin, the antioxidant capacity of the hydrolysates was evaluated after hydrolysis at different incubation times (1, 3, 5, and 6 h) (Table S2). As a result, a hydrolysis time of 1 h was established since there was not a significant increase in the antioxidant capacity after this incubation time. Therefore, the antioxidant capacity of all extracts was evaluated by TEAC and ORAC assays after 1 h of hydrolysis with trypsin.

Table 2 shows that the antioxidant capacity of the extracts increased after the hydrolysis treatments. Particularly, the PLE-NaDES hydrolysates exhibited higher antioxidant capacity than the UAE-NaDES hydrolysates, highlighting those obtained with the Gly:Glu:Bet (4:1:1) NaDES with 50% water. However, the PLE-water hydrolysates presented the highest antioxidant capacity determined by the ORAC assay compared to the PLE-NaDES hydrolysates.

Table 2. Antioxidant capacity of UAE-NaDES, UAE-water, PLE-NaDES, and PLE-water extracts and their respective hydrolysates determined by TEAC (μmol trolox/g sample) and ORAC (IC_{50}, μg/mL sample) assays.

	TEAC (μmol trolox/g Sample)				ORAC (IC_{50} μg/mL Sample)			
	Extracts		Hydrolysate		Extracts		Hydrolysate	
Solvents	UAE	PLE	UAE	PLE	UAE	PLE	UAE	PLE
Gly:Glu, 50% H_2O	14.81 ± 0.02 ^{Bb}	25.64 ± 0.04 ^{Ba}	20.90 ± 0.01 ^{Bb}	35.60 ± 0.02 ^{Ca}	107 ± 7 ^{Ba}	111 ± 9 ^{Bb}	29 ± 2 ^{Bb}	27.8 ± 0.8 ^{Ba}
Gly:Glu:Bet, 50% H_2O	14.39 ± 0.03 ^{Bb}	25.32 ± 0.03 ^{Ba}	19.30 ± 0.01 ^{Cb}	46 ± 1 ^{Aa}	111 ± 4 ^{Ca}	112 ± 8 ^{Ca}	32 ± 2 ^{Cb}	28 ± 3 ^{Ba}
Gly:Glu:Pro, 50% H_2O	13.28 ± 0.07 ^{Cb}	13 ± 0.02 ^{Ca}	18.10 ± 0.02 ^{Db}	40.17 ± 0.02 ^{Ba}	116 ± 5 ^{Da}	116 ± 3 ^{Da}	31 ± 1 ^{Cb}	28 ± 1 ^{Ba}
H_2O	15.74 ± 0.05 ^{Ab}	27.48 ± 0.03 ^{Aa}	22.30 ± 0.01 ^{Ab}	42.05 ± 0.02 ^{Ba}	101 ± 11 ^{Ab}	94 ± 3 ^{Aa}	22 ± 2 ^{Ab}	15.4 ± 0.2 ^{Aa}

^{A,B,C,D} Letters indicate statistically significant differences in the same column ($p \leq 0.05$). ^{a,b} Letters indicate statistically significant differences between extraction techniques ($p \leq 0.05$).

2.1.2. PLE-NaDES Extraction of Phycobiliproteins, Proteins, and Sulfated Polysaccharides (Step 2)

Considering the potential protein and sulfated polysaccharide contents of *P. palmata*, their extraction along with the remaining non-thermolabile phycobiliproteins from the residual biomass of step 1 was considered to obtain high value-added products. For that, the residual biomass from the application of step 1 (the PLE-NaDES composed of Gly:Glu with 50% water) was studied for step 2.

Step 2 was applied considering six different NaDESs at two different PLE extraction temperatures (25 °C and 40 °C), but excluding the NaDESs composed of Gly:Glu:Bet and Gly:Glu:Pro with 25% water, as previously mentioned. The PLE-NaDES extracts were compared with the PLE-water extracts obtained under the same extraction conditions.

Table 3 shows that the extracts exhibited higher phycobiliprotein contents than in step 1 (see Table 1). These results indicated that phycobiliproteins remain retained in the residual biomass of step 1, and additional steps are required to completely exploit the biomass. As can be seen in Table 3, similar phycobiliprotein results were obtained using PLE at 25 °C and 40 °C with NaDESs and water solvents, except when Gly:Glu with 50% water was used, which provided the extracts with the highest phycobiliprotein contents when an extraction temperature of 40 °C was applied. The Gly:Glu NaDES with 50% water was the only one that improved the extraction of phycobiliproteins, showing a protective effect against the degradation of these compounds when an extraction temperature of 40 °C was used compared with the rest of the NaDESs. In fact, the extracts obtained at 40 °C with the other NaDESs and with water showed similar values or even lower values than those obtained at 25 °C. In addition, even though the PLE-water extracts presented higher total protein and sulfated polysaccharide contents than the PLE-NaDES extracts, the PLE-water extracts showed lower phycobiliprotein contents.

Table 3. Total phycobiliprotein contents (μg/mg sample, R-phycocyanin, allophycocyanin, and B-phycoerythrin), total protein content (μg/mg sample), and total sulfated polysaccharide contents (μg/mg sample) from extracts obtained by PLE-NaDES at 25 °C and 40 °C during step 2.

STEP-2	R-Phycocyanin (R-PC) (μg/mg Sample)		Allophycocyanin (APC) (μg/mg Sample)		B-Phycoerythrin (B-PE) (μg/mg Sample)		Total Protein Content (μg/mg Sample)		Total Sulfated Polysaccharide Content (μg/mg Sample)	
Solvents	**25 °C**	**40 °C**	**25 °C**	**40 °C**	**25 °C**	**40 °C**	**25 °C**	**40 °C**	**25 °C**	**40 °C**
Gly:Glu, 50% H_2O	20 ± 1 ^{ABb}	28 ± 2 ^{Aa}	36 ± 2 ^{Ab}	52 ± 8 ^{Aa}	29 ± 1 ^{ABb}	43 ± 4 ^{Aa}	218 ± 8 ^{Db}	268 ± 14 ^{Da}	123 ± 2 ^{Cb}	131 ± 3 ^{Ba}
Gly:Glu:Bet, 50% H_2O	20.1 ± 0.7 ABa	20 ± 3 ^{BCa}	35.4 ± 0.6 Aa	35 ± 4 ^{Ba}	29 ± 1 ^{ABb}	30 ± 4 ^{Ba}	181 ± 10 ^{Ea}	176 ± 3 ^{Ea}	119 ± 3 ^{Db}	124 ± 3 ^{Ca}
Gly:Glu:Pro, 50% H_2O	22 ± 2 ^{Aa}	20.9 ± 0.4 Bb	28 ± 3 ^{Ba}	25.3 ± 0.9 Cb	32 ± 3 ^{Aa}	30.4 ± 0.5 Bb	357 ± 5 ^{Ba}	330 ± 7 ^{Cb}	129.9 ± 0.4 Ba	131 ± 5 ^{Ba}
Gly:Glu, 25% H_2O	18.1 ± 0.4 Ba	17.1 ± 0.4 Cb	18.0 ± 0.9 Ca	15.6 ± 0.9 Db	26.1 ± 0.5 Ba	24.5 ± 0.5 Cb	292 ± 7 ^{Cb}	387 ± 3 ^{Ba}	89 ± 4 ^{Eb}	100 ± 1 ^{Da}
H_2O	22 ± 2 ^{Aa}	20.9 ± 0.4 Bb	28 ± 3 ^{Ba}	25.3 ± 0.9 Cb	32 ± 3 ^{Aa}	30.4 ± 0.5 Bb	431 ± 5 ^{Aa}	410 ± 2 ^{Ab}	146.0 ± 0.7 Aa	141.9 ± 0.4 Aa

[A,B,C,D] Letters indicate statistically significant differences in the same column ($p \leq 0.05$). [a,b] Letters indicate statistically significant differences between extraction temperatures ($p \leq 0.05$).

Considering these results, the PLE-NaDES extraction using Gly:Glu with 50% water at 40 °C was selected as the best to obtain the richest extracts in phycobiliproteins with significant amounts of proteins and sulfated polysaccharides.

2.1.3. PLE-NaDES Extraction of Bioactive Phenolic Compounds (Step 3)

The third and last step of the biorefinery process focused on the recovery of bioactive phenolic compounds from the residual biomass of step 2. For that, the PLE-NaDES extraction with ChCl:Gly (1:2) with 60% water as the extraction solvent at 150 °C for 25 min was applied for the recovery of phenolic compounds according to Domínguez-Rodríguez et al.'s [35] method for the recovery of antioxidant and anticholinergic phenolic compounds from food matrices. In addition, the same PLE extraction conditions were employed, but ethanol/water (70:30, *v*/*v*) was used as the extraction solvent instead of the NaDES in order to compare both extracts in terms of their total phenolic contents and their antioxidant and anticholinergic capacities.

As can be observed in Figure 2, the PLE-NaDES extraction provided higher TPC values (Figure 2A) and a higher antioxidant capacity than the ethanolic PLE extraction, determined by the TEAC assay (Figure 2B). However, the ethanolic extract presented a higher antioxidant capacity evaluated by the ORAC assay (see Figure 2C) as well as a higher anticholinergic capacity (see Figure 2D). This means that the PLE-NaDES extraction with ChCl:Gly (1:2) with 60% water or the ethanolic PLE extraction can be used depending on the final application added to the extract.

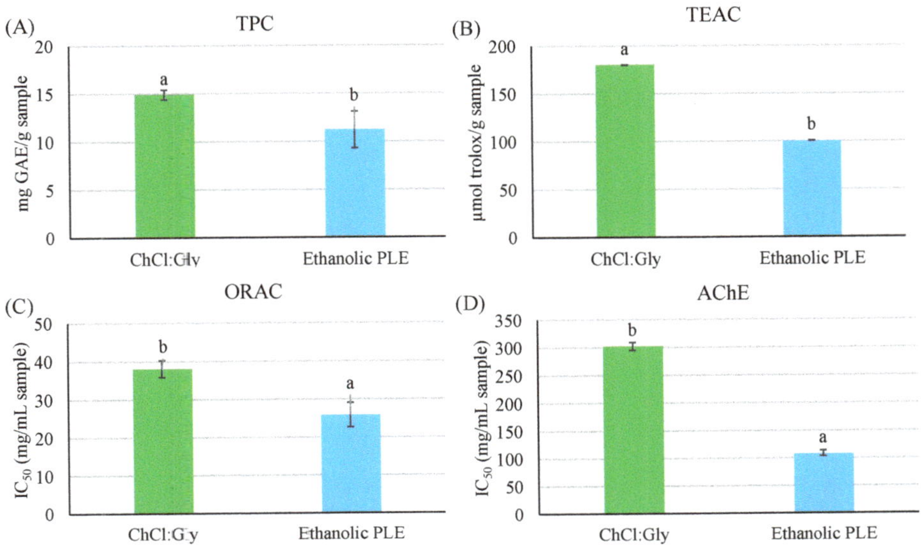

Figure 2. (**A**) Total phenolic content (TPC) determined by Folin–Ciocalteu method, antioxidant capacity measured by (**B**) TEAC and (**C**) ORAC assays, and (**D**) anticholinergic capacity evaluated by the inhibition of AchE enzyme from phenolic extracts obtained by PLE-NaDES with ChCl:Gly (1:2) with 60% water and PLE with ethanol/water (70:30, v/v). [a,b] Letters indicate statistically significant differences between extraction solvents ($p \leq 0.05$).

2.2. Stability Study of PLE-NaDES and PLE-Water Phycobiliprotein Extracts

The selection of an appropriate solvent for the extraction of bioactive compounds significantly impacts its stability post-extraction. Numerous studies have demonstrated that NaDESs are particularly effective in preventing the degradation of bioactive compounds, such as phenolic compounds, under forced storage conditions [36,37]. However, to our knowledge, there are no studies about the stability of phycobiliproteins achieved using NaDESs as the extraction solvent from *P. palmata* algae. Thus, a stability study of the optimal PLE-NaDES extraction (using Gly:Glu (2:1) NaDES) and the PLE-water extracts obtained in step 1 was performed by monitoring the phycobiliprotein contents (B-PE, R-PC, and APC contents), the antioxidant capacity of their hydrolysates (determined by TEAC and ORAC assays), and the color change (measured by CIELAB coordinates) for 30 days. During these 30 days, the extracts were submitted to 40 °C, equivalent to 6 months at room temperature.

As can be observed in Figure 3, the B-PE and R-PC values decrease up to three times in the PLE-water extracts from the first week to the last week compared with the PLE-NaDES extract (see Figure 3A,B).

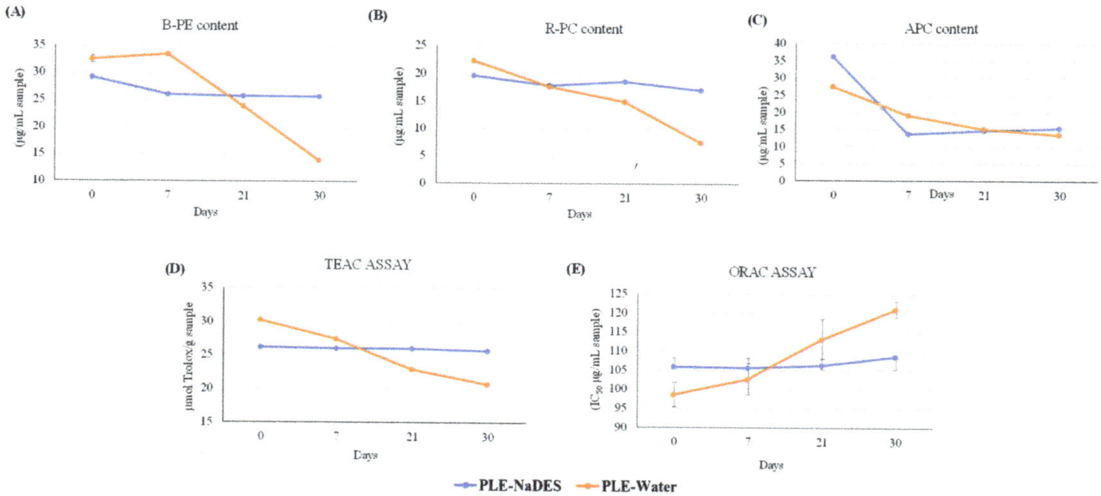

Figure 3. Forced stability study of (**A**) total B-phycoerythrin content, (**B**) total R-phycocyanin content, (**C**) total allophycocyanin content, (**D**) antioxidant capacity determined by TEAC, and (**E**) ORAC assays of PLE-NaDES and PLE-water extracts from step 1 of the biorefinery process submitted to 40 °C for 30 days.

However, the contents of these phycobiliproteins in the PLE-NaDES extracts were slightly reduced over time. By contrast, the low stability of APC was observed because its content was reduced from 36.2 ± 0.1 µg/mg sample to 15.60 ± 0.01 µg/mg sample in the PLE-NaDES extracts, with this reduction being more pronounced in the PLE-water extract (see Figure 3C). This means that the NaDES provided a protective effect on phycobiliproteins' stability, particularly for B-PE and R-PC. This effect was also observed for the antioxidant capacity of hydrolysate extracts, because the TEAC and ORAC values were maintained over time in the PLE-NaDES extracts, while this capacity decreased in the PLE-water extracts (see Figures 3D and 3E, respectively). In fact, even though initially the PLE-water extracts showed a higher antioxidant capacity as determined by the ORAC assay, this capacity was reduced up to 20% at the end of the stability study, presenting higher IC_{50} values than the PLE-NaDES extracts.

On the other hand, as can be seen in Table 4, the color measurements in the PLE-NaDES showed that L* and α* parameters were maintained during the stability study. These results indicated that the NaDES offers a protective effect on the degradation of phycobiliproteins over time, keeping its pink color, as can be observed in the measurement of the α* value. An increase in b* values is noted, indicating a more intense yellow color, particularly at 21 days.

Table 4. Color parameters (L* = luminosity; α* = redness/greenness; b* = yellowness/blueness) of PLE-NaDES and PLE-water extracts during the forced stability study.

	PLE-NaDES				PLE-Water			
Days	**L***	**α***	**b***	**ΔE**	**L***	**α***	**b***	**ΔE**
0	838 ± 1 ^{C}	179 ± 1 ^{B}	69 ± 2 ^{C}	0	760 ± 1 ^{C}	233 ± 1 ^{A}	61 ± 2 ^{D}	0
7	841 ± 1 ^{C}	105 ± 0 ^{D}	51 ± 0 ^{D}	76 ± 0 ^{Ab}	755 ± 0 ^{D}	76 ± 1 ^{B}	112± 1 ^{C}	165.3 ± 1 ^{Ba}
21	864 ± 1 ^{A}	162 ± 1 ^{C}	81 ± 1 ^{B}	33 ± 1 ^{Cb}	974 ± 0 ^{A}	59 ± 1 ^{C}	268 ± 1 ^{B}	344 ± 1 ^{Aa}
30	844 ± 1 ^{B}	183 ± 0 ^{Aa}	125 ± 0 ^{A}	56 ± 2 ^{Bb}	968 ± 0 ^{B}	64 ± 0 ^{D}	278 ± 2 ^{A}	345 ± 3 ^{Aa}

^{A,B,C,D} Letters indicate statistically significant differences in the same column ($p \leq 0.05$). ^{a,b} Letters indicate statistically significant differences between extraction solvents ($p \leq 0.05$).

By contrast, the color measurement of the PLE-water extracts varied significantly over time. The L* values increased from 760 to 968 and b* values from 61 to 278 in the PLE-water extracts, resulting in dark and blue extracts, respectively. Moreover, α* values decreased progressively, favoring the appearance of green colors. In fact, ΔE values indicated a slight color variation in the PLE-NaDES extracts of 56 ± 2, while for PLE-water, this variation was bigger (345 ± 3). This means that the NaDES exerts a protective effect against the degradation of compounds extracted by PLE that is not offered by conventional extraction solvents such as water.

3. Discussion

P. palmata is an underexplored red macroalga that is interesting for its potential and utilization as a source of phycobiliproteins, proteins, sulfated polysaccharides, and polyphenols. Usually, these components have been obtained from *P. palmata* using conventional extraction techniques with water as the extraction solvent [12,13,38]. The extraction solvent selection not only determines the efficiency of the extraction but also the integrity and stability of the compounds of interest. In fact, it is known that the color of phycobiliproteins is unstable with heat, acid, and light [19]. Thus, several authors have focused their efforts on the encapsulation of phycobiliproteins or on the addition of preservatives such as benzoic acid or citric acid, among others, to preserve their color integrity [39,40]. However, these are processes that significantly increase production costs.

In addition, advanced extraction techniques such as EAE have been applied to break down the cell wall of the algae to facilitate its destruction, increasing the extraction of proteins and phycobiliproteins [2]. Nevertheless, EAE can be a complex process, requiring the precise control of temperature, substrate concentration, and pH, which depend on specific enzymes that can be expensive and sensitive to degradation. For this reason, the use of the NaDES as the extraction solvent for the recovery of phycobiliproteins, proteins, and sulfated polysaccharides was proposed for this study. NaDESs are composed of natural compounds such as amino acids, sugars, or organic acids that are easy to obtain, cheap, and biodegradable [25]. In addition, NaDESs have shown an important stabilizing activity against the degradation of bioactive compounds, such as phenolic compounds [41]. However, the stabilizing properties of these solvents against phycobiliprotein degradation have not been studied yet. Taking into account the advantages of NaDES, its use could reduce the environmental impact of extraction processes compared to the use of industrially produced enzymes, the utilization of toxic volatile organic solvents, or other conventional solvents, without preservative properties against the degradation of target compounds. Moreover, the use of NaDES combined with advanced extraction techniques such as UAE or PLE could increase the breakage of algae cell walls by the ultrasound waves as well as by the high pressure applied during the extraction, respectively [42]. However, to our knowledge, this combination has not been applied for the recovery of phycobiliproteins, proteins, sulfated polysaccharides, and polyphenols from *P. palmata*. For these reasons, a biorefinery process was developed to obtain different fractions of high added-value compounds from *P. palmata* by using NaDESs combined with UAE and PLE.

3.1. Extraction of Phycobiliproteins, Proteins, and Sulfated Polysaccharides from P. palmata (Step 1)

The first step of the biorefinery process targeted the extraction of phycobiliproteins, proteins, and sulfated polysaccharides from *P. palmata*. One of the most important parameters that influence the recovery of phycobiliproteins is the extraction temperature [43]. High temperatures could improve solvent penetration into the matrix, increasing the extraction yield of target compounds. However, thermolabile compounds, such as phycobiliproteins, can be degraded at high temperatures. In fact, extraction temperatures below 50 °C are recommended to maintain the stability of the pigments [24]. For this reason, the first step of the biorefinery process was carried out at low extraction temperatures (25 °C) to prevent the pigments' degradation.

In order to select the best extraction technique combined with NaDESs for the recovery of phycobiliproteins, proteins, and sulfated polysaccharides in the first step of the biorefinery process, different NaDESs were tested with UAE and PLE. Moreover, the different NaDESs were synthetized with 25% and 50% water, providing different physicochemical properties (viscosity, density, and polarity) using the same components. Nevertheless, the nature of NaDESs made PLE difficult; for instance, Gly:Glu:Bet and Gly:Glu:Pro NaDESs with only 25% water produced an obstruction during the extraction process. Even though these NaDESs provided lower viscosity values than the rest of the NaDESs (see Table S1), other physicochemical parameters such as the density or the nature of each NaDES component could have produced the obstruction of the PLE instrument. Thus, both NaDESs could not be implemented in step 1 of the biorefinery process using PLE. The results indicated that PLE using the Gly:Glu NaDES with 50% water provided extracts with the highest phycobiliprotein contents (see Table 1). In this sense, the application of a high pressure by PLE along with the physicochemical properties of the Gly:Glu NaDES with 50% water could have provided a better disruption of the cell structure of *P. palmata* compared to the ultrasonic waves of UAE, favoring the release of target compounds into the solvent [44]. Moreover, the addition of high percentages of water in the NaDES (50% instead of 25%) increased the mass transfer of target compounds by a reduction in NaDES viscosity and surface tension, improving the extraction of phycobiliproteins [35]. However, the PLE-water extraction provided extracts with higher protein and sulfated polysaccharide contents compared to the PLE-NaDES, UAE-NaDES, and UAE-water extracts. In fact, the hydrolysate of the PLE-water extracts presented the highest antioxidant capacity, as determined by the ORAC assay (see Table 2). This could be due to the fact that the PLE-water extraction allowed us to obtain a higher content of antioxidant water-soluble proteins. The solubility of proteins is strongly influenced by the molecular weight and the polar and nonpolar amino acids present in their structure [45]. Probably, the use of water submitted to a high pressure allowed us to break the cell wall of *P. palmata,* releasing higher polar protein and sulfated polysaccharide contents to the extraction solvent than with the use of NaDESs. Moreover, the high viscosity of the NaDES could have reduced the diffusion coefficients of proteins and sulfated polysaccharides, producing low mass transfer [27]. In fact, Table S1 shows the high viscosity of the NaDESs at room temperature, which is reduced when a temperature of 40 °C was applied. At moderately elevated temperatures, the solubility of proteins in NaDESs may improve by increasing the kinetic energy of molecules and by modifying the NaDES structure, facilitating its ability to solubilize proteins. Thus, higher extraction temperatures were considered for step 2 of the biorefinery process to maximize the recovery of non-thermolabile phycobiliproteins along with proteins and sulfated polysaccharides from the biomass residue of step 1.

3.2. Maximizing the Recovery of Phycobiliproteins, Proteins, and Sulfated Polysaccharides from *P. palmata* (Step 2)

Taking into account that the PLE-NaDES extractions provided the highest recovery rates of phycobiliproteins in step 1, UAE-NaDES extraction to maximize the recovery of phycobiliproteins, proteins, and sulfated polysaccharides from the residue of step 1 was not considered. In this sense, six different NaDESs were tested in combination with PLE for step 2 of the biorefinery process. Moreover, two PLE extraction temperatures were tested (25 °C and 40 °C) in order to determine their influence on the recovery of target compounds. The results indicated that the NaDES composed of Gly:Glu (2:1) with 50% water at 40 °C provided the extracts with the highest phycobiliprotein contents, as in step 1. This fact could be due to the Gly:Glu NaDES's polarity, viscosity, density, pH, or its sugar composition, which could have improved its interaction with phycobiliproteins through hydrogen bonding and other interactions, improving its solubility and extraction. In fact, the extraction efficiency of this NaDES has been previously demonstrated by Hilali et al. [46], who evaluated the recovery of phycocyanin from *Arthrospira platensis* using UAE combining different glycerol-based NaDESs. Furthermore, the use of higher temperatures

(40 °C) decreases the viscosity of NaDESs (Table S1), allowing for better penetration in the matrix and improving the extraction of target compounds.

On the other hand, comparing Tables 1 and 3, it can be observed that the PLE-NaDES extraction in step 1 probably degraded the cell wall of *P. palmata*, facilitating the release of mainly sulfated polysaccharides, which can be recovered in step 2, as it is confirmed by the higher content of sulfated polysaccharides in the step 2 extracts (up to three times higher than in step 1). This effect was also observed for the extraction of proteins, but to a lower extent. In general, the use of PLE-NaDESs at 40 °C increased the extraction of proteins and sulfated polysaccharides compared with the use of PLE-NaDESs at 25 °C. This means that an increase in the extraction temperature facilitated the solubilization of proteins in the NaDESs [47]. Nevertheless, the PLE-water extracts presented higher total protein and sulfated polysaccharide contents than the PLE-NaDES extract, although with lower contents of phycobiliproteins. Thus, PLE-NaDES extraction using Gly:Glu (2:1) with 50% water was selected as the best extraction technique for the recovery of phycobiliproteins, proteins, and sulfated polysaccharides from *P. palmata* in step 1 and step 2 of the biorefinery process.

3.3. *Recovery of Phenolic Compounds from the Residue of Phycobiliproteins, Protein, and Sulfated Polysaccharide Extractions*

In general, the phenolic content of red algae is low (< 4% dry weight); however, *P. palmata* has demonstrated interesting contents in antioxidant phenolic compounds, although this has not been widely explored [48,49]. Particularly, ChCl:Gly (1:2) NaDES has been widely used for the extraction of phenolic compounds from natural sources [25,35,50]. This favorable behavior might be attributed to the strong interaction of hydrogen bonds between chemical groups of ChCl and Gly with phenolic compounds, increasing its extraction [51]. Nevertheless, its viscosity can reduce the penetration of the NaDES into the matrix, decreasing the extraction efficiency. For this reason, the water percentage in the NaDES is added to reduce its viscosity. In this sense, Domínguez-Rodríguez et al. [35] observed that the extraction of phenolic compounds increased with the addition of water in ChCl:Gly (1:2) NaDES and determined that 60% water in NaDES combined with PLE at 150 °C for 25 min provided extracts with the highest antioxidant and anticholinergic phenolic compound extracts from *Citrus reticulata* leaves. Thus, these extraction conditions were selected to extract the biomass residue obtained after step 2, targeting bioactive phenolic compounds.

Figure 2 shows that TPC values from the PLE-NaDES extract were within the range of the TPC values reported by other authors from a direct extraction of phenolic compounds from *P. palmata* (between 5 and 13 mg GAE/g extract) [52–54]. This means that the biorefinery process developed in this study allowed for the selective separation of different components from *P. palmata*, maximizing the use of biomass by extracting all valuable compounds. First, phycobiliproteins, proteins, and sulfated phycobiliproteins were obtained in step 1 and 2, preserving their degradation, followed by the extraction of phenolic compounds in step 3. As can be seen in Figure 2, TPC values obtained in PLE-NaDES extract were slightly higher than those reported in the literature data. Moreover, this study confirmed also that NaDES interacts with antioxidant phenolic compounds determined by a TEAC assay, increasing its extraction compared with ethanol/water (70:30, *v*/*v*) solvent, obtaining higher TPC values in PLE-NaDES than in ethanolic PLE extracts. However, the ethanolic extracts presented a higher antioxidant capacity determined by an ORAC assay as well as a higher anticholinergic capacity than the PLE-NaDES extract. This means that different phenolic compounds were obtained depending on the extraction solvent. The NaDES provided extracts that were more able to neutralize ABTS radicals, while ethanol/water (70:30, *v*/*v*) allowed us to obtain extracts with a higher capacity to neutralize O_2 species. Probably, the polarity and low viscosity of the ethanol/water solvent promoted the extraction of more polar compounds different from phenolic compounds with a higher antioxidant capacity (as determined by an ORAC assay) and anticholinergic capacity than those obtained with the NaDES.

3.4. Preservative Effect of NaDES against Phycobiliprotein Degradation

Phycobiliprotein extracts and, in particular, the PLE-NaDES extract obtained using Gly:Glu (2:1) NaDES in step 1 were submitted to a forced stability study to determine the potential protective effect of NaDES on the degradation of these compounds; PLE-water extract exposed to the same conditions was employed as a control. The results indicated (see Figure 3) that the PLE-NaDES extract maintained the phycobiliprotein contents, the antioxidant capacity of its hydrolysate, and the color of the extract over time while the PLE-water extract showed a reduction in all the tested parameters. This preservative effect of NaDES against the oxidative and thermal degradation of phycobiliproteins could be due to the high viscosity of this solvent compared with water [55,56]. An increase in the viscosity of NaDES produces a decrease in the mobility of molecules, reducing their exposure time to oxygen and avoiding their degradation [57]. In fact, the PLE-water extract presented a more intense yellow-brown color over time, which could indicate the oxidation of the extract by exposure to oxygen (see Table 4). This stabilizing effect can be adjusted by reducing the water content in the NaDES to increase the formation of hydrogen bonds between the target compounds and the NaDES [56]. However, the reduction in water content could affect the extraction efficiency of the target compounds. Thus, the water content in the NaDES is a crucial parameter to optimize in order to obtain stabilized extracts rich in target compounds.

4. Materials and Methods

4.1. Chemicals and Samples

Gallic acid, ascorbic acid, Trizma hydrochloride (Tris-HCl), trolox, disodium phosphate (Na_2HPO_4), monopotassium phosphate (KH_2PO_4), fluorescein sodium salt, sodium hydroxide (NaOH), sodium carbonate (Na_2CO_3), potassium persulfate ($K_2S_2O_8$), acetylcholinesterase (AChE) Type VI-S from *Electrophorus electricus*, 2,2′-azino-bis(3-ethylbenzothiazoline-6-slphonic acid) (ABTS), toluidine blue, bovine serum albumin, and Bradford Reagent were supplied by Sigma-Aldrich (Madrid, Spain). Ethyl acetate (ETAC), ethanol (EtOH), methanol, and formic acid were purchased from VWR Chemicals (Barcelona, Spain). Folin–Ciocalteu reagent was acquired from Merck (Darmstadt, Germany) while acetylthiocholine iodide (ATCI), galantamine hydrobromide, 4-(amino-sulfonyl)-7-fluoro-2,1,3-benzoxadiazole (ABD-F), 2,2-azobis(2-aminodinopropane) dihydrochloride (AAPH), 2,2-difenil-1-picrilhidracilo (DPPH), choline chloride (ChCl), glucose, betaine, and proline were purchased from TCI Chemicals (Tokyo, Japan). Glycerol was provided by Labkem (Barcelona, Spain). Fucoidan (from Fucus serratus algae) was acquired from Carbosynth Limited, Berkshire, UK). Trypsin was purchased from MP Biomedical (Santa Ana, CA, USA).

The ultrapure water used (18.2 MΩ/cm) was obtained from a Millipore system (Millipore, Billerica, MA, USA).

Dried *Palmaria palmata* was provided by Porto Muiños (Cerceda, A Coruña, Spain). *P. palmata* powder was vacuum-packed and stored at −20 °C.

4.2. Proposed Biorefinery Process for the Valorization of P. palmata

In order to recover bioactive compounds from *P. palmata* with green solvents, two different approaches were used: UAE and PLE, both combined with green solvents such as water and NaDES. Figure 1 (in the Results section) illustrates a scheme of the proposed processes for the valorization of the algae.

A sequential process composed of three steps was designed for the extraction of phycobiliproteins, sulfated polysaccharides, and phenolic compounds from *P. palmata* as follows.

Step 1: The first step involved a comparative study between PLE and UAE to select the best extraction technique for the recovery of phycobiliproteins and sulfated polysaccharides from the alga. In this step, different NaDESs were tested and compared with water as extraction solvent. For this, a DIONEX ASE 200 (Dionex, Sunnyvale, CA, USA) was used for PLE extractions. PLE extractions were achieved in 11 mL extraction cells, which were filled with 1 g of *P. palmata* using 10.5 MPa for 20 min at 25 °C following Gallego et al. [24]'s method for the recovery of phycobiliproteins and sulfated polysaccharides from *Porphyridium cruentum* biomass. In order to compare PLE with UAE, 100 mg of *P. palmata* was mixed with 10 mL NaDES or water and sonicated at a frequency of 40 kHz at 25 °C for 50 min according to the optimized extraction methods of Domínguez-Rodríguez et al. [35] and Hilali et al. [46] for the extraction of bioactive compounds and phycobiliproteins from *Citrus reticulata* leaves and *Arthrospira platensis*, respectively.

Step 2: The residual biomass of the best extraction in terms of phycobiliprotein contents from step 1 was employed to extract the remaining phycobiliproteins and sulfated polysaccharides from *P. palmata*. In this step, the same NaDESs from the first step were tested and compared with water as extraction solvent. In addition, two temperatures were tested (25 °C and 40 °C) to obtain phycobiliproteins and sulfated polysaccharides.

Step 3: Phenolic compounds were recovered from the residual biomass of step 2 by PLE-NaDES using choline chloride:glycerol (ChCl:Gly) in a 1:2 molar ratio with 60% water in NaDES for 25 min at 150 °C and 10.5 MPa, according to Domínguez-Rodríguez [35]'s protocol. Additionally, to determine the efficiency of the use of NaDESs on the recovery of phenolic compounds from the residual biomass of step 2, the same PLE extraction conditions were applied but using ethanol:water (70:30, v/v) as solvent extraction instead of NaDES.

All extracts were centrifuged at 12,000× g for 15 min at 10 °C, the supernatant was removed, and they were stored at −20 °C until their use.

4.3. Preparation of Natural Deep Eutectic Solvents (NaDESs)

According to NaDESs employed in the literature data for the extraction of proteins and phycobiliproteins from algae, NaDESs presented in Table 5 were selected and formed following the protocol of Rajha et al. [58]. Each NaDES was synthesized using 25 and 50% water to obtain NaDESs with different viscosities. The mixture was heated for 1 h at 80 °C until a clear liquid was obtained.

Table 5. Hydrogen bond acceptors (HBAs) and hydrogen bond donors (HBDs) used in the NaDESs' compositions.

Abbreviations	HBA	HBD	Molar Ratio	Percentage of Water in NaDES	Reference
Gly:Glu	Glycerol	Glucose	2:1	25 and 50%	[46]
Gly:Glu:Bet	Glycerol	Glucose and Betaine	4:1:1	25 and 50%	[46]
Gly:Glu:Pro	Glycerol	Glucose and Proline	4:1:1	25 and 50%	[46]
ChCl:Gly	Choline chloride	Glycerol	1:2	60%	[35]

4.4. Hydrolysis of Protein Fraction for In Vitro Assays

UAE-NaDES and PLE-NaDES extracts from step 1 were hydrolyzed using trypsin enzyme for obtaining bioactive peptides following the protocol described by Liu et al. [14]. Briefly, each 1 mL of extract was homogenized with 1 mL of phosphate buffer at pH of 8 for 10 min. Then, trypsin was added according to the total extract amount so that the enzyme/substrate ratio would be 4% (w/w). This mixture was incubated in a thermomixer (Eppendorf AG, Hamburg, Germany) at 37 °C to initiate the digestion process. The hydrolysate was recovered at 1, 3, 5, and 6 h of incubation in order to determine the optimal hydrolysis time. After incubation periods, hydrolysis was stopped by heating them at 95 °C for 10 min, then they were placed on ice, followed by cooling them to room temperature. Finally, the hydrolysates were centrifuged at 8000× g for 15 min, and the supernatants were removed and stored until their analysis.

4.5. Preparation of Phenolic Extracts for In Vitro Assays

To avoid NaDESs interfering with the analytical methods employed in this investigation for the study of phenolic compounds, phenolic extracts were purified by employing solid-phase extraction (SPE) according to Domínguez-Rodríguez et al. [25]'s method to remove NaDESs from the extracts. Briefly, C-18 cartridges (Strata C18-T, 500 mg) were placed in a vacuum system and equilibrated with 2.5 mL methanol (100%), followed by 7.5 mL of acidified water with formic acid (0.35%, *v*/*v*). After loading 2.5 mL of the sample, the cartridges were flushed with 2.5 mL of acidified water with formic acid (0.35%, *v*/*v*) to remove NaDESs. Then, phenolic compounds were eluted with 5.0 mL of ethyl acetate and 2.0 mL of acidified methanol with formic acid (0.1%, *v*/*v*). The phenolic fraction was dried with nitrogen and stored at −20 °C.

4.6. Spectrophotometric Analysis

4.6.1. Determination of Total Protein Content

Bradford protein assay was employed to determine the total protein content of *P. palmata* extracts from steps 1 and 2 following the method described by Bradford [59]. Briefly, 5 µL of extract was mixed with 5 µL NaOH (1 M, pH: 8.0), and 250 µL of Bradford reagent was added. After 10 min in the dark at room temperature, absorbance was measured at 595 nm. Protein concentration was calculated by interpolation with a calibration curve carried out with bovine serum albumin (BSA) standard, and the results are expressed as mg protein/g sample.

4.6.2. Determination of Phycobiliprotein Contents

Phycobiliprotein (B-Phycoerythrin (B-PE), Allophycocyanin (APC), and R-Phycocyanin (R-PC)) contents in the extracts of *P. palmata* from steps 1 and 2 were calculated using Roman et al. [60]'s method. The extracts were diluted at 1 mg/mL with water and the absorbance was measured at 620, 650, and 565 nm to determine the R-PC, APC, and B-PE contents, respectively. The results were expressed in mg phycobiliprotein/mL sample and calculated with the following equations:

$$\text{R-phycocyanin [R-PC]} = (\text{Abs 620 nm} - 0.7 \times \text{Abs 650 nm})/7.38 \quad (1)$$

$$\text{Allophycocyanin: [APC]} = (\text{Abs 650 nm} - 0.19 \times \text{Abs 620 nm})/5.6 \quad (2)$$

$$\text{B-Phycoerythrin: [B-PE]} = (\text{Abs 565 nm} - 2.8 \times \text{[R-PC]} - 1.34 \times \text{[APC]})/12.27 \quad (3)$$

4.6.3. Determination of Sulfated Polysaccharides

The quantification of sulfated polysaccharides was carried out using the method described by Beutler et al. [61] and Albano et al. [62]. The extract (200 µL) was mixed with 1 mL of 0.01 mg/mL toluidine blue solution. After 10 min at room temperature, the absorbance of the mixture was measured at 620 nm. A calibration curve was utilized with fucoidan, and the results are expressed as mg sulfated polysaccharides/g sample.

4.6.4. Determination of Total Phenolic Content

The total phenolic content in the phenolic extracts obtained by PLE-NaDES in step 3 was measured utilizing the Folin–Ciocalteu method, based on the procedure established by Singleton et al. [63]. A standard curve was generated using gallic acid in the range of 0.05–2 mg/mL to present the results as milligrams of gallic acid equivalents (GAE)/ sample.

4.7. Biological Activities

4.7.1. Antioxidant Capacity

Reactive oxygen species (ROS) scavenging capacity according to ORAC assay: The antioxidant capacity of the extracts was determined by ORAC method described by Qu et al. [64]. Briefly, 100 μL of extracts at different concentrations was added to a mixture containing 100 μL of AAPH (590 mM) prepared in 30 mM phosphate buffer at a pH of 7.5 and fluorescein at a concentration of 10 μM in 25 μL phosphate buffer. The reaction was started at 37 °C, and fluorescence measurements were recorded every 5 min for 1 h (λexcitation = 485 nm; λemission = 530 nm). The peroxyl radical scavenging capacity of the extracts was calculated using the difference between the area under the curve (AUC) of fluorescence reduction and the percent inhibition obtained in the presence (AUCextract) or absence (AUCcontrol) of the extract according to the following equation:

$$\%\text{Inhibition} = \frac{\text{AUCcontrol} - \text{AUCsample}}{\text{AUCcontrol}} \times 100 \quad (4)$$

AUC was calculated by mean equation below:

$$\text{AUC} = 0.5 + \sum f_i/f_0 \quad (5)$$

where f_0 and f_i are fluorescence measurements at t = 0 min and every 5 min, respectively.

Trolox equivalent antioxidant capacity (TEAC) assay: TEAC assay was carried out using the method described by Re et al. [65]. ABTS stock solution was used, mixing 7 mM ABTS with 2.45 mM potassium persulfate. It was maintained under darkness for 12–16 h at room temperature. After that, the ABTS working solution was prepared by mixing 5 mM phosphate buffer (pH 7.4) with ABTS stock solution until absorbance at 734 nm reached values of 0.70 AU. Then, 10 μL of extract was added to 990 μL of ABTS working solution. Absorbance was measured at 734 nm after 45 min. A calibration curve was made employing Trolox as reference standard to express the results as TEAC (mmol Trolox/g sample). TEAC values were obtained from a calibration curve of each sample achieved from four different concentrations, which showed a liner response between 20 and 80% compared with the initial absorption.

4.7.2. Anticholinergic Activity

To determine the inhibitory effect on acetylcholinesterase (AChE) activity, a fluorescent enzyme kinetics assay based on a modified version of Ellman et al. [66]'s method was applied [67]. The extracts were prepared at seven different concentrations ranging from 25 to 250 μg/mL by dissolving them in EtOH/H_2O (1:1, *v*/*v*). A total of 100 μL of Tris-HCl buffer (150 mM, pH 8), 25 μL of AChE enzyme (0.8 U/mL), and 100 μL of extract were added to each reaction well, and the mixture was incubated at room temperature for 10 min. After incubation, 25 μL of ABD-F (125 μM) and 50 μL of acetylthiocholiniodide (ATCI) at the concentration calculated by Michaelis–Menten constant (KM) were added to each well. The reaction mixture was monitored by taking fluorescence measurements at 389 nm excitation and 513 nm emission wavelengths every minute using a microplate reader (Cytation 5, BioTek Instruments, Winooski, VT, USA) for 15 min at 37 °C. The percentage of enzyme inhibition was calculated using the mean velocities measured for AChE enzyme in the absence (V0) and presence (V1) of the sample according to the following equation:

$$\%\text{Inhibition} = \frac{\text{V0} - \text{V1}}{\text{V0}} \times 100 \quad (6)$$

The concentration of the extract that inhibited the enzyme activity by 50% (IC_{50}) was determined in μg/mL, and it was observed that higher IC_{50} values indicated lower anticholinergic capacity. Galantamine hydrobromide at a concentration of 0.0125 mg/mL was used as a positive control. All measurements were performed in triplicate, and the results were reported as mean ± standard deviation (SD).

4.8. Stability Study

In order to observe the preservation effect of NaDESs on phycobiliproteins' contents and the antioxidant capacity of their hydrolysates, a stability study following the protocol of Hilali et al. [46] was performed. The NaDES extract with the highest antioxidant phycobiliprotein content and water extracts were stored and submitted to accelerated aging conditions at 40 °C for 30 days, equivalent to 6 months at room temperature. Every 7 days, aliquots of extracts were collected and the phycobiliprotein concentrations (determined following the protocol described in Section 4.6.2), the antioxidant capacity of their hydrolysates (measured by TEAC and ORAC assays), and the color change of the extracts were monitored.

The color measurements were carried out during the stability test according to Idowu et al. [68]'s protocol using a Konica Minolta portable colorimeter (model CR-400), with D65 illuminant and an observation angle of 2°. Results were expressed according to CIELAB model, in which L* represents lightness (L* = 0 corresponds to the darkest, while L* = 100 is the brightest), α* represents the range color from red with positive values to green with negative values, and b* represents the color channel from the yellow positive values to the blue negative values. The Chroma Meter was initially calibrated in the CIELAB color space system employing a white tile. Three readings were taken for each sample. Color differences between the initial extract and the extract during the stability study were determined according to the following equation:

$$\Delta E^{*}_{Lab} = \sqrt{(L2 - L1)^2 + (\alpha 2 - \alpha 1)^2 + (b2 - b1)^2} \quad (7)$$

where $L1$ represents the luminosity of the initial extract, $L2$ provides the lightness/darkness of the extract during each week of the stability study, α is the redness or greenness of the initial extract, and $\alpha 2$ the redness or greenness of the extract in each week of the stability study, while $b1$ is the yellowness/blueness of the initial extract and $b2$ is the yellowness/blueness of the extract in each week of the stability study.

4.9. Statistical Analysis

Statistical analysis was carried out employing Statgraphics Centurion version XVII software (Statistical Graphics Corp, The Plains, VA, USA) to compare the total phycobiliprotein, protein, and total sulfated polysaccharide contents as well as the antioxidant and anticholinergic capacities and color changes of the extracts. To determine statistically significant differences ($p \leq 0.05$) between mean values for different extracts at a 95% confidence level, an analysis of variance (ANOVA) with Fisher's exact test was utilized.

5. Conclusions

The potential of the pressurized NaDES extraction process was demonstrated for the sequential recovery of different fractions of valuable compounds from *P. palmata*. A pressurized NaDES composed of Gly:Glu (2:1) with 50% water improved the selectivity of thermolabile phycobiliprotein contents in the first step of the biorefinery process, compared to UAE-NaDES extraction. This pressurized NaDES allowed us to maximize the recovery of phycobiliproteins using 40 °C as the extraction temperature in comparison with 25 °C in the second step of the biorefinery process, as well as to obtain interesting protein and sulfated polysaccharide contents. The efficiency of PLE-NaDES extraction in the recovery of phycobiliproteins, proteins, and sulfated polysaccharides was corroborated by comparison with PLE-water extracts, with water being the extraction solvent usually employed for the extraction of these compounds. Moreover, a preservative effect of the NaDESs against oxidative damage and thermal exposure was confirmed with a forced stability study compared to water extracts. Finally, the extraction of the residual biomass of the second step was performed using a PLE-NaDES with ChCl:Gly (1:2) compared to PLE with ethanol:water (70:30, v/v); this corresponded to the third step of the biorefinery process and provided extracts enriched in antioxidant and anticholinergic phenolic compounds. In summary, the results obtained demonstrated the efficiency of pressurized NaDESs compared with the use of UAE-NaDESs and conventional solvents as a green alternative for the valorization of *P. palmata* biomass through a new biorefinery process.

Supplementary Materials: The following supporting information can be downloaded at: https://www.mdpi.com/article/10.3390/md22100467/s1, Table S1: Viscosity values (mPas·s) of NaDES employed in this study with 25% and 50% of water measured at 25 °C and 40 °C. Table S2: Antioxidant capacity of PLE-Water and PLE-NaDES (Gly:Glu, 50% H_2O) extract according to hydrolysis time determined by ORAC (IC_{50}, µg/mL sample) analyses and TEAC (µmol trolox/g sample).

Author Contributions: Conceptualization, M.C., G.D.-R., E.I. and A.C.; methodology, M.C., G.D.-R., E.I. and A.C.; validation, G.D.-R., H.K., E.I. and A.C.; formal analysis, M.C. and G.D.-R.; investigation, G.D.-R., H.K., E.I. and A.C.; resources, M.C., G.D.-R., E.I. and A.C.; data curation, M.C., G.D.-R. and E.I.; writing—original draft preparation, M.C. and G.D.-R.; writing—review and editing, M.C., G.D.-R., E.I. and A.C.; visualization, G.D.-R., H.K., E.I. and A.C.; supervision, G.D.-R., H.K., E.I. and A.C.; project administration, H.K., E.I. and A.C.; funding acquisition, E.I. and A.C. All authors have read and agreed to the published version of the manuscript.

Funding: This research was supported by projects PID2020-113050RB-I00, PDC2021-120814-I00, and EQC2021-007112-P funded by the Ministry of Science and Innovation (MCIN/AEI/10.13039/501100011033) and The European Union Next GenerationEU/PRTR. Moreover, this work was funded by the Ministry of Science and Innovation with the project number AGL2017-89417R. In addition, this work was supported by a "Margarita Salas" grant from the University of Alcalá for G.D-R. M.C. was funded by the Ministry of National Education, Turkey (scholarship program: YLSY-2018).

Institutional Review Board Statement: Not applicable.

Data Availability Statement: The original contributions presented in this study are included in the article/Supplementary Materials; further inquiries can be directed to the corresponding authors.

Acknowledgments: The authors would like to acknowledge Porto Muiños (Cerceda, A Coruña, Spain) for providing the dried *Palmaria palmata* to carry out the study.

Conflicts of Interest: The authors declare no conflict of interest.

References

1. Amchova, P.; Siska, F.; Ruda-Kucerova, J. Food Safety and Health Concerns of Synthetic Food Colors: An Update. *Toxics* **2024**, *12*, 466. [CrossRef] [PubMed]
2. Dumay, J.; Clément, N.; Morançais, M.; Fleurence, J. Optimization of Hydrolysis Conditions of *Palmaria palmata* to Enhance R-Phycoerythrin Extraction. *Bioresour. Technol.* **2013**, *131*, 21–27. [CrossRef] [PubMed]
3. Harnedy, P.A.; Soler-Vila, A.; Edwards, M.D.; FitzGerald, R.J. The Effect of Time and Origin of Harvest on the in Vitro Biological Activity of *Palmaria palmata* Protein Hydrolysates. *Food Res. Int.* **2014**, *62*, 746–752. [CrossRef]
4. Irvine, L.M.; Chamberlain, Y.M. Seaweeds of the British Isles. Volume 1. Rhodophyta. Part 2B. Corallinales, Hildenbrandiales. *J. Mar. Biol. Assoc. U. K.* **1994**, *74*, 986.
5. Stévant, P.; Schmedes, P.S.; Le Gall, L.; Wegeberg, S.; Dumay, J.; Rebours, C. Concise Review of the Red Macroalga Dulse, *Palmaria palmata* (L.) Weber & Mohr. *J. Appl. Phycol.* **2023**, *35*, 523–550.
6. Liboureau, P.; Pampanin, D.M. Effects of Vegetative Propagation on Protein Content and Bioactivity of the Red Seaweed *Palmaria palmata*. *Food Chem.* **2024**, *455*, 139929. [CrossRef]
7. Schmedes, P.S.; Nielsen, M.M.; Petersen, J.K. Improved *Palmaria palmata* Hatchery Methods for Tetraspore Release, Even Settlement and High Seedling Survival Using Strong Water Agitation and Macerated Propagules. *Algal Res.* **2019**, *40*, 101494. [CrossRef]
8. Holdt, S.L.; Kraan, S. Bioactive Compounds in Seaweed: Functional Food Applications and Legislation. *J. Appl. Phycol.* **2011**, *23*, 543–597. [CrossRef]
9. Ma, J.; Hu, J.; Sha, X.; Meng, D.; Yang, R. Phycobiliproteins, the Pigment-Protein Complex Form of Natural Food Colorants and Bioactive Ingredients. *Crit. Rev. Food Sci. Nutr.* **2024**, *64*, 2999–3017. [CrossRef]
10. Kovaleski, G.; Kholany, M.; Dias, L.M.S.; Correia, S.F.H.; Ferreira, R.A.S.; Coutinho, J.A.P.; Ventura, S.P.M. Extraction and Purification of Phycobiliproteins from Algae and Their Applications. *Front. Chem.* **2022**, *10*, 1065355. [CrossRef]
11. Ji, L.; Qiu, S.; Wang, Z.; Zhao, C.; Tang, B.; Gao, Z.; Fan, J. Phycobiliproteins from Algae: Current Updates in Sustainable Production and Applications in Food and Health. *Food Res. Int.* **2023**, *167*, 112737. [CrossRef]
12. Lee, D.; Nishizawa, M.; Shimizu, Y.; Saeki, H. Anti-Inflammatory Effects of Dulse (*Palmaria palmata*) Resulting from the Simultaneous Water-Extraction of Phycobiliproteins and Chlorophyll a. *Food Res. Int.* **2017**, *100*, 514–521. [CrossRef] [PubMed]
13. Furuta, T.; Miyabe, Y.; Yasui, H.; Kinoshita, Y.; Kishimura, H. Angiotensin I Converting Enzyme Inhibitory Peptides Derived from Phycobiliproteins of Dulse *Palmaria palmata*. *Mar. Drugs* **2016**, *14*, 32. [CrossRef] [PubMed]
14. Liu, J.; Bai, X.; Fu, P. In Silico and in Vitro Assessment of Bioactive Peptides from *Arthrospira platensis* Phycobiliproteins for DPP-IV Inhibitory Activity, ACE Inhibitory Activity, and Antioxidant Activity. *J. Appl. Phycol.* **2022**, *34*, 1497–1511. [CrossRef]

15. Gomes-Dias, J.S.; Teixeira-Guedes, C.I.; Teixeira, J.A.; Rocha, C.M.R. Red Seaweed Biorefinery: The Influence of Sequential Extractions on the Functional Properties of Extracted Agars and Porphyrans. *Int. J. Biol. Macromol.* **2024**, *257*, 128479. [CrossRef] [PubMed]
16. Premarathna, A.D.; Ahmed, T.A.E.; Kulshreshtha, G.; Humayun, S.; Shormeh Darko, C.N.; Rjabovs, V.; Hammami, R.; Critchley, A.T.; Tuvikene, R.; Hincke, M.T. Polysaccharides from Red Seaweeds: Effect of Extraction Methods on Physicochemical Characteristics and Antioxidant Activities. *Food Hydrocoll.* **2024**, *147*, 109307. [CrossRef]
17. Mittal, R.; Tavanandi, H.A.; Mantri, V.A.; Raghavarao, K.S.M.S. Ultrasound Assisted Methods for Enhanced Extraction of Phycobiliproteins from Marine Macro-Algae, *Gelidium pusillum* (Rhodophyta). *Ultrason. Sonochem.* **2017**, *38*, 92–103. [CrossRef]
18. Castro-Varela, P.; Celis-Pla, P.S.M.; Figueroa, F.L.; Rubilar, M. Highly Efficient Water-Based Extraction of Biliprotein R-Phycoerythrin from Marine the Red-Macroalga *Sarcopeltis skottsbergii* by Ultrasound and High-Pressure Homogenization Methods. *Front. Mar. Sci.* **2022**, *9*, 877177. [CrossRef]
19. Nowruzi, B.; Konur, O.; Anvar, S.A.A. The Stability of the Phycobiliproteins in the Adverse Environmental Conditions Relevant to the Food Storage. *Food Bioproc. Technol.* **2022**, *15*, 2646–2663. [CrossRef]
20. Spain, O.; Hardouin, K.; Bourgougnon, N.; Michalak, I. Enzyme-Assisted Extraction of Red Seaweed *Solieria chordalis* (*C. agardh*) J. Agardh 1842—The Starting Point for the Production of Biostimulants of Plant Growth and Biosorbents of Metal Ions. *Biomass Convers. Biorefinery* **2024**, *14*, 1621–1635. [CrossRef]
21. Choi, W.Y.; Lee, H.Y. Effect of Ultrasonic Extraction on Production and Structural Changes of C-Phycocyanin from Marine *Spirulina maxima*. *Int. J. Mol. Sci.* **2018**, *19*, 220. [CrossRef]
22. Tavanandi, H.A.; Raghavarao, K.S.M.S. Ultrasound-Assisted Enzymatic Extraction of Natural Food Colorant C-Phycocyanin from Dry Biomass of *Arthrospira platensis*. *LWT* **2020**, *118*, 108802. [CrossRef]
23. Le Guillard, C.; Dumay, J.; Donnay-Moreno, C.; Bruzac, S.; Ragon, J.Y.; Fleurence, J.; Bergé, J.P. Ultrasound-Assisted Extraction of R-Phycoerythrin from *Grateloupia turuturu* with and without Enzyme Addition. *Algal Res.* **2015**, *12*, 522–528. [CrossRef]
24. Gallego, R.; Martínez, M.; Cifuentes, A.; Ibáñez, E.; Herrero, M. Development of a Green Downstream Process for the Valorization of *Porphyridium cruentum* Biomass. *Molecules* **2019**, *24*, 1564. [CrossRef] [PubMed]
25. Domínguez-Rodríguez, G.; Amador-Luna, V.M.; Benešová, K.; Pernica, M.; Parada-Alfonso, F.; Ibáñez, E. Biorefinery Approach with Green Solvents for the Valorization of *Citrus reticulata* Leaves to Obtain Antioxidant and Anticholinergic Extracts. *Food Chem.* **2024**, *456*, 140034. [CrossRef]
26. Plaza, M.; Domínguez-Rodríguez, G.; Sahelices, C.; Marina, M.L. A Sustainable Approach for Extracting Non-Extractable Phenolic Compounds from Mangosteen Peel Using Ultrasound-Assisted Extraction and Natural Deep Eutectic Solvents. *Appl. Sci.* **2021**, *11*, 5625. [CrossRef]
27. Hikmawanti, N.P.E.; Ramadon, D.; Jantan, I.; Mun'im, A. Natural Deep Eutectic Solvents (Nades): Phytochemical Extraction Performance Enhancer for Pharmaceutical and Nutraceutical Product Development. *Plants* **2021**, *10*, 2091. [CrossRef]
28. Mišan, A.; Pojić, M. Applications of NADES in Stabilizing Food and Protecting Food Compounds against Oxidation. In *Advances in Botanical Research*; Academic Press: Cambridge, MA, USA, 2021; Volume 97.
29. Bertolo, M.R.V.; Martins, V.C.A.; Plepis, A.M.G.; Bogusz, S. Utilization of Pomegranate Peel Waste: Natural Deep Eutectic Solvents as a Green Strategy to Recover Valuable Phenolic Compounds. *J. Clean. Prod.* **2021**, *327*, 129471. [CrossRef]
30. Abdallah, M.M.; Cardeira, M.; Matias, A.A.; Bronze, M.R.; Fernández, N. Lactic Acid-Based Natural Deep Eutectic Solvents to Extract Bioactives from Marine By-Products. *Molecules* **2022**, *27*, 4356. [CrossRef]
31. Gkioni, M.D.; Andriopoulos, V.; Koutra, E.; Hatziantoniou, S.; Kornaros, M.; Lamari, F.N. Ultrasound-Assisted Extraction of *Nannochloropsis oculata* with Ethanol and Betaine: 1,2-Propanediol Eutectic Solvent for Antioxidant Pigment-Rich Extracts Retaining Nutritious the Residual Biomass. *Antioxidants* **2022**, *11*, 1103. [CrossRef]
32. García-Roldán, A.; Piriou, L.; Jauregi, P. Natural Deep Eutectic Solvents as a Green Extraction of Polyphenols from Spent Coffee Ground with Enhanced Bioactivities. *Front. Plant Sci.* **2023**, *13*, 1072592. [CrossRef] [PubMed]
33. Munier, M.; Jubeau, S.; Wijaya, A.; Morançais, M.; Dumay, J.; Marchal, L.; Jaouen, P.; Fleurence, J. Physicochemical Factors Affecting the Stability of Two Pigments: R-Phycoerythrin of *Grateloupia turuturu* and B-Phycoerythrin of *Porphyridium cruentum*. *Food Chem.* **2014**, *150*, 400–407. [CrossRef] [PubMed]
34. Dussan, K.; Huijgen, W.J.J.; de Vrije, T.; van der Wal, H.; Capella, H.; van Doorn, J.; López-Contreras, A.M.; van Hal, J.W. Biorefinery of Red Seaweed *Palmaria palmata* for Production of Bio-Based Chemicals and Biofuels. *Algal Res.* **2024**, *82*, 103608. [CrossRef]
35. Domínguez-Rodríguez, G.; Amador-Luna, V.M.; Mendiola, J.A.; Parada-Alfonso, F.; Ibanez, E. *Development of a Sustainable Extraction and Storage Stability of Antioxidant and Anticholinergic Pressurized Natural Deep Euteectic Solvent Extracts from Citrus reticulata Leaves*; Institute of Food Science Research: Madrid, Spain, 2024; *submitted*.
36. Gómez-Urios, C.; Viñas-Ospino, A.; Puchades-Colera, P.; Blesa, J.; López-Malo, D.; Frígola, A.; Esteve, M.J. Choline Chloride-Based Natural Deep Eutectic Solvents for the Extraction and Stability of Phenolic Compounds, Ascorbic Acid, and Antioxidant Capacity from *Citrus sinensis* Peel. *LWT* **2023**, *177*, 114595. [CrossRef]
37. Jeong, K.M.; Ko, J.; Zhao, J.; Jin, Y.; Yoo, D.E.; Han, S.Y.; Lee, J. Multi-Functioning Deep Eutectic Solvents as Extraction and Storage Media for Bioactive Natural Products That Are Readily Applicable to Cosmetic Products. *J. Clean. Prod.* **2017**, *151*, 87–95. [CrossRef]

38. Miyabe, Y.; Furuta, T.; Takeda, T.; Kanno, G.; Shimizu, T.; Tanaka, Y.; Gai, Z.; Yasui, H.; Kishimura, H. Structural Properties of Phycoerythrin from Dulse *Palmaria palmata*. *J. Food Biochem.* **2017**, *41*, e12301. [CrossRef]
39. Pradeep, H.N.; Nayak, C.A. Enhanced Stability of C-Phycocyanin Colorant by Extrusion Encapsulation. *J. Food Sci. Technol.* **2019**, *56*, 4526–4534. [CrossRef]
40. Kannaujiya, V.K.; Sinha, R.P. Thermokinetic Stability of Phycocyanin and Phycoerythrin in Food-Grade Preservatives. *J. Appl. Phycol.* **2016**, *28*, 1063–1070. [CrossRef]
41. Usmani, Z.; Sharma, M.; Tripathi, M.; Lukk, T.; Karpichev, Y.; Gathergood, N.; Singh, B.N.; Thakur, V.K.; Tabatabaei, M.; Gupta, V.K. Biobased Natural Deep Eutectic System as Versatile Solvents: Structure, Interaction and Advanced Applications. *Sci. Total Environ.* **2023**, *881*, 163002. [CrossRef]
42. Guzmán-Lorite, M.; Marina, M.L.; García, M.C. Successive Extraction Using Natural Deep Eutectic Solvents and Pressurized Liquids for a Greener and Holistic Recovery of Proteins from Pomegranate Seeds. *Food Res. Int.* **2022**, *161*, 111862. [CrossRef]
43. Chentir, I.; Hamdi, M.; Li, S.; Doumandji, A.; Markou, G.; Nasri, M. Stability, Bio-Functionality and Bio-Activity of Crude Phycocyanin from a Two-Phase Cultured Saharian *Arthrospira* sp. Strain. *Algal Res.* **2018**, *35*, 395–406. [CrossRef]
44. Perez-Vazquez, A.; Carpena, M.; Barciela, P.; Cassani, L.; Simal-Gandara, J.; Prieto, M.A. Pressurized Liquid Extraction for the Recovery of Bioactive Compounds from Seaweeds for Food Industry Application: A Review. *Antioxidants* **2023**, *12*, 612. [CrossRef] [PubMed]
45. Navaf, M.; Sunooj, K.V.; Aaliya, B.; Sudheesh, C.; Akhila, P.P.; Mir, S.A.; Nemtanu, M.R.; George, J.; Lackner, M.; Mousavi Khaneghah, A. Contemporary Insights into the Extraction, Functional Properties, and Therapeutic Applications of Plant Proteins. *J. Agric. Food Res.* **2023**, *14*, 100861. [CrossRef]
46. Hilali, S.; Wils, L.; Chevalley, A.; Clément-Larosière, B.; Boudesocque-Delaye, L. Glycerol-Based NaDES as Green Solvents for Ultrasound-Assisted Extraction of Phycocyanin from *Arthrospira platensis*—RSM Optimization and ANN Modelling. *Biomass Convers. Biorefinery* **2022**, *12*, 157–170. [CrossRef]
47. Hu, R.S.; Yu, L.; Zhou, S.Y.; Zhou, H.F.; Wan, H.T.; Yang, J.H. Comparative Study on Optimization of NADES Extraction Process by Dual Models and Antioxidant Activity of Optimum Extraction from Chuanxiong-Honghua. *LWT* **2023**, *184*, 114991. [CrossRef]
48. Gallagher, J.A.; Adams, J.M.M.; Turner, L.B.; Kirby, M.E.; Toop, T.A.; Mirza, M.W.; Theodorou, M.K. Bio-Processing of Macroalgae *Palmaria palmata*: Metabolite Fractionation from Pressed Fresh Material and Ensiling Considerations for Long-Term Storage. *J. Appl. Phycol.* **2021**, *33*, 533–544. [CrossRef]
49. Wang, T.; Jónsdóttir, R.; Kristinsson, H.G.; Hreggvidsson, G.O.; Jónsson, J.Ó.; Thorkelsson, G.; Ólafsdóttir, G. Enzyme-Enhanced Extraction of Antioxidant Ingredients from Red Algae *Palmaria palmata*. *LWT* **2010**, *43*, 1387–1393. [CrossRef]
50. de Lima, N.D.; da Silva Monteiro Wanderley, B.R.; Andrade Ferreira, A.L.; Pereira-Coelho, M.; da Silva Haas, I.C.; Vitali, L.; dos Santos Madureira, L.A.; Müller, J.M.; Fritzen-Freire, C.B.; de Mello Castanho Amboni, R.D. Green Extraction of Phenolic Compounds from the by-Product of Purple Araçá (*Psidium myrtoides*) with Natural Deep Eutectic Solvents Assisted by Ultrasound: Optimization, Comparison, and Bioactivity. *Food Res. Int.* **2024**, *191*, 114731. [CrossRef]
51. Vilková, M.; Płotka-Wasylka, J.; Andruch, V. The Role of Water in Deep Eutectic Solvent-Base Extraction. *J. Mol. Liq.* **2020**, *304*, 112747. [CrossRef]
52. Yuan, Y.V.; Bone, D.E.; Carrington, M.F. Antioxidant Activity of Dulse (*Palmaria palmata*) Extract Evaluated In Vitro. *Food Chem.* **2005**, *91*, 485–494. [CrossRef]
53. Yuan, Y.V.; Carrington, M.F.; Walsh, N.A. Extracts from Dulse (*Palmaria palmata*) Are Effective Antioxidants and Inhibitors of Cell Proliferation In Vitro. *Food Chem. Toxicol.* **2005**, *43*, 1073–1081. [CrossRef] [PubMed]
54. Idowu, A.T.; Amigo-Benavent, M.; Whelan, S.; Edwards, M.D.; FitzGerald, R.J. Impact of Different Light Conditions on the Nitrogen, Protein, Colour, Total Phenolic Content and Amino Acid Profiles of Cultured *Palmaria palmata*. *Foods* **2023**, *12*, 3940. [CrossRef] [PubMed]
55. Rebocho, S.; Mano, F.; Cassel, E.; Anacleto, B.; Bronze, M.d.R.; Paiva, A.; Duarte, A.R.C. Fractionated Extraction of Polyphenols from Mate Tea Leaves Using a Combination of Hydrophobic/Hydrophilic NADES. *Curr. Res. Food Sci.* **2022**, *5*, 571–580. [CrossRef] [PubMed]
56. Varriale, S.; Delorme, A.E.; Andanson, J.M.; Devemy, J.; Malfreyt, P.; Verney, V.; Pezzella, C. Enhancing the Thermostability of Engineered Laccases in Aqueous Betaine-Based Natural Deep Eutectic Solvents. *ACS Sustain. Chem. Eng.* **2022**, *10*, 572–581. [CrossRef]
57. Queffelec, J.; Beraud, W.; Dolores Torres, M.; Domínguez, H. Advances in Obtaining Ready to Use Extracts with Natural Solvents. *Sustain. Chem. Pharm.* **2024**, *38*, 101478. [CrossRef]
58. Rajha, H.N.; Mhanna, T.; El Kantar, S.; El Khoury, A.; Louka, N.; Maroun, R.G. Innovative Process of Polyphenol Recovery from Pomegranate Peels by Combining Green Deep Eutectic Solvents and a New Infrared Technology. *LWT* **2019**, *111*, 138–146. [CrossRef]
59. Bradford, M.M. Determinación de Proteínas: Método de Bradford. *Anal. Biochem.* **1976**, *254*, 248–254. [CrossRef]
60. Román, R.B.; Alvárez-Pez, J.M.; Fernández, F.G.A.; Grima, E.M. Recovery of Pure B-Phycoerythrin from the Microalga *Porphyridium cruentum*. *J. Biotechnol.* **2002**, *93*, 73–85. [CrossRef]
61. Beutler, J.A.; Mckee, T.C.; Fuller, R.W.; Tischler, M.; Cardellina, J.H.; Snader, I.K.M.; Mccloud, T.G.; Boyd, M.R. Frequent Occurrence of HIV-Inhibitory Sulphated Polysaccharides in Marine Invertebrates. *Antivir. Chem. Chemother.* **1993**, *4*, 167–172. [CrossRef]

62. Albano, R.M.; Mourao, P.A.S. Isolation, Fractionation, and Preliminary Characterization of a Novel Class of Sulfated Glycans from the Tunic of Styela Plicata (*Chordata tunicata*). *J. Biol. Chem.* **1986**, *261*, 758–765. [CrossRef]
63. Singleton, V.L.; Orthofer, R.; Lamuela-Raventós, R.M. Analysis of Total Phenols and Other Oxidation Substrates and Antioxidants by Means of Folin-Ciocalteu Reagent. *Methods Enzymol.* **1999**, *299*, 152–178. [CrossRef]
64. Ou, B.; Hampsch-Woodill, M.; Prior, R.L. Development and Validation of an Improved Oxygen Radical Absorbance Capacity Assay Using Fluorescein as the Fluorescent Probe. *J. Agric. Food Chem.* **2001**, *49*, 4619–4626. [CrossRef] [PubMed]
65. Re, R.; Pellegrini, N.; Proteggente, A.; Pannala, A.; Yang, M.; Rice-Evans, C. Antioxidant Activity Applying an Improved ABTS Radical Cation Decolorization Assay. *Free Radic. Biol. Med.* **1999**, *26*, 1231–1237. [CrossRef] [PubMed]
66. Ellman, G.L.; Courtney, K.D.; Andres, V.; Featherstone, R.M. A New and Rapid Colorimetric Determination of Acetylcholinesterase Activity. *Biochem. Pharmacol.* **1961**, *7*, 88–95. [CrossRef]
67. Sanchez-Martinez, J.D.; Bueno, M.; Alvarez-Rivera, G.; Tudela, J.; Ibanez, E.; Cifuentes, A. In Vitro Neuroprotective Potential of Terpenes from Industrial Orange Juice By-Products. *Food Funct.* **2021**, *12*, 302–314. [CrossRef]
68. Idowu, A.T.; Amigo-Benavent, M.; Santos-Hernández, M.; Whelan, S.; Edwards, M.D.; FitzGerald, R.J. Impact of Growth Conditions on the Nitrogen, Protein, Colour and Amino Acid Profiles of the Cultured Macroalga, *Palmaria palmata*. *J. Appl. Phycol.* **2023**, *35*, 2397–2411. [CrossRef]

MDPI AG
Grosspeteranlage 5
4052 Basel
Switzerland
Tel.: +41 61 683 77 34

Marine Drugs Editorial Office
E-mail: marinedrugs@mdpi.com
www.mdpi.com/journal/marinedrugs

* 9 7 8 3 7 2 5 8 7 0 5 2 3 *